Community Health Analysis

Global Awareness at the Local Level

Second Edition

G. E. Alan Dever, PhD, MT

Professor, Department of Family and Community Medicine
Director, Clinical Epidemiology and Biostatistics
Director, Office of Health Policy
Mercer University School of Medicine
Macon, Georgia

AN ASPEN PUBLICATION ®
Aspen Publishers, Inc.
Gaithersburg, Maryland
1991

Library of Congress Cataloging-in-Publication Data

Dever, G. E. Alan.
Community health analysis : global awareness at the local level /
G. E. Alan Dever — 2nd ed.
p. cm.
Includes bibliographical references and index.
ISBN: 0-8342-0191-7
1. Health planning. 2. Community health services—
Evaluation. 3. Epidemiology. 4. Holistic medicine.
[DNLM: 1. Community Health Services. 2. Holistic Health. WA 546.1
D491c]
RA393.D49 1991
362.1—dc20
DNLM/DLC
for Library of Congress
90-14495
CIP

Editorial Services: Lorna Perkins

Library of Congress Catalog Card Number: 90-14495
ISBN: 0-8342-0191-7

Printed in the United States of America

1 2 3 4 5

Half of the fun of doing this book was the thought that I would be able to give a copy to Jim Alley and watch the smile appear on his face. I won't be able to do that this time. But I can do it in spirit and with all my heart. So Jim, this book is for you.

To
James W. Alley, M.D.
1929–1990

Table of Contents

Preface

"Our planet, our health; think globally, act locally"[1]

Community Health Analysis is designed to bring to the health care sector philosophical concepts and methodological tools that encompass the many dimensions of health. The above phrase reflects a major theme in this book—a holistic analysis that encompasses a healthy public policy (think globally), but analyzes the problems by applying methods and techniques at the community level (act locally).

The broad base of subject material and the several analytical approaches discussed in this book reflect the theme of holistic planning and analysis.

This edition is greatly expanded and updated in several key areas—readers may quite easily perceive this as a new book. Chapter 1 is the foundation for the concepts expressed throughout the book. Our belief systems as they relate to health care are examined in Chapter 1, along with the changing nature of disease patterns. It argues that our health beliefs, both as individuals and as a community must be altered. Chapter 2 examines health policy issues and suggests a need for redirection toward a healthy public policy. Chapter 3 focuses on strategic planning and evaluation, particularly on planning for change, assessing change and the barriers to change. Basic statistical measures, epidemiological methods, and demographic analysis as applied to community health problems are outlined in Chapters 4, 5, and 6. Chapter 6 is a new chapter, and much of the material in Chapters 1 through 5 has undergone significant revision.

Chapter 7's focus on applications of health status indicators and indexes is much expanded and updated. Chapter 8, "Marketing Community Health," and Chapter 9, "Ethics and Social Justice in Community Health Analysis," are new chapters. They reflect the growing emphasis on making prevention a salable product (marketing) and the need for rational and ethical approaches to allocating resources (social justice). Chapter 10, "Computer Graphics," is updated and ex-

ix

panded. The proliferation of products and vendors for graphics has been explosive, yet their use in community health analysis is still in its infancy.

This edition of the book was written in response to the many students, educators, planners, analysts, researchers, policy makers, and community activists who embraced the first edition. I, indeed, thank all of you who believe in the merits of the approach presented in this volume. Certainly, if not for you, this second edition would not have become a reality.

NOTE

1. American Association for World Health, *Our Planet, Our Health; Think Globally, Act Locally. An Activities Background and Resources Guidebook* (Washington, DC: AAWH, 1990).

Acknowledgments

As I was finishing this book, a man who has been a major influence in my life and to my way of thinking died unexpectedly. James W. Alley, M.D., 1929–1990, Director of Public Health in Georgia from 1973 to 1990, was convinced that the community is the key to dealing with the major problems in our society, such as racism, sexism, and ageism. I thank him for sharing his perspective with me and his persistence in dealing with these public and community health problems. He was a dear friend and a compelling mentor.

Another man who played a leading role in the completion of this book, believed in me, and provided me with support is Douglas W. Skelton, M.D., Dean of the Mercer University School of Medicine. He is a man of science who possesses both vision and insight, a powerful mixture. His confidence in this project has been unfailing, and I am indebted to him.

Also, I especially want to thank Mark Sceigja, who like me, grew as a result of the influence of Jim Alley. Much of the material on justice and ethics was developed while Mark and I wrote together. Tom Wade also influenced the material on justice issues and played a major role in the development and writing of this topic.

In addition, Terri Lofton and Michael Lavoie have been important to my writing and opinions for several years and regularly have provided constructive feedback.

Further, I am indebted to another friend and colleague, Richard Cunningham, who consistently supported my needs.

Walter Treadwell, M.D., Chairman of the Department of Family Medicine, has always been a sensitive friend and has regularly provided me with support.

Many others have helped to complete this book. They are Sandy Coxon, Charlotte Nolan, Nohemy Brewer, Susan Deaver, Ray Seabolt, and Dee Thomas-Hanson. Variously, they retrieved data, typed manuscripts, edited material, and provided effective and productive feedback on a regular basis.

The most important person in my life, my wife, Georgie, has always given me the strength, love, and commitment to complete my work. Georgie, your laughter and caring makes me a fortunate man. My children, James and Tammy have always known how to humor Dad when he is writing. Thanks kids.

Finally, the Aspen team members have been clearly committed to the author, and they have kept everything on course. They have been most encouraging in some unusual situations. Thank you, Lorna Perkins, Neal Poema, Trudi Court, and Jack Bruggeman.

Introduction: Status of Prevention in the United States

A strange paradox exists in the U.S. health care system. Within the government ranks, especially the Department of Health and Human Services (DHHS), prevention, as noted by Secretary Sullivan, "must become a national obsession."[1] Yet, also within the government bureaucracy, especially in the Medicare and Medicaid systems and the Health Care Financing Administration, reimbursement for prevention activities and/or procedures is almost nonexistent. Furthermore, major third-party payers offer limited reimbursement for preventive procedures. In 1988, only 4 percent of our health care dollar was allocated to prevention efforts and the remainder to the medical care system and research.[2] We as a country have not put our money where the most benefit is to be obtained—our national resources continue to be drained by the medical care system. The 1990s must usher in a new era of prevention.

PREVENTION TODAY

Most people in the United States believe that health care should be a basic right—a social justice to be allocated according to various distributive principles. In reality, however, health care is a privilege. deVise has stated,

> If you are either very poor, blind, disabled, over 65, male, female, white, or live in a middle- or upper-class neighborhood in a large urban center, you belong to a privileged class of health care recipients, and your chances of survival are good. . . . But, if you are none of these, if you are only average poor, under 65, female, black, or live in a low-income urban neighborhood, small town, or rural area, you are a disenfranchised citizen as far as health care rights go, and your chances of survival are not good."[3]

These statements were made in 1973, and the situation has not changed. The facts and statistics in this book make it clear that the problems of today in the health care system reflect these same disparities.

Thus, how sick one is in the United States depends on the following factors:

ISSUE	PROBLEM
How poor you are	Distribution of wealth
How old you are	Ageism
Where you live	Locationalism
If you are in a minority group	Racism
What sex you are	Sexism
How sick you are	Health status
How educated you are	Literatism

For example, Table I-1 shows how these factors are reflected in the percentages of adults who try to maintain a recommended weight. A profile develops. Those who live in the South or Midwest (rural); are black, over age 50, and not high-school graduates; earn less than $15,000 a year; work as blue-collar or labor (service) workers; and are in fair or poor health status have a diminished ability to follow this preventive measure of maintaining weight.

The resolution of these issues/problems requires the development of two major strategies: a healthy public policy and prevention. Clearly, these issues cannot be resolved by traditional health care concerns and a limited public health policy. The transition from a public health policy to a healthy public policy is not only crucial to the resolution of the issues of locationalism, racism, sexism, ageism, literatism, distribution of wealth, and health status but is also a major factor in the development of the strategy of prevention. We are on the brink of a new era of prevention, and our sickness-oriented system is an ideology that is failing.[4]

Prevention Magazine has prepared a report card on the nation's health since 1983.[5] It measures the percentage of the adult population aged 18 and over who practice 21 key health behaviors. Table I-2 lists the 21 health-promoting behaviors, the percentage of adults practicing those behaviors, the experts' rating scale, and the value contributed to the index. The sum of these values produces the prevention index. Simply stated, 65.4 percent of our nation's population practice preventive health behaviors, only a modest increase from 61.5 percent recorded in 1984, the year of the second survey. Some of the behaviors are practiced by more than 80 percent of our population, however. For example, avoiding smoking in bed, avoiding driving after drinking, having a smoke detector in the home, socializing regularly, drinking alcohol moderately, avoiding home accidents, and taking annual blood pressure tests have above 80 percent compliance. The two poorest percentages are 21 percent and 36 percent for maintaining proper weight and engaging in frequent strenuous exercise, respectively. Table I-3 demonstrates the trends in the preventive behavior items from 1983 to

Table I-1 Percent of Adults Who Keep Their Weight Within the Recommended Range Classified According to Factors Affecting How Sick One Is in the United States

Factor	Base*	%
Locationalism		
Region		
East	258	27
South	315	17
Midwest	258	16
West	200	26
Urbanism		
Central city	307	18
Rest of metropolitan area	479	25
Outside metropolitan area	245	17
Sexism		
Sex		
Male	476	20
Female	555	22
Racism		
Race		
White	898	22
Black	64	16†
Hispanic	47	22†
Ageism		
Age		
18–29 years	161	22
30–39 years	287	27
40–49 years	190	24
50–64 years	234	15
65 and over	159	15
Literatism		
Educational level		
Not high school graduate	143	16
High school graduate	358	18
Some college	249	20
Four-year college graduate	280	28
Distribution of wealth		
Household income		
$7,500 or less	67	19†
$7,501–$15,000	116	9
$15,001–$25,000	194	22
$25,001–$35,000	231	20
$35,001–$50,000	171	23
$50,001 and over	161	29
Occupation		
Blue-collar labor, service	249	18
Clerical, sales	146	29
Professional, manager or proprietor	290	25

continues

Table I-1 continued

Factor	Base*	%
Health status		
Self-described health status		
Excellent	257	27
Very good or good	611	21
Fair or poor	160	14
Preventive habits		
Those who practice 76% to 100%	278	29
Those who practice 51% to 75%	556	19
Those who practice 0% to 50%	197	15
Total	1031	21

*Base: Adults aged 25 and older whose recommended weight could be calculated given their height/build/sex data. Metropolitan Life Insurance Company tables were used for the classification.
†Caution needed in interpreting data because of small base.

Source: Adapted from *The Prevention Index, Summary Report: A Report Card on the Nation's Health,* a project of Prevention Magazine, p.13, with permission of Rodale Press, Inc., © 1989.

Table I-2 Prevention Index, 1989

Health-Promoting Behavior	Adults Practicing (%)	Experts' Rating Scale (1–10)	Value Contributed to Index
1. Do not smoke	74	9.78	4.4
2. Avoid smoking in bed	90	9.24	5.0
3. Wear seatbelt	60	9.16	3.3
4. Avoid driving after drinking	81	9.03	4.4
5. Smoke detector in home	81	8.53	4.2
6. Socialize regularly	84	8.31	4.2
7. Frequent strenuous exercise	36	8.20	1.8
8. Drink alcohol moderately	90	8.15	4.4
9. Avoid home accidents	82	8.07	4.0
10. Limit fat in diet	54	7.82	2.5
11. Maintain proper weight	21	7.71	1.0
12. Obey speed limit	56	7.65	2.6
13. Annual blood pressure test	83	7.62	3.8
14. Control stress	69	7.58	3.1
15. Consume fiber	60	7.41	2.7
16. Limit cholesterol in diet	48	7.15	2.1
17. Adequate vitamins/minerals	57	7.12	2.4
18. Annual dental examination	71	7.08	3.0
19. Limit sodium in diet	48	7.04	2.0
20. Limit sugar in diet	47	6.90	2.0
21. 7–8 hours sleep/night	62	6.71	2.5
		Prevention Index	65.4

Source: Reprinted from *The Prevention Index, Summary Report: A Report Card on the Nation's Health,* a project of Prevention Magazine, p.3, with permission of Rodale Press, Inc., © 1989.

Table I-3 Trends in 24 Preventive Behavior Items (1983–1988)*

Behaviors	1983 Survey (%)	1984 Survey (%)	1985 Survey (%)	1986 Survey (%)	1987 Survey (%)	1988 Survey (%)	Percentage Point Change from 1983 Survey
Nonsmoking and restricted use of alcohol							
Do not smoke cigarettes	70	72	70	72	72	74	+4
Drink alcohol moderately	54	57	55	56	50	51	−3
(Drink moderately or do not drink at all)	89	87	88	88	86	90	+1
Exercise and weight control							
Get strenuous exercise 3 or more days a week	34	33	31	33	35	36	+2
Are within the weight range recommended for height, build, and sex†	23	22	21	23	24	21	−2
(Are not overweight)	42	39	38	41	40	36	−6
Diet and nutrition							
Try a lot to get enough vitamins and minerals	63	57	63	63	59	57	−6
Try a lot to eat enough fiber	59	58	59	59	60	60	+1
Try a lot to avoid eating too much fat	55	59	56	56	54	54	−1
Try a lot to avoid eating too much salt or sodium	53	54	54	57	54	48	−5
Try a lot to avoid eating too much sugar and sweet food	51	52	50	49	49	47	−4
Try a lot to get enough calcium	50	45	57	57	54	53	+3
Try a lot to avoid eating too many high-cholesterol foods	42	43	42	46	42	48	+6
Control of stress							
Socialize with friends or relatives once a week or more	84	85	85	81	83	84	0
Get 7 or 8 hours of sleep most nights	64	63	64	65	61	62	−2
Take specific steps to control or reduce stress	59	70	69	64	68	69	+10

continues

Table I-3 continued

Behaviors	1983 Survey (%)	1984 Survey (%)	1985 Survey (%)	1986 Survey (%)	1987 Survey (%)	1988 Survey (%)	Percentage Point Change from 1983 Survey
Periodic examinations and tests							
Have a blood pressure reading at least once a year	82	85	85	81	83	84	+2
Have a dental checkup at least once a year	71	73	74	76	75	71	0
Women have a Pap smear test every 1 or 2 years	75	77	78	80	75	79	+4
Women examine their breasts at least once each month for signs of cancer	37	42	48	45	42	51	+14
Safety precautions							
Say that no one in their home smokes in bed	88	89	91	91	92	90	+2
Say they take specific steps to avoid accidents in and around the home	72	81	80	80	81	82	+10
Say they have a smoke detector in their home	67	74	76	77	82	81	+14
Drivers who say they drive at or below the speed limit all the time	56	52	50	51	50	51	−5
Drivers who say they either never drive after drinking or do not drink at all	68	68	72	74	74	78	+10
Say they wear seat belts all the time when in the front seat of a car	19	27	41	55	57	60	+41

*Total number of adults participating in each survey: 1254 (1983), 1253 (1984), 1256 (1985), 1250 (1986), 1250 (1987), and 1250 (1988).

†Based on those aged 25 and above whose recommended weight could be calculated given their height/build/sex data. Metropolitan Life Insurance Company tables were used for the classification. Bases vary slightly across the years; 995 (1983), 1061 (1985), 1022 (1986), 1008 (1987), 1031 (1988).

Source: Reprinted from *The Prevention Index, Summary Report: A Report Card on the Nation's Health,* a project of Prevention Magazine, p.9, with permission of Rodale Press, Inc., © 1989.

Table I-4 Issues of the 1990s Reflecting a Need for a Healthy Public Policy

National Issues	Problems
Medical dilemmas	Health costs: Modern medicine's spectacular results in curing sick people are producing equally spectacular costs. Cost problems are intensifying as the population ages and as scientists develop more ways to keep people alive and functioning.
	Screening: People often are unaware that they have serious medical problems that need treatment.
	Drugs to boost intelligence: Should they go only to the rich, who can pay whatever the manufacturer charges, or should the government pay for drugs so that poor people can improve their intelligence and perhaps climb out of poverty?
	Rationing human organs: People are dying today because there are not enough hearts and kidneys available for transplantation to all those who need them.
	AIDS: This dread disease, which threatens to take more lives than the Black Death of the Middle Ages, will pose numerous painful questions: What steps should governments take to stop people who have the disease from passing it on to others? Who should pay for the expensive drugs needed by people with AIDS?
	Abortion: Abortion promises to be one of the hottest issues in the United States during the 1990s.
	Infanticide: Neonatologists are succeeding in saving the lives of infants at ever younger ages. Often, they are forcibly kept alive despite the wishes of the parents and at enormous cost to the taxpayers.
	Choosing the sex of one's children: Physicians are currently developing various means whereby parents can choose to have a boy or a girl. What can be done to prevent the proportion of one sex from becoming unbalanced?
Drug crisis	Narcotics: Controlling cocaine and other narcotics has emerged recently as a top concern of the American people. Halting the drug trade, now that it has become pervasive, will likely require very stern and costly measures.
	Crime: Addicts commit crimes to support their drug habits. Dealers pay off officials to stay in business, thereby corrupting government even at high levels.
	Legalization of drugs: Frustrated at the consequences of rampant drug trafficking, some people have suggested that drugs should be "decriminalized." Advocates say the legalization of narcotics would greatly reduce the

continues

Table I-4 continued

National Issues	Problems
Drug crisis	crime and violence associated with drug trafficking. But which drugs should be legalized and under what circumstances?
	Addicted mothers: Mothers who use crack cocaine produce babies with deformed hearts, lungs, digestive systems, or limbs. The babies are also born addicted and begin life experiencing the agonies of withdrawal. Pregnant women who drink alcohol may give birth to babies who are permanently damaged mentally (fetal alcohol syndrome).
	Alcohol: Alcohol is perhaps the largest single cause of automobile and other accidents. People driving under the influence of alcohol kill thousands of people every year. Alcohol is also implicated in train, airplane, industrial, and other types of accidents.
	Tobacco: Tobacco products shorten lives all over the world, but the industry fights efforts aimed at reducing the use of this drug. In recent years, medical authorities have focused attention on the "passive smokers"— people who must breathe the air polluted by tobacco smoke—and smoking has been forbidden in many workplaces and public areas.
Struggle against poverty	Destitution: Even wealthy nations have people who are not merely poor but destitute—lacking the basic essentials needed to sustain life. Reducing their misery will be a major issue of the 1990s.
	Starvation: Inadequate nutrition leads to stunted physical and mental growth among children, a high rate of illness, and shortened life-spans.
	Homelessness: Millions in wealthy as well as poor nations have no home of their own. They may sleep on the streets, in automobiles, in abandoned packing boxes, or in caves. The causes of homelessness include loss of income, mental illness, alienation from family, and the poverty of the community.
	Unemployment: Educational requirements for jobs have risen steadily in recent years, but many workers have lagged behind in acquiring new skills and find themselves unemployable or nearly so. Other workers become unemployed due to economic recessions or factory closings attributed to automation or imported goods.
	Poverty as a lifestyle: Much poverty stems from socioeconomic conditions, but much results from

Table I-4 continued

National Issues	Problems
Struggle against poverty	individual behavior. Reducing poverty depends heavily on changing the behavior patterns that contribute to it, but getting people to change is not easy.
	Reforming education: Despite rising expenditures for education, millions of young people leave schools without the basic skills required to function effectively in modern society. But there is little agreement on just what needs to be done to improve education.
	The distribution of wealth: Living standards have risen greatly during the twentieth century, but wealth remains unequally distributed, both among individuals and among nations.
Collapsing family	Divorce: Divorce has increased steadily in the twentieth century, with a sharp rise during the 1970s. Today, nearly one out of every two marriages ends in divorce. The rise of divorce has fractured the family, the institution charged with rearing children to be good workers and citizens. Following a divorce, many children see their fathers only occasionally and suffer a loss in their standard of living. Family breakdown is widely recognized as contributing to crime, school failure, and other problems. Efforts to help families may intensify in the 1990s.
	Unmarried motherhood: Changing mores and welfare payments have led to a dramatic rise in the percentage of unmarried teenage girls and women who become pregnant and keep their babies, rather than putting them up for adoption. Many of these unmarried mothers are woefully unprepared to provide a good home for a child. In the 1990s, efforts may intensify to break the cycle of unmarried pregnancy and children having children.
	Single-parent homes: The prevalence of divorce and unmarried parenthood means that very large numbers of children now have only one parent to care for them. As a result, they often get inadequate love and discipline and grow up psychically immature. Many such children are left on their own and drift into idleness, drugs, and crime.
	Child negligence: Many parents abandon their children completely. Other parents provide far less support than the children need for proper development. Millions of children fail to get the basic training from their parents that they need to succeed in school, work, and life. Many children who are viewed as runaways are actually "throwaways"; their parents did not want them around.

continues

Table I-4 continued

National Issues	Problems
Collapsing family	Social isolation: Besides divorce, increasingly late marriage and celibacy have meant that more and more adults live by themselves. As a result, many people have no one at home to help them when they become ill or incapacitated. They may also find themselves increasingly cut off from the larger community.
Population problems	Population growth: In many Third World nations, population growth is devastating the natural environment and driving down living standards; yet, most nations are doing little to curb births. Halving high birth rates in poor countries will be a major challenge during the decade ahead.
	Birth dearth: Some advanced nations now have negative population growth (except for immigration). In the United States and a number of European countries, native-born women in the childbearing years are not having enough children to replace themselves. The low birth rates, especially among highly educated women, have begun to concern a number of scholars.
	Migration: People moving from one region to another can pose problems both for the countries, states, and counties they leave and the countries, states, and counties they enter. The areas they leave may experience a "brain drain" as the brightest and most energetic people depart for better opportunities elsewhere. At the same time, the recipient areas may face problems assimilating newcomers.
	Deadly demographics: Migration and differentials in birth rates often change the demographic makeup of a nation because the percentage of people belonging to one ethnic group or religion rises as that of another declines. Such a change may upset the political balance in a nation and even lead to civil war, because a group with a growing percentage of the population will begin demanding changes in long-established practices—wider use of its language, more benefits for its religion, etc.—and resistance to such changes can bring bloodshed.
	Extending the human life-span: If current research on aging proves successful, the human life-span may be lengthened far beyond the 70 to 90 years that is considered normal today. Some people alive today may conceivably live to be 200 or more years old. But if it becomes possible to extend life-span dramatically, innumerable new problems will emerge: What will

Table I-4 continued

National Issues	Problems
Population problems	happen to pension funds if people continue to retire in their sixties but then live on for many decades drawing benefits?
Environmental problems	Air pollution: Motor vehicles and factories pour smoke and noxious gases into the atmosphere. These pollutants cause breathing difficulties and other health problems for millions of people, resulting in serious illnesses and deaths. The pollutants also damage equipment, ruin crops, and coat buildings and outside structures with grime. Despite widespread concern in recent years, air quality worldwide continues to decline.
	Water pollution: Rain washes soil, fertilizer, insecticides, and other pollutants into rivers, while factories and cities are adding sewage and chemicals. Airborne dust and chemicals also fall into lakes, killing fish and other wildlife.
	Depletion of the ozone layer: The upper atmosphere of the earth contains a region where the gas ozone acts as a shield to protect the planet from the sun's deadly ultraviolet radiation. This ozone layer has been weakened by the release of chlorofluorocarbon gases, which are used in refrigerants and as propellants in spray cans. As the ozone layer weakens, more people will succumb to the effects of ultraviolet radiation, which include skin cancer and blindness. In addition, many food crops, such as wheat, rice, and potatoes, will be harmed.
	The greenhouse effect: The buildup of carbon dioxide and other gases in the atmosphere (due to the burning of coal and other factors) may cause melting of the ice at the North and South Poles, flooding coastal areas around the world.
	Noise: The noise level has risen steadily in the twentieth century, increasing both stress and hearing loss in individuals. Cities and suburbs seem to become ever noisier with pneumatic drills, lawnmowers, motorcycles, and other noisy equipment. Experts report that loud music already is causing permanent damage to the hearing of many young people.
	Solid-waste problems: Many cities are running out of space in nearby landfills and are searching for places to dump their garbage. In some cases, barges laden with garbage have wandered from port to port seeking permission to dump their loads.

continues

Table I-4 continued

National Issues	Problems
Environmental problems	Oceans: Oil spills from tankers, rivers of garbage and chemicals, and the dumping of garbage at sea are killing sea life and littering or damaging large areas of beach and ocean. Beaches may have to be closed as oil and sewage wash up on the sand.

Source: Adapted from E. Cornish, "Issues of the 1990s. A Short List of Global Concerns" in *The Futurist,* Vol. 24, No. 1, pp. 29–36, with permission of the World Future Society, © 1990.

The percentage of adults engaging in those behaviors increased in 15, decreased in 7, and showed no change in 2. In sum, the authors of the prevention project state, "Our progress in prevention has not been dramatic. If our index score were a grade, we'd still barely pass. But we are going in the proper direction."[6]

Our problems internationally, nationally, and locally are interrelated in ways that make it impossible to deal with one problem in isolation from the others.[7] Thus, a healthy public policy seems reasonable and responsible for dealing with the issues of the 1990s. Community health planners and analysts must assume responsibility for and advocate resolution of these issues.

Cornish has prepared a short list of global concerns that are, indeed, quite significant to our future generally and to our health specifically.[8] Table I-4 lists some of these future concerns. Certainly, making progress toward solving these problems will require a change in values, beliefs, ideologies, and priorities. Possibly, the 1990s will be the decade when we see these changes. In any event, as health professionals who develop plans, make decisions, and set policies, we have much to resolve, much to accomplish, and a healthy future to help form.

NOTES

1. "President's Column. A New Era for Prevention," *The Nation's Health* (January 1990): 2.

2. J.O. Wiener, "Year 2000 Objectives: Altering the Medical Model" *Medicine and Health Perspectives* (October 23, 1989).

3. P. deVise, *Misuses and Misplaced Hospitals and Doctors. A Locational Analysis of the Urban Health Care Crisis,* Resource Paper No. 2 (Commission on College Geography, 1973), 1.

4. "President's Column," 2.

5. *The Prevention Index Summary Report. A Report Card on the Nation's Health* (Rodale Press, Inc., 1989), 32.

6. Ibid., 2.

7. E. Cornish, "Issue of the 1990s. A Short List of Concerns," *The Futurist* 24 (January/February 1990): 29–36.

8. Ibid.

Chapter 1

Health and Our Belief Systems

During the 1970s, the traditional health care concerns of regulation, cost containment, accessibility, availability, quality, continuity, and acceptability were emphasized. In the 1980s, the focus shifted from such legislative and technological issues to methods of disease prevention and health promotion. The pursuit of health, as reflected by individuals' personal awareness or self-actualization in physical activity, nutrition, stress management, and overall individual lifestyle, led to the development of holistic centers, wellness resource centers—both independent and hospital based—health spas and resorts, and a population more concerned about its physical and mental condition. Jogging, tennis, basketball, swimming, vitamins, health foods, and coping skills were often major items of the community public health agenda in the 1980s, as the emphasis moved from illness to wellness.

What will happen in the 1990s and the first decade of the twenty-first century? What forces will shape the trends in health care? It seems likely that, during the 1990s, new and compelling issues that require tough decisions will arise in the health care field. Such issues may include

- prevention—the burden of illness
- resource allocation
- distributive justice
- quality of life
- social justice
- ethics
- building community capacity
- inequalities and inequities in health care
- program accountability
- challenge of demographic change[1]

- internationalization of the United States[2]
- knowledge revolution[3]
- challenge of change

Community health analysts must focus on these issues if they are to address current health care problems. Indeed, they must create an environment or community in which the issues of the 1990s become an integral part of each individual's knowledge base.

The major barriers to the creation of such a community are in today's belief systems. In the 1970s, people were guided by the philosophy that physicians and the medical care system would enable them to overcome their life-death crises and make them well by doing everything humanly possible in the areas of curative and treatment services. In the 1980s, beliefs changed as people embraced the concepts of health promotion and disease prevention, which included the self-improvement movement. Expectations of medical practitioners were reduced. People realized that they could not continue to abuse their bodies and then expect a medical team to make repairs time after time after time. Thus, people came to see wellness as a function of prevention and maintenance, and to accept responsibility for their own health.

In the 1990s, people must begin to balance the physician/medical care system and wellness/preventive medicine with the social issues of justice, ethics, resource allocation, and the quality of life. Thus, the challenge of the 1990s is to develop a belief system that melds the concepts encompassed by preventive medicine, wellness, and quality of life. Doing so will require the involvement of all sectors of society—health, energy, transportation, education, agriculture, economics, technology, and the environment. The role of the health care sector must be to advocate and coordinate policy positions that focus on healthy public policy to promote health. In the 1990s, people are changing direction, and those in the public health field must be in a position to direct this change.

BELIEF SYSTEMS AND EPIDEMIOLOGY

Belief systems, the concepts that people use to run their lives, are created by knowledge or data without experience. Problems occur when people become "stuck" in their beliefs. Most people persist in thinking and doing what they learned long ago, rather than acting from experience.

A young bride regularly cut off the ends of the ham before putting it in the pan to bake. After watching her do this several times, her husband asked her why. She answered that her mother always did it that way. So the husband asked his mother-in-law why she cut off the ends of the ham. She replied, "Because my mother always did it that way." When the husband visited the old grandmother one day, he asked the same question. "I cut off the ends of the ham," she explained, "because we were poor and had only one pan for all our baking. To get a large ham into the small pan, we had to cut off the ends.[4]

Most people continue to cut off the ends of something in their lives to fit into a pan that is no longer too small.

Epidemiology is the study of the determinants and distribution of diseases in human populations. It is linked to concepts of health and causality, as the evolution of these concepts reflects shifts in disease patterns. Medical/clinical epidemiology focuses on the study of patients in clinics, whereas community/social epidemiology is concerned with the study of populations in communities.

CAUSALITY AND ASSOCIATION

Models of Causality

Over the past 100 years, three generalized causal models have directed epidemiological studies. The models are intrinsically related to the concepts of health and health measurement, as well as to the shift in disease patterns (Exhibit 1-1).

Single-Cause/Single-Effect Model

The simplest epidemiological causal model is the single-cause/single-effect pattern, in which a single cause produces an observed effect (Fig. 1-1). This model is quite logical, but operates only rarely. Epidemiologists used this approach in the late 1800s and early 1900s to characterize infectious disease patterns in which a single bacterium or virus was sufficient to produce disease.

Multiple-Cause/Single-Effect Model

Although it is more complex, the multiple-cause/single-effect model is an obvious extension of the single-cause/single-effect model (Fig. 1-2). The multiple-cause/single-effect approach is valid when disease patterns are in a transitory state; for example, it is useful in communities or areas where the incidence of infectious diseases is declining and that of chronic disease is increasing. Thus, patterns of chronic disease such as heart disease, cancer, and stroke may be ana-

Exhibit 1-1 Epidemiology, Concepts of Health, and Health Measurement: Evolution and Relationships

Time	Epidemiological Methods	Concepts of Health	Health Measurement
1900 1920	Single-Cause Model (Infectious Diseases)	Ecology Model (Agent-Host-Environment)	Mortality from Infectious Diseases (Death Rates: Crude, Specific, Adjusted)
	Multiple-Cause Model (Infectious/Chronic Diseases, Transition Cycle)	Social Ecological Model (Host, Environment, Personal Factors)	Morbidity Measurement (Incidence, Prevalence)
1940		W.H.O. Model (Physical, Mental, Social)	Disability Measurement (Work Loss, Disability Days)
   1970	Multiple-Cause/ Multiple-Effect Model (Chronic Disease Cycle)	Holistic Model (Life Style, Environment, Biology, Health Care System) High-Level Wellness Model (Physical Exercise, Stress Management, Nutrition, Self-Responsibility)	Holistic and Wellness Measurement (HHA, RADAR, Prospective Measures)
1980		Content/Context Model (What's in Health/How to Hold on to Health)	Measurement of the Content and Context of Health (Mind/Body Relationships)
1990 2000	Multiple-Cause/ Multiple-Effect Model (Social Transformation Disease Cycle)	Model Achieving Health for All of Community and Self (Development of a Healthy Public Policy)	Measurement of Quality of Life, Resource Allocation, and Distributive Justice Measurement in All Sectors of Society (Social, Economic, Education, Environment, Technology)

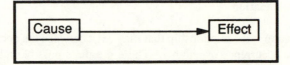

Figure 1-1 Single-Cause/Single-Effect Model

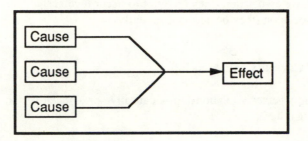

Figure 1-2 Multiple-Cause/Single-Effect Model

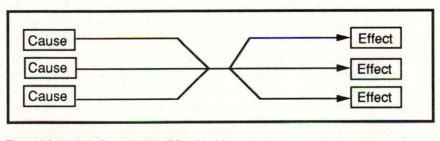

Figure 1-3 Multiple-Cause/Multiple-Effect Model

lyzed through the multiple-cause/single-effect model. Some infectious diseases, such as Legionnaire's disease, may also be investigated by means of this model.

Multiple-Cause/Multiple-Effect Model

The model of causality for situations in which several causes produce many observed effects is extremely complex (Fig. 1-3). This multiple-cause/multiple-effect model closely embraces the health concepts of holism and wellness (self and community) and is quite applicable to the disease patterns of the 1980s, 1990s, and 2000s. For instance, air pollution, smoking, and specific forms of radiation may produce lung cancer, emphysema, and bronchitis.

Models of Association

An association is the relationship that may exist between the occurrence of one thing and the occurrence of another.[5] There are three possible relationships between the risk factor and the disease.

1. a positive association (they tend to occur together)
2. a negative association (they tend not to occur together)
3. no association (they occur independently)

Criteria of Causality and Association

In judging whether a relationship is causative or associative, an analyst uses the following criteria:

- *temporal relationship*. If *A* causes *B*, logically *A* should occur first.
- *specificity*. With high specificity, a cause leads to a single effect; with low specificity, a cause may be associated with multiple effects. In the latter case, for example, cigarette smoking can cause both lung cancer and bronchitis; low socioeconomic status can be associated with both illness and disability.
- *strength or intensity of the association or the degree of correlation between the cause and the effect*. The strength of the association between a pathogen and an infectious disease process is usually high. In the case of chronic disease, however, the association is statistical or probabilistic; thus, there is a certain degree of uncertainty, as in the association of exercise and diet with lower rates of cardiac disease. The three causal models are not quite logical in dealing with this problem, which requires statistical probability tests and broader concepts of health.
- *consistency*. When the same type of association consistently appears in research studies of different designs, it is likely to be a real, causative relationship.
- *coherence*. A supposed causal relationship should make sense in the light of existing biological facts. Contrary evidence suggests, however, that this point should not be heavily weighted; there is some doubt, for example, about the relationship between sugar consumption and such conditions as cancer and hypoglycemia.

These subjective criteria are highly variable and operate quite effectively with the infectious disease cycle. The criteria do not, however, describe well the interactions within the holistic approach or the social transformation disease model. To understand this, it is necessary to explore the changing nature of our disease patterns.

SHIFTING DISEASE PATTERNS: 1900–2000

Agricultural and industrial changes in our society have resulted in a shift in disease patterns. The transition currently under way from an industrial and even postindustrial society to a service and information transfer society (knowledge/ information revolution) brings with it new patterns of disease. The leading causes of illness and death have changed significantly over the past 90 years and will undergo a dramatic shift in the next 10 years (Table 1-1).

The turning point for deaths from infectious and chronic diseases in the United States occurred about 1925 (Fig. 1-4). Collectively, deaths due to infectious diseases declined from approximately 650 deaths per 100,000 population in 1900 to approximately 20 deaths per 100,000 in 1970, a decline of 96 percent. (Because of a major epidemic of influenza that occurred in 1918, the death rate from infectious diseases mounted to 850 deaths per 100,000 population at that time.)

Table 1-1 The Ten Leading Causes of Illness and Death in the United States, 1900–2000

	1900*	1950*	1985*	2000†
1.	Tuberculosis	Diseases of the heart	Diseases of the heart	Diseases of the heart
2.	Pneumonia	Cancer	Cancer	Cancer
3.	Diarrhea and enteritis	Cerebrovascular disease	Cerebrovascular disease	Cerebrovascular disease
4.	Diseases of the heart	Accidents	Accidents	Accidents
5.	Nephritis	Pneumonia/influenza	Chronic obstructive pulmonary disease	AIDS
6.	Accidents/violence	Tuberculosis	Pneumonia/influenza	Obesity/nutritional disorders
7.	Cerebrovascular disease	Arteriosclerosis	Suicide	Suicide
8.	Cancer	Nephritis	Diabetes mellitus	Drugs/alcoholism
9.	Bronchitis	Diabetes mellitus	Chronic liver disease	Aging/mental illness
10.	Diphtheria	Suicide	Arteriosclerosis	Coping/adaptability

*Health United States, 1987. U.S. DHSS. PHS. National Center for Health Statistics, Hyattsville, Maryland, March 1988, pp. 10–11.

†Dever, G.E. Alan. "The Future of Health Services in Georgia" paper presented at Armstrong State College, Savannah, Georgia, 1974, p. 13 and Epp, J. "Achieving Health for All: A Framework for Health Promotion." Canadian Journal of Public Health. Vol. 77, No. 6 Nov/Dec. 1986 pp. 394–407.

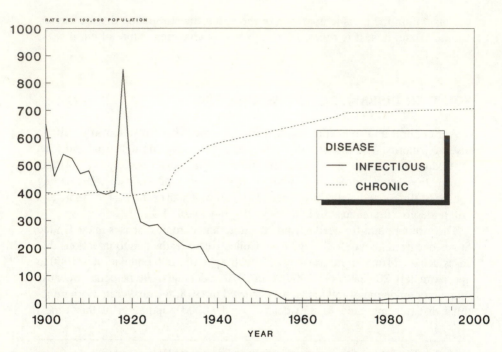

Figure 1-4 Infectious and Chronic Disease Death Rates in the United States, 1900–2000. *Source:* Reprinted from *Dynamics of Health and Disease* by C.L. Marshall and D. Pearson, p. 131, with permission of Appleton & Lange, © 1972.

Chronic diseases, on the other hand, collectively accounted for approximately 350 deaths per 100,000 population in 1900 and increased to approximately 690 deaths per 100,000 in 1970, an increase of 97 percent. Since 1970, specifically since about 1980, deaths from infectious diseases (namely, acquired immune deficiency syndrome [AIDS]) have increased, whereas deaths from chronic diseases have remained relatively stable. This disease transition—not unlike a demographic transition—was caused by the societal shift from an agrarian to an industrialized society.

Infectious Disease Cycle

The agrarian society generated a cycle of events that is portrayed in the infectious disease model (Fig. 1-5). The fertility rate was high in the agricultural era, as large families were essential to harvest food from the land. Thus, in 1900, 52 percent of the population was under 21 years of age, and only 3 percent was over

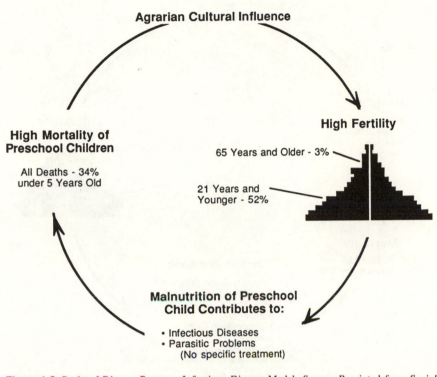

Figure 1-5 Cycle of Disease Patterns, Infectious Disease Model. *Source:* Reprinted from *Social Indicators Research,* Vol. 4, p. 485, with permission of Kluwer Aademic Publishers, © 1977.

65. (This type of population pyramid is typical of today's inner cities, rural counties, and developing countries where the infectious disease model is still applicable.) With no specific medical treatment available, however, parasitic diseases, infectious diseases, and malnutrition contributed to high infant and preschool mortality. In fact, 34 percent of all deaths occurred between birth and 5 years of age.

Chronic Disease Cycle

The cycle of disease during the industrial period is demonstrated by the chronic disease model (Fig. 1-6). Deleterious social, physical, emotional, and environmental ways of life have resulted from affluence, changing values, and increased leisure time. With this overall societal change, the fertility has dropped; the population under 21 years decreased to 40 percent, and the population over 65 years increased to 8 percent in 1970. Consequently, the diseases of

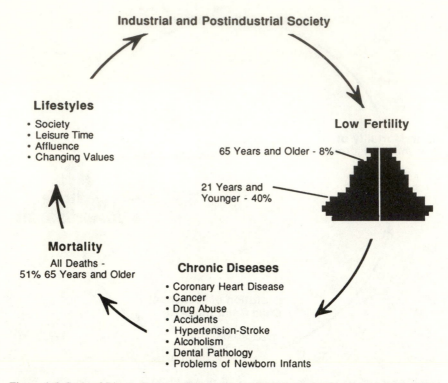

Figure 1-6 Cycle of Disease Patterns, Chronic Disease Model. *Source:* Reprinted from *Social Indicators Research,* Vol. 4, p. 486, with permission of Kluwer Aademic Publishers, © 1977.

an older age group became more prevalent, and 51 percent of all deaths occurred among those 65 and older. The big three—heart disease, cancer, and stroke—accounted for a little more than 60 percent of all deaths in 1970 and a little less than 70 percent in 1985.

Presently, society is undergoing a knowledge/information revolution in which intellectual capital is becoming the key to strength, prosperity, and social well-being. This is in stark contrast to the material- and labor-intensive products and processes that characterized the industrial revolution.[6] As a result of these changes, a new cycle is emerging—the social transformation disease model—that has several parallels to the infectious and chronic disease models.

Social Transformation Disease Cycle

Analysts now need a conceptual framework that goes beyond the infectious and chronic disease models. The social transformation model has been developed

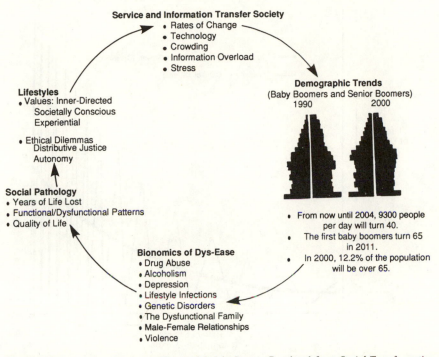

Figure 1-7 Social Transformation Disease Model. *Source:* Reprinted from *Social Transformation Model: Human Development and Disease Patterns,* Datalog File No. 87–1153 by J.W. Alley, G.E.A. Dever, and T.E. Wade, p. 9, with permission of SRI International, © 1986

to reflect the new disease patterns (Fig. 1-7).[7] It outlines societal and demographic patterns that produce "dys-ease" and social pathology. It assumes that society will face an increasing number of social dysfunctions, environmental dislocations and disasters, and major demographic challenges. Completing the cycle of the social transformation model are societal values and ethical dilemmas.

A Service and Information Transfer Society

The move from an industrial manufacturing economy to a service, information transfer society (knowledge/information revolution) is reflected in changing employment patterns. In 1978, 21 million people held manufacturing jobs, and 16.5 million performed jobs in the service industry; by 1983, however, 19.2 million worked in service jobs, and 18 million worked in manufacturing.[8] By the year 2000 and beyond, this continuing shift to service occupations will play a major role in formulating disease patterns.

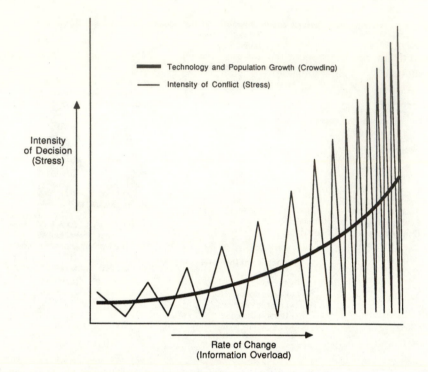

Figure 1-8 Characteristics of a Service and Information Transfer Society. *Source:* Modified from G.E. Alan Dever, "Future Shock and You" (1974), unpublished paper.

The interaction of the increasing rate of change, technology shifts, greater crowding (density), information overload, and stress—all characteristics of the service and information transfer society—plays a role in creating new disease patterns (Fig 1-8).[9] As Lesse noted,

> Clinically, some adolescents have demonstrated significant emotional illness secondary to the current rate of sociocultural change. Decompensation occurred when the adolescents, after attaining certain goals, found that they were no longer applicable. Their world had been changing at a rate that was in excess of their projections.[10]

Of course, change and conflict will not be limited to adolescents; demographic shifts may further accelerate problems and illnesses.

Crowding accompanies increasing urbanization. In the United States, the population density is 64 people per square mile, yet in 1980, 74 percent of the population lived in urban areas.[11] In New York's Manhattan, the density exceeds

60,000 people per square mile, leading to numerous problems. Lesse suggested that overcrowding will create a conflict between the individual's need for privacy and desire for group security.[12] No one knows, however, at what level of population density societal breakdown is likely to occur, if at all.

Associated with crowding (density) and urbanization is information overload, a problem in many U.S. cities. Information overload requires people to make endless choices among options, causing stress and eventually social shock. Nonetheless, restricting the opportunity for choice transforms the desire to choose into the "need" to choose.

Demographic Trends: The Baby Boom/Senior Boom

Between 1946 and 1964, 76.4 million babies were born in the United States; these individuals now make up one-third of the current population. The post–World War II increase in the fertility rate also occurred in many other countries, including Canada, New Zealand, Australia, and the Soviet Union. This "baby boom" created birth cohorts considerably larger than the Great Depression cohort (i.e., those between ages 45 and 49) and the "baby bust" cohort (i.e., those under age 20). The population distribution of people over age 50 resembles a typical population pyramid, as deaths decrease the size of older age groups.

The great upsurge in fertility between 1946 and 1964 still affects all aspects of contemporary society. Because of its relatively small size, the Depression cohort has experienced relative abundance. The large baby boom cohort can expect continued frustrations as it passes through life, however. For example, this group encountered overcrowded classrooms and a shortage of teachers during the 1960s and 1970s, and faced school closings and unemployment problems throughout the 1980s.

The recent increase in the number of births and in the crude birth rate is an "echo" effect of the baby boom that reflects the arrival of the cohort's female members at the prime childbearing ages of 20 to 29. Analysts expected this rise in the number of annual births in the 1980s, even with a continued fertility rate of approximately 1.8 births per woman. The number of births will remain high during the early 1990s, but should then decrease (fertility rates remaining constant) as the females in the baby bust cohort reach childbearing age from 1995 to 2005. From the early 1990s on, the number of births should remain constant because the age-sex profile will change from a pyramid to a stationary rectangular profile.

As the baby boom generation ages and as fertility remains low, the median age of the population will increase. In fact, as a result of declining birth rates and a progressively aging population, people 65 and over (particularly those 85 and over) are the fastest growing group in the United States. Because the Depression cohort is small, this growth will slow in the 1990s and in the first decade of the next century. Thereafter, however, the baby boom of the 1950s will become a senior boom, and the proportion of the population over 65 will grow rapidly to 15 percent in 2020 and 18 percent in 2030. After 2030, that group's relative size probably will decrease sharply again as the baby bust cohorts of the 1960s and 1970s become 65 and over.

The Bionomics of "Dys-ease"

Disease in a society usually results from the convergence of preconditions, or bionomics. For example, the preconditions set by demographics and the service and information transfer society are partially responsible for the current cycle of disease. The "dys-eases" typical of this cycle can be grouped as psychological, lifestyle, genetic, and social problems.

Psychological Problems. Drugs, alcohol, and depression will be the major causes of psychological problems in the future. These problems have already begun to increase dramatically and could easily reach epidemic proportions.

Increasing use of marijuana and cocaine is particularly notable (Table 1-2). Marijuana use has increased from 1974 to 1982 in all groups, except for the current users aged 12 to 17. The greatest increase is in the adult group (26 and older)—a 4.6 percent increase in the current user group and a 13.1 percent increase in the ever used group. Young adults (18 to 25) show the greatest percentage of current users (25.2 percent) and people who have ever used drugs (64.1 percent). Substantial increases occur in all age groups for both types of cocaine use.

Depression and associated psychological disturbances often occur with the advent of middle age. In 1986, approximately 9,300 persons per day reached the age of 40, and this rate will continue until the year 2004. For the 15-to-44 age group, 1983 hospital discharge records listed neurosis as the most common problem for males and the second most common problem for females. For the 45-to-64 age group, neurosis dropped to third and fourth positions, respectively, for males and females.[13]

From 1974 to 1982, all age groups increased their use of stimulants, sedatives, and tranquilizers, the prescribed drugs of choice to combat neurosis and depression. Selby suggested the following reason for this enormous consumption of psychotropic drugs:

> [They are] taken more as a means of defense than for a therapeutic effect; they provide momentary escape or support rather than cure, relief from fatigue, monotony, anguish, frustration, or even minor anxieties arising in everyday life. Curiously, as the stresses of modern life increase, so is the threshold of tolerance to them becoming progres-

Table 1-2 Percentage Drug Use by Type of Drug and Age Group, 1974 and 1982

Type of Drug	12- to 17-Year-Olds				18- to 25-Year-Olds				Adults 26 or Older			
	Ever Used		Current User*		Ever Used		Current User*		Ever Used		Current User*	
	1974	1982	1974	1982	1974	1982	1974	1982	1974	1982	1974	1982
Marijuana	12.0	26.7	12.0	11.5	52.7	64.1	25.2	27.4	9.9	23.0	2.0	6.6
Cocaine	3.6	6.5	1.0	1.6	12.7	28.3	3.1	6.8	0.9	8.5	<.5	1.2
Stimulants	5.0	6.7	1.0	2.6	17.0	18.0	3.7	4.7	3.0	6.2	<.5	<.5
Sedatives	5.0	5.8	1.0	1.3	15.0	18.7	1.6	2.6	2.0	4.8	<.5	<.5
Tranquilizers	3.0	4.9	1.0	0.9	10.0	15.1	1.2	1.6	2.0	3.6	<.5	<.5
Alcohol	54.0	65.2	34.0	26.9	81.6	94.6	69.3	67.9	73.2	88.2	54.6	56.7

*Those who used drugs at least once within a month before this study.

Source: Statistical Abstract of the U.S. 1986, 106th Edition, U.S. Department of Commerce, Bureau of the Census, Washington, D.C., page 118.

sively lower, so that substances which at one time were taken only for some pressing cause, such as severe insomnia or profound anxiety, are now ingested almost routinely in anticipation of such minor stresses as starting school or occasional insomnia. These drugs are too often looked on as a panacea, as a chemical screen behind which to escape from the stress of everyday life, as the ultimate recourse in the face of conflict situations.[14]

Alcohol use in the United States has contributed to many diseases and will continue to do so in the future. Violence, such as motor vehicle accidents, homicide, and suicide, is often a result of alcohol use. Table 1-2 shows that 65.2 percent of youths and 94.6 percent of young adults have used alcohol at least once. The corresponding figure for adults is 88.2 percent. These percentage increases are dramatic, although the percentage of current users has declined.

Psychological patterns of disease (depression, drug use, and alcohol) are fueled by the stresses of the service and information transfer society, as well as by demographic pressures. Most frightening, the age groups that use mind-altering drugs will grow rapidly over the next 15 to 20 years, creating a potentially volatile situation.

Lifestyle Problems. Both infectious and chronic diseases may stem from destructive lifestyles. The social transformation disease cycle, however, suggests that two of the major diseases plaguing U.S. society—AIDS and violence—are bionomically unique. AIDS has reached epidemic proportions among homosexuals and intravenous drug users, and it is now spreading to the general population. Social conditions and time/space clustering have contributed to the evolution and eventual spread of AIDS in the United States. Furthermore, homophobia and ignorance have frightened some groups, causing some regression to medieval values of control and prevention. AIDS could become even more devastating in the next 15 years, as the number of AIDS cases has increased approximately 150 percent per year since 1981.[15]

Violence, the other major lifestyle disease pattern, threatens the social fabric of the United States; it is the fourth leading cause of death in this country. In many instances, suicide, homicide, and motor vehicle accidents can be traced to depression, alcohol abuse, and drug use. Again, societal and demographic preconditions have led to these disease patterns. For the most part, the rates of violence show a downward trend, but they remain persistently high (Table 1-3). Violence, however, will have more impact in the next 5 to 10 years.

Genetic Problems. Scientific change has occurred most dramatically in the field of genetics. In 1970, scientists had identified only a few genes on any chromosome; by 1975, more than 100 genes had been mapped on human chromo-

Table 1-3 Number of Deaths per 100,000 Population from Accidents and Violence

	White				Black			
Cause of Death	*1960*	*1970*	*1975*	*1982*	*1960*	*1970*	*1975*	*1982*
Male, total	91.3	101.9	95.8	88.1	137.1	183.2	163.2	133.8
Motor vehicle accidents	31.5	39.1	31.8	30.1	33.2	44.3	32.4	25.9
All other accidents	38.6	38.2	35.1	27.8	60.8	63.3	51.8	38.7
Suicide	17.6	18.0	19.9	20.7	6.4	8.0	9.9	10.1
Homicide	3.6	6.8	9.0	9.6	36.7	67.6	69.0	59.1
Female, total	38.3	42.4	33.4	33.4	50.8	51.7	45.3	36.3
Motor vehicle accidents	11.2	14.8	11.3	11.0	9.7	13.4	9.1	7.6
All other accidents	20.4	18.3	16.5	13.2	29.1	22.5	18.6	14.6
Suicide	5.3	7.1	7.3	6.1	1.6	2.6	2.7	2.1
Homicide	1.4	2.1	2.9	3.1	10.4	13.3	14.9	12.0

Note: Beginning in 1970, rates include only deaths of residents of the United States. Beginning in 1979, deaths are classified according to the ninth revision of the *International Classification of Diseases.*

Source: U.S. National Center for Health Statistics, *Vital Statistics of the United States* (annual); unpublished data.

somes.[16] It has been estimated, however, that there may be as many as 100,000 genes in a single human chromosome.

This rapid growth in genetic research has important consequences for biological medicine. Clearly, genetic mapping or engineering introduces enormous risks and ethical dilemmas. Because it could lead to mishaps comparable to the thalidomide crisis, some degree of control is essential. On the one hand, too much change at too rapid a pace could produce dysfunctional products with overwhelmingly destructive consequences. On the other hand, genetic engineering promotes greater understanding of human development, facilitates the diagnosis of birth defects, and may make it possible to predict inherent susceptibility to disease.[17] Interferon, which helps to arm the body against viral infections, is one positive outcome of genetic engineering. Furthermore, the ability to combine segments of deoxyribonucleic acid (DNA) to produce hybrid molecules could contribute to scientists' understanding of cancer and several other diseases. Lesse underscored the ethical dilemmas that are some of the many "stop/go" decisions that society must make.

The potentialities of genetic manipulations are theoretically endless. . . . The prevention of or effective treatment of a variety of diseases that have hereditary propensities (diabetes mellitus, hemophilia, hematologic ailments, renal and cardiac problems) are valid possibilities.[18]

Lesse also noted the potential for minor or even cataclysmic problems if recombinant DNA research proceeds without controls.[19]

The dilemma is to control genetic engineering so that it produces positive outcomes while preventing the negative effects of re-engineered bacteria or genetically changed human, animal, or plant life. Society has a responsibility to temper its desire for scientific research with careful exploration, and control, of the possible outcomes.

Social Problems. In the social pathology of dysfunctional families and male-female relations, the most telling statistic is the divorce rate. In 1970, the rate was 41 per 1,000 people; by 1984, it had increased to 89 per 1,000 people. One of every two marriages ends in divorce.[20] The health of a community depends on the quality of family life, and increasing divorce rates jeopardize the family's ability to act as a force for stability.

The number of people in prison is another indicator of family breakdown. The number of adults under correctional supervision (jail, prison, parole, or probation) increased dramatically from 1979 to 1983—from 113 per 10,000 adults over age 18 in 1979 to 143 per 10,000 in 1983.[21] The number of prisoners in all institutions has jumped drastically since 1950, with the greatest increase occurring between 1980 and 1984.[22] In 1950, the rate was 110 prisoners per 100,000 people. In 1980, the rate had climbed to 139 per 100,000, and by 1984, it had reached 188 per 100,000.

In the future, relationships between men and women will be in a state of flux and will be a major source of stress. During the industrialization era, men increasingly participated in hierarchical organizations, whereas women, as a group, did not. One result is that men are more likely to speak as "we," reflecting their group orientation and their power. Women, on the other hand, have traditionally had the status of the "other," while those individuals with power made decisions affecting them.[23] Between 1948 and 1985, the percentage of women in the labor force rose from 29 to 55 percent, however, and it may reach 60% by 2000.[24] Greater conflict is likely as women show greater psychological similarity to men, becoming "we"-oriented. Friction will result from role shifts[25] and women's refusal to accept "other" or "object" status.

Future Issues: Measurement and Lifestyles

The measurement of these new bionomic problems clearly requires new criteria. In analyzing dys-ease, quality of life becomes the basic concern. Thus, years of life lost, workdays lost to disability, functional health status, and an overall index for the quality of life are essential measures for understanding the bionomics of disease. In addition, the social transformation model requires new data systems to track new disease patterns. Thus, it offers an opportunity to develop more function-, morbidity-, and ecology-oriented data sets that pertain to the development of a healthy public policy.

The dominance of services in the economy, the proliferation of information, and the subsequent changes in disease patterns will all affect individual and community lifestyles. Questions about social and individual behavior will create ethical dilemmas. Furthermore, values, which will emphasize turning inward in the next two decades, will influence how people live.

In the mid-1980s, the health care industry attempted to provide quality health care with relatively fewer resources. An aging population will continue to make increasing demands on the health care system. Allocating resources judiciously, through efficiency measures or even voluntary restraint, may partially resolve this dilemma, but resource allocation will require ethical decisions that take into account human rights, equity, equality, and justice.

Lifestyle intervention will continue to be necessary to prevent some diseases, and society will have to make difficult decisions about an individual's freedom to behave in a manner that threatens health, right to receive health care, and responsibility for personal health care. What is the individual's responsibility for making lifestyle changes? What is society's responsibility for providing care to individuals who have chosen lifestyles that contribute to poor health? How far does the individual's right to health care extend, given moral issues and inadequate resources?[26]

People's values affect their lifestyles or behaviors.[27] Certainly, the pressures of contemporary society require that individuals learn to adapt and cope.[28] In the past 20 years, the United States has seen a major shift in the values and, therefore, lifestyles of its citizens; moreover, this trend will continue at least through the year 2000. People are moving toward "lifestyles focused on the inner world rather than the external world of tangibles," according to Mitchell.[29]

MODELS OF HEALTH

Ecological Model

A model that is essential to the investigation of infectious diseases, the ecological model is based on the traditional concept of ecological balance in which the host, the environment, and the agent are in dynamic equilibrium (Fig. 1-9). When the balance is upset, disease occurs. Upsets may happen when (1) the environment changes, (2) the agent's ability to infect humans increases, and/or (3) the proportion of susceptible hosts increases in the population. Drug therapy, sanitation, immunization, or surgery may be used to tip the balance in favor of the host (humans) and thereby control infectious diseases. This model is a natural

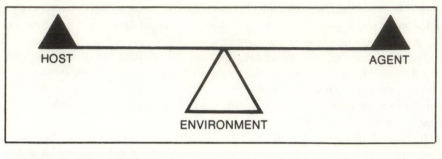

Figure 1-9 The Ecological Model

consequence of the acceptance of the "germ theory" postulated by Koch.[30] It assumes a single causative agent (single-cause/single-effect model) based on statistically absolute correlations. It is questionable, however, whether this assumption is valid for the new disease patterns. Because this model's methods of control are borrowed from infectious disease epidemiology, the approach is outmoded or less important for today's disease patterns and those of the future. Yet, despite its inherent limitations, the ecology model has been applied to a great many new illnesses, diseases, and hazards.

Social-Ecological Model

A major improvement over the ecology model is the social-ecological model developed by Morris[31] (Fig. 1-10). It replaces the agent (an infectious disease consideration) with personal behavior factors. The model suggests that, because many factors influence a person's health, there may be no specific etiological agent (multiple-cause/multiple-effect or multiple-cause/single-effect) for a disease. Thus, medical care services are not considered an influence on health; iatrogenesis (illness caused by physicians), for example, is not considered a factor. With this model, behavioral factors have a greater impact than does the physical environment, but all aspects are believed to contribute to a dynamic balance.

Holistic Model

The concept of health held by the World Health Organization (WHO) is an expansion of the social-ecological model. The WHO constitution states, "Health is a state of complete physical, mental, and social well-being and not merely the absence of disease and infirmity."[32] This approach adds the dimension of mental

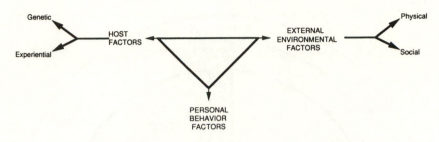

Figure 1-10 The Social-Ecological Model. *Source:* Adapted from *Uses of Epidemiology*, 3rd ed., by J.N. Morris, p. 177, with permission of Churchill Livingstone Inc., © 1975.

well-being while retaining the social and physical characteristics of the social-ecological model. The basic difference is that the WHO model defines health in terms of what should be, rather than in terms of the components or factors that constitute health. The WHO concept has been a major impetus toward changing beliefs about the dimensions of health. Unrestricted by a specific definition of health, it has led to the development of multidimensional models that have broadened the framework of what constitutes health. These models can be described as holistic.

> Holistic means . . . viewing a person and his/her wellness from every perspective, taking into account every available concept and skill for the person's growth toward harmony and balance. It means treating the person, not the disease. The holistic approach promotes the interrelationship and unity of body, mind, and spirit. A holistic approach differs from simply following an "alternative" therapy. It is not an alternative to conventional medical practice. Rather, it includes judicious use of the best of modern Western medicine combined with the best health practices from East and West, old and new.[33]

The holistic model has fostered nontraditional approaches to health planning and policy making in an era of new disease patterns. Its basic assumption is that health, with its many dimensions, has four fundamental attributes: (1) environment, (2) lifestyle, (3) human biology, and (4) system of health care. Blum called it the "environment of health" (Fig. 1-11);[34] Lalonde termed it the "health field concept" (Fig. 1-12);[35] and Dever, building on Lalonde's model, labeled it "an epidemiological model for health policy analysis" (Fig. 1-13).[36]

In Blum's model (see Fig. 1-11), the width of the four attributes, or inputs, indicates assumptions about the relative importance of their contributions to health. The four inputs relate to and affect one another by means of an encompassing wheel made up of population, cultural systems, mental health, ecologi-

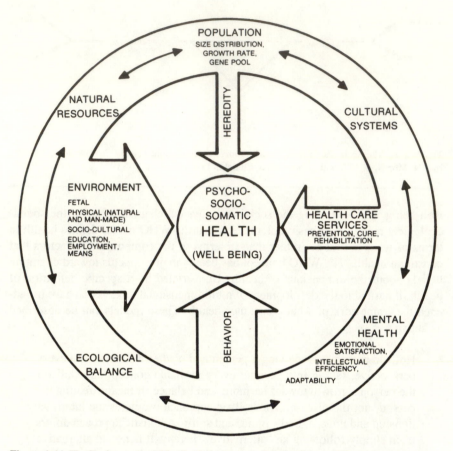

Figure 1-11 The Environment of Health Model. *Source:* Reprinted from *Planning for Health: Developmental Application of Social Change Theory* by H.L. Blum, p. 3, with permission of Human Sciences Press, © 1974.

cal balance, and natural resources. In contrast, Lalonde and Dever assumed that the four inputs are weighted equally and must be in balance for health to occur. The important question to answer is, How do these four inputs operate in the presence of specific diseases or, alternatively, in the absence of disease, that is, in a state of wellness? The analysis of risk factors for disease categories within the framework of Dever's epidemiological model for policy analysis provides results similar to those hypothesized by Blum.[37]

These holistic models have engendered a new belief system about what constitutes health, but many people still retain the belief that, in order to feel better, they must go to the physician. This belief is an outgrowth of the single-cause/

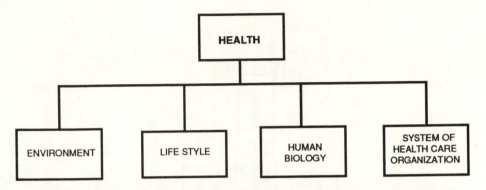

Figure 1-12 The Health Field Concept. *Source:* Adapted from *A New Perspective on the Health of Canadians* by M. Lalonde, p. 31, Office of the Canadian Minister of National Health and Welfare, 1974.

single-effect model associated with the ecological concept of health. The concepts of what constitutes health have changed, but people have not let go of the medical care system as the only means to make them feel better. The alternative means to survival is the concept of wellness.

Wellness Model

Travis made the distinction between holism and wellness quite clear: "The primary orientation of holistic health is still towards healing conditions of illness. In contrast, the primary orientation of wellness is on increasing conditions of wellness."[38] Specifically, the wellness model focuses on four dimensions: (1) physical activity, (2) nutritional awareness, (3) stress management, and (4) self-responsibility.

Travis developed the concept of an illness-wellness continuum (Fig. 1-14).[39] The neutral point indicates no illness or wellness. Movement to the left shows poorer conditions of illness; movement to the right shows better levels of wellness. For instance, it is possible to be not quite physically ill, yet to experience depression, anxiety, frustration, and an overall dissatisfaction with life. Although traditional medicine may eliminate discernible physical illness, wellness goes beyond this point and deals with aliveness and enlightenment.

ACHIEVING HEALTH FOR ALL—2000

Thinking about the components of health care and ways to achieve health for all has shifted from the "self-centered" activities of the holistic models in the

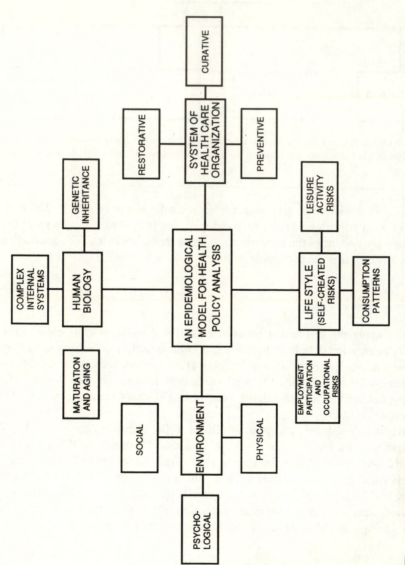

Figure 1-13 An Epidemiological Model for Health Policy Analysis. *Source:* Reprinted from *Social Indicators Research,* Vol. 2, p. 455, with permission of Kluwer Aademic Publishers, © 1976.

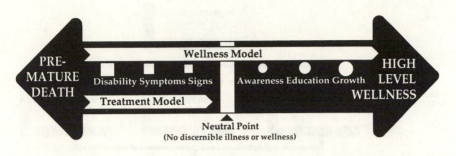
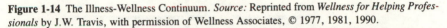

Figure 1-14 The Illness-Wellness Continuum. *Source:* Reprinted from *Wellness for Helping Professionals* by J.W. Travis, with permission of Wellness Associates, © 1977, 1981, 1990.

1980s to an approach that embraces communities yet supports the tenets of individual participation in achieving health. This new vision of health requires an understanding of the changing nature of society as portrayed in the social transformation disease model. Many countries, as well as the WHO, have embraced this shift in focus to a more balanced policy that promotes health by supporting communities and fostering individual participation.[40–51]

In the United States, efforts have been directed toward establishing health objectives for the year 2000[52] (e.g., reducing tobacco use and improving surveillance and data systems[53]) and studying the future of public health.[54] Despite these efforts, public health in the United States is in a state of disarray. Although there is a focus on issues, such as preventive services, health protection, health promotion, objectives for vulnerable groups, expansion of access, social and physical correlates of disease, data collection needs, the objective process, and funds for health promotion and disease prevention,[55] there is no framework for action—no overall strategy or policy. Similarly, there is no strategy for dealing with the health care priorities of the Bush Administration: human immunovirus (HIV) infection, drug abuse, health problems of the poor and minorities, the high cost of health care, and long-term care and health care for the uninsured and underinsured.[56]

Given the fragmented situation in the United States, the Canadian experience is to be emulated. Epp outlined a model with components that are not topical or issue based, but are concepts, challenges, and strategies for achieving health for all Canadians by the year 2000 (Fig. 1-15).[57]

The health *challenges* identified in Epp's model are (1) reducing inequities in the health of low- versus high-income groups in Canada, (2) increasing the prevention effort to find new and more effective ways of preventing the major cripplers and killers (e.g., estimated 45 percent reduction in mortality through lifestyle changes alone),[58] and (3) enhancing people's capacity to cope with chronic

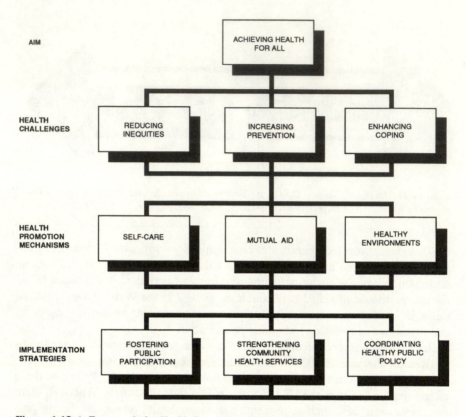

Figure 1-15 A Framework for Health Promotion. *Source:* Reprinted from *Canadian Journal of Public Health,* Vol. 77, No. 6, p. 402, with permission of Canadian Public Health Association, © 1986.

problems, disabilities, and mental health problems. The latter requires a capacity-building strategy at the individual level in contrast to traditional services-building policies that can be incapacitating or can foster dependency.[59,60] This point is critical to health care in the twenty-first century as the baby boom becomes the senior boom.

These critical challenges of the twenty-first century can be met through a broadened application of health promotion and disease prevention efforts. In the process of enabling people to increase control over and to improve their health, self-care, mutual aid, and healthy environments are the mechanisms to be promoted. Self-care comprises the decisions and actions that *individuals* take in the interest of their own health or simply healthy choices. Mutual aid, on the other hand, involves groups, such as families, neighborhoods, communities, voluntary organizations, self-help groups, in which people work together; support each other emotionally; and share ideas, information, and experiences. Thus, informal networking is a basic resource in the promotion of health. The value of such mutual aid is that it enables people to live interdependently within a community while maintaining their independence. Ironically, the third health promotion mechanism, the healthy environment, was all but discarded during the transition from infectious diseases to chronic diseases. Now, in the 1990s and in the twenty-first century, the environment is seen as a major and critical component of health and well-being. This perspective must broaden to include social and economic, not just physical, elements. Education, labor, transportation, and health agencies must come together to promote legislation that will achieve a healthy environment.

To meet these health challenges and ensure that the health promotion mechanisms are implemented, Epp identified a set of strategies: (1) fostering public participation, (2) strengthening community health services, and (3) coordinating healthy public policy.[61] Health is a function of participation, and a strategy that is directed toward public participation is of paramount importance to the improvement in disease patterns. Individuals must participate not only to improve their own health, but also to deal with such societal problems as drug abuse, homelessness, illiteracy, AIDS, social injustice, inequity, and ecological threats.

Community health services must be strengthened in two ways. First, public health professionals must strengthen and expand their services to promote health. Second, communities must build their capacity to resolve their own health problems. This concept of capacity building versus service assistance in communities will emerge in the 1990s as a major policy shift that will be essential to our aim of ensuring conditions in which people can be healthy.

The third strategy—coordinating healthy public policy—will be the most critical in ensuring health for all in the 1990s. It will require changes in thinking about ways to improve and promote health in the next 10 to 20 years. This change in direction will result in our directing change.[62] In the 1980s, health was recognized as a function of lifestyle, environment, biology, and health care delivery system. This model, which is still useful, was initially adopted in the United States in the public health arena. Yet, outside this arena, it has seldom been recognized. This lack of recognition cannot continue in the 1990s and into the 2000s. It is essential to coordinate policies among various sectors, which obviously do not share the same priorities. For example, a chemical company that dumps toxic waste into a river may argue that it would have to release employees if forced to clean up the pollution. This creates a dilemma, as a community needs both clean water and jobs. This type of ethical conflict will dominate the 1990s and will require health-promoting policy in such fields as energy, transportation, food, agriculture, economics, environment, education, and technology, not only in the health care sector. Thus, the challenge will be to advocate and coordinate healthy public policy.

The health promotion framework outlined by Epp will be of value to the United States in formulating a health policy. Epp stated

> Use it to visualize the kinds of mechanisms and strategies that are needed to support and encourage *Americans* as they strive to live healthy full lives. The framework links together a set of concepts, providing us with a particular way of thinking about and taking action toward achieving our aim of health for everyone in this country.[63]

NOTES

1. J. John Dundustadt, "The State of the University—Leadership for the Twenty-First Century," *Michigan Alumnas* (November/December 1988): 22–28.

2. Ibid., 22–28.

3. Ibid.

4. Adelaide Bry, *EST* (New York: Avon Books, 1976).

5. I have not discussed the concept of association as it relates to causation; however, the reader may find a brief, but excellent, comparison of association and causation in Donald F. Austin and S. Benson Werner, *Epidemiology for the Health Sciences* (Springfield, Ill.: Charles C. Thomas, 1974). For a more sophisticated interpretation of causality in epidemiology, *see* P.O. Woolley et al., *Syncrisis: The Dynamics of Health* (Washington, D.C.: U.S. Government Printing Office, June 1972) and M. Susser, *Causal Thinking in the Health Sciences* (New York: Oxford University Press, 1973).

6. Dundustadt, "State of the University," 22–28.

7. James W. Alley, G.E. Alan Dever, and Thomas E. Wade, "Social Transformation Model: Human Development and Disease Patterns," Stanford Research International (SRI), Menlo Park, Calif., Datalog File 87-1153 (October 1986): 1–29.

8. Foundation of the American College of Health Care Executives, *Health Care Consumers; Demographic Analysis of the Market for Health Services* (Ann Arbor, Mich.: Health Administration Press, 1985).

9. G.E. Alan Dever, "Future Shock and You." 1974.

10. Stanley Lesse, *The Future of the Health Sciences: Anticipating Tomorrow* (New York: Irvington Publishers, 1981), 98.

11. U.S. Bureau of the Census, *Statistical Abstract of the United States: 1986,* 106th ed. (Washington, D.C.: U.S. Government Printing Office, 1985), 15.

12. Lesse, *Future of the Health Sciences,* 100.

13. U.S. Bureau of the Census, *Statistical Abstract,* 10.

14. Philip Selby, *Health in 1980–1990: A Predictive Study Based on an International Inquiry* (New York: S. Karger, 1974), 38.

15. Division of Public Health, *Disease Patterns of the 1980's* (Atlanta: Georgia Department of Human Resources, 1986), 124.

16. Lesse, *Future of the Health Sciences,* 89.

17. Ibid.

18. Ibid., 90.

19. Ibid.

20. U.S. Bureau of the Census, *Statistical Abstract,* 35.

21. Ibid., 185.

22. Ibid., 184.

23. Simone de Beauvoir, *The Second Sex* (New York: Alfred A. Knopf, 1952), 28.

24. David E. Bloom, "Women and Work," *American Demographics* (September 1986): 25–30.

25. Lesse, *Future of the Health Sciences,* 104.

26. Tom L. Beauchamp and James F. Childress, *Principles of Biomedical Ethics* (New York: Oxford University Press, 1983), 59.

27. Arnold Mitchell, *The Nine American Lifestyles* (New York: Warner Books, 1984), 25.

28. Dever, "Future Shock and You," 8.

29. Mitchell, *Nine American Lifestyles,* 16.

30. Austin and Werner, *Epidemiology for the Health Sciences,* 42.

31. J.N. Morris, *Uses of Epidemiology,* 3rd ed. (Edinburgh: Churchill Livingstone, 1975), 173–180.

32. *Basic Documents,* 15th ed. (Geneva: World Health Organization, 1964).

33. D.B. Ardell, *High Level Wellness, An Alternative to Doctors, Drugs, and Disease* (Erasmus, Pa.: Rodale Press, 1977), 5.

34. Henrich L. Blum, *Planning for Health: Development and Application of Social Change Theory* (New York: Human Sciences Press, 1974), 31–34.

35. Marc Lalonde, *A New Perspective on the Health of Canadians* (Ottawa: Office of the Canadian Minister of National Health and Welfare, 1974), 31–34.

36. G.E.A. Dever, "An Epidemiological Model for Health Policy Analysis," *Social Indicators Research* 2 (1976): 453–466.

37. G.E.A. Dever, *Community Health Analysis: A Holistic Approach* (Gaithersburg, Md.: Aspen Publishers, 1980).

38. J.W. Travis, *Wellness for Helping Professionals* (Mill Valley, Calif.: Wellness Associates, 1977, 1981, 1990).

39. Ibid.

40. J. Epp, "Achieving Health for All: A Framework for Health Promotion," *Canadian Journal of Public Health* 77 (November/December 1986): 393–407.

41. Secretariat for Future Studies, *Care and Welfare at the Crossroads* (Stockholm: 1982).

42. The Swedish Ministry of Health and Social Affairs, *Health in Sweden. The Swedish Health Services in the 1990's* (Stockholm: 1982).

43. *Healthy People—The Surgeon General's Report on Health Promotion and Disease Prevention,* DHEW (PHS) Publ. No. 79550712, 1979.

44. Department of Health and Social Security, *Care in Action. A Handbook of Policies and Priorities for the Health and Personal Social Services in England* (London: Her Majesty's Stationery Office, 1981).

45. World Health Organization, *Global Strategy for Health for All by the Year 2000* (Geneva: 1981).

46. *Research in Health Promotion Priorities, Strategies, Barriers.* Report of a Joint WHO/SHEG Working Group, Edinburgh, Scotland, November 5–7, 1984.

47. *Working Group on Concepts and Principles of Health Promotion,* Summary report on a Working Group, Health Education Unit, WHO Regional Office for Europe (Copenhagen: 1981).

48. *Study Group on Health Promotion,* EURO.WHO Regional Office for Europe (Copenhagen, May 28–31, 1985).

49. U.S. Department of Health and Human Services, "National Guidelines for Health Planning: Proposed Rules," *Federal Register,* November 25, 1980.

50. U.S. Department of Health and Human Services, Public Health Service, *Promoting Health/Preventing Disease Objectives for the Nation* (Washington, D.C.: U.S. Government Printing Office, 1980).

51. "Promoting Health/Preventing Disease. Public Health Service I Implementation Plans for Attaining the Objectives for the Nation," *Public Health Reports* supplement (September-October 1983).

52. M.A. Stoto, Memorandum to Members of the Year 2000 Health Objectives Consortium. Update on the Year 2000 Objectives. National Academy of Sciences, June 14, 1988, p. 10.

53. Ibid.

54. Institute of Medicine, "Committee for the Study of the Future of Public Health," National Academy of Sciences (1988): 225.

55. Stoto, Memorandum to Members of the Year 2000 Health Objectives Consortium, 10.

56. L.W. Sullivan, "Shattuck Lecture—The Health Care Priorities of the Bush Administration," *New England Journal of Medicine* (July 13, 1989): 125–128.

57. Epp, "Achieving Health for All," 393–407.

58. Dever, "An Epidemiological Model for Health Policy Analysis," 456–461.

59. John Stewart and Michael Clarke, "The Public Service Orientation: Issues and Dilemmas," *Public Administration* 65 (Summer 1987): 161–177.

60. John McKnight, "Why 'Servanthood' is Bad," *The Other Side* (January/February 1989): 38–41.

61. Epp, "Achieving Health for All," 393–407.

62. G.L. Siler-Wells, *Directing Change and Changing Direction—A New Health Policy Agenda for Canada* (Ottawa: Canadian Public Health Association, 1988), 131.

63. Epp, "Achieving Health for All," 393–407.

Chapter 2

Health Policy:
A Need for Redirection

In the 1970s and mid-1980s, the elements of lifestyle, environment, and biology were raised to a level of categorical importance equal to that of the health care delivery system. In the 1990s, the goal will be to expand our health policy beyond these four traditional elements of the health field concept to establish a *healthy public policy*. To achieve this goal will require that much of health programming be carried out independently of health care and that public health professionals adopt an advocacy role in promoting health.

HEALTH FIELD CONCEPT REVISITED

In his model—the health field concept—Lalonde made a clear statement about the factors that contribute to the health status of a community: lifestyle, biology, environment, and the health care delivery system.[1] The Lalonde effort has become a landmark study that has provided the impetus for changing the direction of health policy. From the Lalonde model, Dever developed an epidemiological model for health policy analysis that addresses the problems concerned with changing disease patterns.[2] This model was developed in an era when infectious diseases were giving way to chronic diseases. Now, however, the chronic diseases are giving way to diseases and community problems related to social, environmental, and economic factors. This change makes it necessary to go beyond the Lalonde model.

The Lalonde model is an epidemiological model that supports a broad and comprehensive health policy analysis. It has four primary divisions: (1) system of medical care organization; (2) lifestyle, that is, self-created risks; (3) environment; and (4) human biology (see Fig. 1-12). This epidemiological model provides a more balanced approach to the development of health policy than do the limiting, traditional divisions of prevention, diagnosis, therapy, and rehabilitation, or public health, mental health, and clinical medicine.

31

Lalonde cited these advantages of his model:

1. This model raises Life Style, Environment, and Human Biology to a level of categorical importance equal to that of the System of Medical Care Organization.
2. The model is comprehensive. Any health problem can be traced to one or a combination of the four divisions.
3. The model allows a system of analysis by which a disease or pattern may be examined under the four divisions in order to assess relative significance and interaction (i.e., what percentage or proportion of Life Style, Environment, Human Biology, and System of Medical Care Organization contributes to suicide?).
4. This model permits further subdivision of the four major factors; for example, Environment is subdivided into physical, social, and psychological.
5. This model provides a new perspective (a new tunnel) on health that creates a recognition and exploration of previously neglected fields.[3]

System of Medical Care Organization

The availability, quality, and quantity of resources to provide health care make up the system of medical care organization. The system has three types of elements: restorative, curative, and preventive. The system's restorative elements include hospital, nursing home, and ambulance services. Its curative elements include medical drugs, dental treatments, and medical professionals. The system has a very limited input of preventive elements.

Efforts and expenditures to improve health in the United States have been directed almost totally toward the system of medical care organization. Yet, the morbidity and mortality patterns of today are deeply entrenched in the other three divisions of the epidemiological model. Lalonde concluded that the huge sums of money spent for restoring and curing should be earmarked for prevention of disease in the population.

Lifestyle

The self-created risks associated with lifestyles are divided into three elements: leisure activity risks, consumption patterns, and employment occupational risks. This division of the epidemiological model comprises the decisions of individuals that affect their health and over which they have more or less control. Poor or incorrect decisions contribute to an increased level of illness or premature death.

The lifestyle component of the epidemiological model is a major contributing factor to present and future disease patterns. The possibility of changing this component, however, is viewed with considerable pessimism, primarily because destructive lifestyles are based on the principle of self-pleasure. A change in hedonistic behavior occurs only after a life-death event, and even this change wanes considerably as the length of time after the critical event increases. The consequence of this pleasure principle is that the lifestyle component at best will change little and at worst will not change at all, thereby effecting little change in major disease patterns. Thus, it is necessary to alter belief systems and realize that the solutions to current disease patterns lie in "new tunnels" to achieve wellness.

Leisure Activity Risks

Some self-imposed destructive modes of health are the result of leisure activities. For instance, lack of recreation is strongly associated with hypertension and coronary heart disease. Similarly, lack of exercise leads to obesity and a total lack of physical fitness. These examples (and there are many more) pinpoint the need to focus more specifically on the other divisions of the epidemiological model. Indeed, such a shift in focus is imperative to reduce disability and promote a better quality of life.

Consumption Patterns

Another kind of self-imposed risk is in the area of "consumption patterns," which include (1) overeating, leading to obesity and its subsequent consequences; (2) cholesterol intake, contributing to heart disease; (3) alcohol addiction, leading to cirrhosis of the liver; (4) alcohol consumption, leading to motor vehicle accidents; (5) cigarette smoking, causing chronic obstructive pulmonary disease (chronic bronchitis, emphysema) and lung cancer, and aggravating heart disease; (6) drug dependency and social drug use, leading to suicide, homicide, malnutrition, accidents, social withdrawal, and acute anxiety attacks; and (7) abundant glucose (sugar) intake, contributing to dental caries, obesity, and hyperglycemia with its concomitant problems.

Employment/Occupational Risks

Destructive lifestyles associated with employment and occupational risks are equally significant, but far more difficult to identify. Work pressures lead to stresses, anxieties, and tensions that, in turn, may cause peptic ulcers and hypertension. Other habits such as careless driving lead to accidents, whereas sexual promiscuity often results in syphilis, gonorrhea, or AIDS.

Environment

In the epidemiological model, the environment is defined as events external to the body over which the individual has little or no control. This element is subdivided into physical, social, and psychological dimensions. Many environmental conditions create risks that pose a far greater threat to health than any present inadequacy of the system of medical care organization. The resulting health problems will be resolved only by imposing standards and controls on the responsible agencies and industries.

Physical Dimension

In the physical environment, certain hazards are closely related to the use of energy (oil) by an expanding population. Per capita energy consumption is increasing concomitantly with the population and the standard of living. Thus, the health hazards that stem from air, noise, and water pollution will almost assuredly increase steadily. The resulting problems and diseases include hearing loss, infectious diseases, gastroenteritis, cancer, emphysema, and bronchitis. Ionizing and ultraviolet radiation have health implications in terms of skin cancer and genetic mutation.

Social and Psychological Dimensions

The major factors in the social and psychological dimensions of environmental health encompass behavior modification, perceptional problems, and interpersonal relationships. For example, crowding, isolation, rapid and accelerated rates of change, and social interchange may contribute to homicide, suicide, decisional stress, and environmental overstimulation.

Human Biology

Focusing on the human body, the human biology component of the epidemiological model is concerned with each individual's basic biological and organic makeup. Thus, the genetic inheritance of the individual may result in genetic disorders, congenital malformation, and mental retardation. The maturation and aging process is a contributing factor in arthritis, diabetes, atherosclerosis, and cancer. Obvious disorders of the skeletal, muscular, cardiovascular, endocrine, and digestive systems can be included in a subcomponent of complex internal systems. Disease categories related to human biology must be weighted in accordance with the other divisions of the epidemiological model.

EPIDEMIOLOGICAL MODEL FOR HEALTH POLICY

In 1976, Dever polled health care professionals in Georgia to estimate the contribution of lifestyle, environment, human biology, and the health care system to the top 13 causes of death in Georgia.[4] It was found that the major contributing factors to the selected diseases are deeply rooted in lifestyle, environment, and human biology (Table 2-1). Furthermore, the system of medical care organization has a limited impact on disease prevention. In fact, inadequacies in the health care system accounted for only about 11 percent of the deaths, whereas problems in lifestyle, environment, and human biology accounted for 43, 19,

Table 2-1 An Epidemiological Model for Health Policy Analysis—Disease Evaluation

Percent Distribution of Total Deaths 1973	Cause of Mortality	Percentage Allocation of Mortality to the Epidemiological Model*			
		System of Medical Care Organization	Life-style	Environ-ment	Human Biology
34.0	Disease of the heart	12	54	9	28
14.9	Cancer	10	37	24	29
13.4	Cerebrovascular disease	7	50	22	21
4.2	Motor vehicle accidents	12	69	18	1
3.8	All other accidents	14	51	31	4
3.8	Influenza and pneumonia	18	23	20	39
2.7	Disease of the respiratory system	13	40	24	24
2.6	Disease of the arteries, veins, and capillaries	18	49	8	26
2.2	Homicides	0	66	30	5
1.9	Birth injuries and other diseases of early infancy	27	30	15	28
1.8	Diabetes mellitus	6	26	0	68
1.4	Suicides	3	60	35	2
0.8	Congenital anomalies	6	9	6	79
	Percentage allocation—average	11	43	19	27

*Due to rounding, the percent allocation may not add to 100%.

Source: Reprinted from *Social Indicators Research,* Vol. 2, p. 462, with permission of Kluwer Academic Publishers, © 1976.

and 27 percent, respectively. The analysis revealed an important message—that most diseases that are killing and crippling Georgians are not amenable to changes in the health care delivery system. In a recent report, La Force noted, "I still remember the sense of correctness that came over me as I was reading their paper because they coincided so well with what I was seeing clinically."[5]

In 1976, the federal government allocated 90.7 percent of its health care dollars to the system of medical care organization, whereas lifestyle, environment, and human biology received 1.1, 1.5, and 6.7 percent, respectively (Table 2-2).[6] In the next decade, the situation did not change. "In 1985, 425 billion dollars were spent on health care in the United States. Public Health and Research made up 2.8 and 1.7 percent of the budget, respectively, while 73.7 percent of health dollars was paid to hospitals, physicians, nursing homes and for drugs."[7] Thus, a disproportionate amount of money has been allocated for the system of medical care organization, despite the fact that the means for reducing mortality and morbidity are deeply rooted in lifestyle, environment, and human biology elements and that only minimal reductions in mortality and morbidity can be expected from the system of medical care organization (Table 2-3).

Table 2-2 Allocation of Federal Health Expenditures in Accordance with the Epidemiological Model for Health Policy Analysis: 1974, 1975, and 1976

Elements of the Epidemiological Model for Health Policy Analysis	Federal Outlay (in millions)		
	1974 Actual	1975 Estimate	1976 Estimate
Total federal health expenditures	29,189	35,044	37,699
Systems of medical care organization	26,216	31,601	34,197
Training and education	1,146	1,324	1,145
Construction of health care facilities	761	967	1,108
Improving organization and delivery	392	527	596
Provision of hospital and medical services	23,918	28,783	31,348
Direct federal services	4,797	5,390	5,828
Indirect services	19,120	23,393	25,520
Percent of total federal health expenditures	89.8%	90.1%	90.7%
Lifestyle	420	458	405
Disease prevention and control	420	458	405
Percent of total federal health expenditures	1.4%	1.3%	1.1%
Environment	468	561	583
Environmental control	90	129	137
Consumer safety	378	432	446
Percent of total federal health expenditures	1.6%	1.6%	1.5%
Human biology	2,085	2,424	2,512
Health research	2,085	2,424	2,512
Percent of total federal health expenditures	7.1%	6.9%	6.7%

Table 2-3 Comparison of Federal Health Expenditures to the Allocation of Mortality in Accordance with the Epidemiological Model for Health Policy Analysis

Epidemiological Model for Health Policy Analysis	Federal Health Expenditures 1974–1976 (%)	Allocation of Mortality to the Epidemiological Model (%)
System of medical care organization	90.2	11
Lifestyle	1.3	43
Environment	1.6	19
Human biology	6.9	27

Source: Reprinted from *Social Indicators Research,* Vol. 2, p. 465, with permission of Kluwer Academic Publishers, © 1976.

The conclusion is obvious. Unless there is a dramatic shift in U.S. health policy from current procedures for reducing mortality and morbidity, there will be little or no change in disease patterns. Furthermore, with the aging of the population, there may well be dramatic increases in mortality and morbidity. It is clear that present policies do not support the methods most likely to improve health status.

A major effort should be undertaken to develop a holistic and wellness policy. Without such an effort, the present tunnel vision analysis will lead to even greater dependence on the system of medical care organization, with its growing medical technology and concomitant increase in specialized personnel. This is a very mechanistic and reductionistic avenue to medical care at a time when there is an essential need for a return to the community.[8]

PUBLIC HEALTH POLICY TO HEALTHY PUBLIC POLICY

Although there have been many criticisms of the Lalonde report,[9-11] its publication was a watershed event in community health, as noted by Hancock:

> In spite of its faults, the Lalonde report was a truly significant milestone in the renaissance of public health. Perhaps the best tribute to its authors is to accept it for what it is—the signpost pointing the way at the start of a journey—and to move off in our more sophisticated promotional vehicles down the road to improve health for all to which the Lalonde report was pointing.[12]

Clearly, the Lalonde report has expanded the vision of public health professionals so that they are willing to go beyond the biomedical health care system (a sick care system). The health policy of the future will be even broader than that which Lalonde envisioned.

Public health is now in a process of change.[13] Siler-Wells recommended a new health policy agenda that has as one of its priorities the expansion of the health policy framework.[14] This expansion would include (1) the health network, in which the primary focus is on health enhancement; (2) the health context, in which the focus is on a healthy public policy, especially on the social, economic, and physical environments and how they affect the individual and community health status; and (3) the health care system, in which the primary focus is on sickness treatment.

The governments of Canada and the United States now recognize the need for an expanded health policy. A Canadian conference on healthy public policy in 1984 suggested that it is essential to look beyond health care.[15] In the United States, Shannon described the Institute of Medicine *Report on the Future of Public Health* as a framework for reassessment in public health. She noted, "It has implications for those involved directly in public health, and for those involved indirectly, particularly in the development of public health policy, and for the community-at-large."[16]

Such complex social, economic, and environmental problems as teenage pregnancy, drugs, infant mortality (e.g., "crack babies"), violence, and homelessness can no longer be solved within the medical world alone, nor even within the world of health alone.[17] The solutions transcend health and include social, economic, and environmental components. For example, the "war on drugs" that President Bush declared when he made a forceful appeal to the major European countries for help in combatting this devastating problem transcends the field of public health.

Bonham noted four areas of prevention, two of which go beyond the traditional health arenas: the political/social arena, the lifestyle arena, the traditional public health arena, and the traditional medical office arena.[18] It is in the political/social arena that a shift to a healthy public policy will be made. "Prosperity and political action in the social arena provides or stimulates better nutrition, housing, and the abatement of most environmental hazards."[19] *All of this is carried out independently of health care.* Legislation on seatbelts, distribution of income, pasteurization, pollution control, and safety in the workplace all relate to political action, social action, or prosperity itself. The players include politicians and citizens' groups.[20] Thus, public health officials need to move into positive and active advocacy for health. Epp and Mahler pointed out the need for these officials to help individuals and communities to develop their health potential; instead of building service systems, they should enable communities to build on their capacities.[21,22]

Hancock made an important distinction between public health policy and healthy public policy (Exhibit 2-1).[23] Public health policy accepts the "what is"

Exhibit 2-1 Public Health Policy vs. Healthy Public Policy

Public Health Policy	*Healthy Public Policy*
1. Chiefly concerned with the health care system	1. Chiefly concerned with creating a healthy society
2. Dominated by the hard health path	2. Dominated by the soft health path
3. Sectoral/analytic	3. Holistic
4. Present oriented	4. Future oriented
5. Accepts the givens	5. Questions the givens

Source: Reprinted from *Canadian Journal of Public Health*, Vol. 76, p. 10, with permission of Canadian Public Health Association, © 1985.

about the present system, which is dominated by technology planned around an individual/group, illness/service care system—a sick care system that is mechanistic and reductionistic. In contrast, healthy public policy, or perhaps more accurately holistic public policy, questions the "what is" and asks "what should be." By emphasizing the building of capacity in communities to solve the local problems, rather than allowing them to continue to rely on service systems that build on people's deficiencies,[24] it involves not only the individual, but also the local community (Fig. 2-1). It sets a social goal and moves health from an outcome measure of social development to one of its major resources.[25] Whereas the Lalonde model was directed (holistically) to the health of the individual, a healthy public policy is directed (holistically) to the individual/community/ global health of the ecosystem. Thus, all public policies (e.g., those in education, housing, business, industry, and environment) become health-related public policies. Therefore, it is necessary to raise the awareness of policy makers, planners, researchers, analysts, and evaluators that public policy has health implications—hence, a healthy public policy.

The current approach to public health policy is directed toward individuals and their diseases with little or no regard for the cause of those diseases, except to note the needs to change lifestyles and environments, check biological markers, and depend less on the medical care system. The current service system builds on people's deficiencies. McKnight pointed out, however, that he has "never seen service systems that brought people to well-being. . . . Peddling services instead of building communities is the one way you can be sure not to help. . . . Service systems teach people their value lies in deficiencies. They are built on inadequacies, called illiteracy, visual deficit, and teenage pregnancy."[26] McKnight noted three reasons that service systems do not work.[27]

1. Service systems constantly get more than the poor people get. For example, of the money apportioned for services to the poor in Chicago, 63

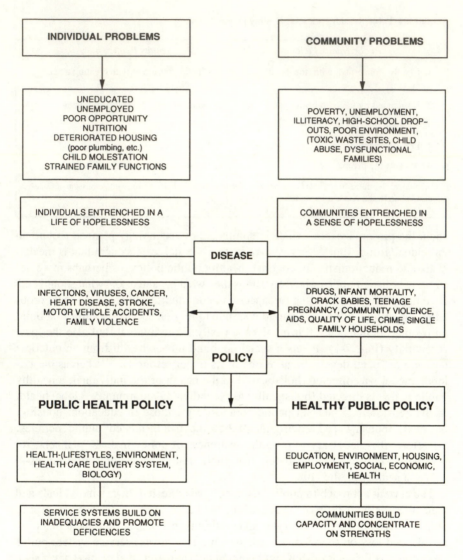

Figure 2-1 Difference between Public Health Policy and Healthy Public Policy

percent went to provide services, and 37% went to provide financial aid. If a family of four was to be allocated $24,000, $15,000 would go to service providers, while the family would receive $9,000. Bureaucracy is not the problem; bureaucrats receive 6 percent of the 63 percent. It is the service system—professionals, nurses, social sorkers, public housing administrators, and welfare workers—that receives the bulk of the funds.

2. Service systems base programs on deficiencies. For example, the antipoverty program case workers focus on the deficiencies of a poor mother who is a high-school dropout, not on her strengths—that she completed 10 years of school, could read a little, and raised five children, one of whom was a teenage mother. The result is a referral to a dropout training center, an illiteracy program, and a new teenage pregnancy counseling program. The poor woman is a gold mine for services. Thus, she received a minimal service, while the service system got the rest.
3. "The service system displaces the capacity of people's organizations to solve problems. The proliferation of therapy and service as 'what you need' has weakened associations and organizations of citizens across the United States."[28]

Table 2-4 summarizes the evolution of health care since 1900 and how it has shaped disease patterns and our concepts of health. Societal changes in the coming decades will continue to affect health care. These include[29-33]

- the increasing proportion of the elderly population
- communication revolution
- increasing number of women in the workplace
- environmental and economic disasters and dislocations
- shift from party to issue politics
- the health promotion and wellness movements and holism
- dependence on a global economy
- rapid rate of change
- technology pressures and information overload

CONCLUSION

In moving toward a healthy public policy, it is essential to consider these significant and persistent challenges.

- Ageism, racism, and sexism impede our progress toward a healthier nation. Each reflects inequalities in health status and health access. The involvement of policy sectors beyond our public health model is required to overcome these impediments.
- Ethical dilemmas occur when there are insufficient resources to meet the needs of all the citizens.

Table 2-4 Eras/Trends and Events That Shape Health

Eras/Trends	Years	Events	Disease Patterns
Building of the monopoly	1900–1910	The Flexner Report—Allopathy Monopolizes	I N F E C T I O U S D I S E A S E
	1920	Sulfa, Sepsis, and Surgery The Great Depression and the rise of the	
Medicine to market	1930	"Blues"	
Rise of the private insurer		Antibiotics available	
	1940	First hearings on Medicare and Medicaid	
	1950	The Salk Vaccine	
Growth of medicine—the "Golden Era" of biomedical research	1960		
Medicine public		The passage of Medicaid and Medicare	
Heights of medical power and influence	1970	Publication of *Limits to Growth, End of Medicine*	C H R O N I C D I S E A S E
	1974	The Lalonde Report	
The era of Limits	1980	*Medical Nemesis*	
The era of lifestyle, self-responsibility, and the promotion of health	1984	*Who Shall Live?* The rise of health promotion and wellness *Vitality and Health* (Fries)	
The era of me-ness		*The Social Transformation of Medicine* (Starr)	
The era of service systems		Public health policy Service and Information Transfer Society	
The era of we-ness	1990	(Social Transformation Disease Cycle)	S O C I A L D Y S - E A S E
The era of community and capacity building		Healthy Public Policy	
Domination of social, economic, education environment, technology and political sectors that promote policies for health	2000	Health no longer an outcome measure of social, economic development, but becomes one of its major resources	

Data from 1900 to 1984 is from R. Carden. Healthy People. *Canadian Journal of Public Health* Supplement 1, Vol. 76, May/June 1985, p. 28. Information from 1984 to 2000 is prepared by the author.

- Allocation of scarce resources evokes the critical question of who will benefit from these resources. In an era of apparently scarce resources, methods for allocation that are just and equitable must be found.
- Social justice is achieved by the equitable distribution of resources. Methods and policies that foster the just distribution of resources are necessary to attain health for all by the year 2000.

Each of these challenges must be considered in the development of the future policies for our nation's health. These prevailing issues confound and often override the social, economic, educational, environmental, and technological sectors of our country.

NOTES

1. Marc Lalonde, *A New Perspective on the Health of Canadians* (Ottawa: Office of the Canadian Minister of National Health and Welfare, 1974), 76.

2. G.E. Alan Dever, "An Epidemiological Model for Health Policy Analysis," *Social Indicators Research* 2 (1976): 453–466.

3. Lalonde, *A New Perspective,* 76.

4. Dever, "An Epidemiological Model for Health Policy Analysis."

5. F. Marc La Force, "Disease Prevention: One Chief's Odyssey." Paper presented at the Mid-Atlantic Meeting of the Society of General Internal Medicine. Baltimore, February 24, 1989, p. 20.

6. Dever, "An Epidemiological Model for Health Policy Analysis," 464.

7. La Force, "Disease Prevention," 7.

8. As used here, the term *reductionistic* refers to an attempt by the medical establishment to reduce the physical, social, and mental well-being of individuals into very specific entities and an attempt to explain causes of disease by simple means when, in fact, the causes are quite complex.

9. R. Evans, "A Retrospective on the New Perspective," *Journal of Health Politics, Policy and Law* 7 (Summer 1982).

10. C. Buck, "Beyond Lalonde—Creating Health," *Canadian Journal of Public Health* 76, supplement 1 (May/June 1985): 19–24.

11. M. Terris, "Newer Perspective on the Health of Canadians: Beyond the Lalonde Report," *Journal of Public Health Policy* (September 1984) 5:327–337.

12. T. Hancock, "Lalonde and Beyond: Looking Back at "A New Perspective on the Health of Canadians," *Health Promotion* 1 (1986): 100.

13. H. Mahler, "Towards a New Public Health," *Health Promotion* 1 (1986): 1.

14. G.L. Siler-Wells, *Directing Change and Changing Direction—A New Health Policy Agenda for Canada* (Ottawa: Canadian Public Health Association, 1988), 131.

15. T. Hancock,"Beyond Health Care: From Public Health Policy to Healthy Public Policy," *Canadian Journal of Public Health* 76, supplement 1 (May/June 1985).

16. I.R. Shannon, "The Challenges of the IOM Report on Public Health," President's Column, *The Nation's Health* (February 1989): 2.

17. Mahler, "Towards a New Public Health," 1.

18. G.H. Bonham, "The Four Areas of Prevention," editorial, *Canadian Journal of Public Health* 76 (January/February 1985): 8–10.

19. Ibid., 9.

20. Ibid., 8–10.

21. J.E. Epp, "Achieving Health for All: A Framework for Health Promotion," *Canadian Journal of Public Health* 77 (November/December 1986): 393–407.

22. Mahler, "Towards a New Public Health," 1.

23. Hancock, "Beyond Health Care."

24. John McKnight, "Why 'Servanthood' Is Bad," *The Other Side* (January/February 1989): 38–41.

25. Mahler, "Towards a New Public Health," 1.

26. McKnight, "Why 'Servanthood' Is Bad," 38–39.

27. Ibid., 38–41.

28. Ibid., 40.

29. C. Bezold, "Health Care in the U.S. Four Alternative Futures," *The Futurist Report* (1982): 14–18.

30. Ropers, "The Public Pulse—Getting Ready for the 1990's," *The Prospects and Problems of 29 Industries* 4 (January 1989): 5.

31. R. Carlos, "Healthy People," *Canadian Journal of Public Health* 76, supplement 1 (May/June 1985): 27–31.

32. J.W. Alley, G.E.A. Dever, and Thomas E. Wade, "Social Transformation Model: Human Development and Disease Patterns." Stanford Research International (SRI), Menlo Park, Calif., Datalog File 87–1153 (October 1986): 1–29.

33. Siler-Wells, *Directing Change and Changing Directions.*

Chapter 3

Planning and Evaluation
for Health

Just as holism and wellness evolved from concern with the entire well-being of the individual, so must planning and evaluation for health take into account the entire fabric of society and its institutions—in essence, the community. Planning for one institution or for one component of health requires full consideration of its interdependency with other parts of society, as the institution or component is part of a larger system. Van Gigch defined a system as "an assembly or set of related elements,"[1] such as concepts (as in language), objects (like a typewriter), and subjects (as in a human-machine system). A hospital, for example, has concepts (e.g., in medical care), objects (e.g., medical equipment), and subjects (e.g., health care workers, patients, and administrators). Such a system can be further divided into subsystems that, in turn, may become subsystems of some other larger system. Each part of the system plays a role in maintaining the equilibrium of the whole in order to reach the objectives of the system.

Ackoff defined the systems approach as focusing on "systems taken as a whole, not on their parts taken separately."[2] In such an approach, properties of the system can be analyzed correctly only from a holistic, total system performance point of view. Even though every part of a system performs perfectly, an imperfectly organized total system will not be able to attain its maximum effectiveness because of the incompatible relationships among the parts.

Health, then, can be considered an element of a system called life. Indeed, as WHO has recognized, the holistic approach to health and health planning "conceives of health as the essence of productive life."[3] The medical care system is one element, or subsystem, within society that seeks to ensure the health of society's members. This subsystem interacts with other subsystems in carrying out society's goals. In planning for the health system, therefore, the interactions both within the system (medical care) and with other systems (lifestyle, environment, and biology) require examination.

45

PLANNING—A SYSTEMS APPROACH TO CHANGE

According to Jantsch, the "new" systems approach to health planning has three essential features.

1. The general introduction of *normative thinking* and *valuation* into planning, making it nondeterministic and futures-creative, and placing emphasis on invention through forecasting.
2. The recognition of *system design* as the central subject of planning, making it nonlinear (i.e., acting upon structures rather than variables of systems) and simultaneous in its general approach; and, following from the two preceding points:
3. The conception of three levels—normative or policy planning (the "ought"), strategic planning (the "can"), and tactical or operational planning (the "will")—in whose interaction the "new," futures-creative planning unfolds.[4]

With the use of these three features as a framework, it is possible to develop a holistic approach to health planning.

1. Health planning should be an attempt to define the ideal system rather than simply the identification of problems.
2. Health planners should strive to free themselves from an incremental, systems improvement attitude and move to a creative, systems design approach. As Van Gigch indicated, the systems improvement attitude implies that the system has been designed and that norms or standards—that is, belief systems—have been set and accepted. In contrast, systems design is a creative process that questions the assumptions on which old forms have been built.[5] The systems design approach blends the incremental approach into a holistic approach to health care that emphasizes prevention, productive living, and the well-being of the whole person in relation to his or her environment.
3. Health planners need to identify the level of planning appropriate to a given situation. Planning needs are defined by the particular subject, by the organizations involved (both in planning and in carrying out the plans), and by the requirements for successful change. Thus, depending on the situation, a health planner can focus on one or more of the three levels of planning.

Policy Planning: What Should Be

The policy level of planning is the most conceptual and the most important in establishing the system design. It deals with society's value structure, or what society considers to be important. Planning at this level is normative, idealistic, or futures-creative, dealing with what ought to be. Both the desired ends and the means to these ends are emphasized. According to Bailey, a policy analysis model involves "a careful, logical analysis of a complex of different problems at the policy level . . . for the purpose of making all assumptions more explicit, recognizing constraints more clearly, drawing conclusions from the assumptions in a more reliable manner, and so on."[6]

Several models may be used for policy planning, including the following:[7]

- Technical models are attempts to provide a scientific understanding of behavior—for example, the population dynamics of disease—and to forecast possible outcomes of intervention with the goals of optimum health. Demographic, marketing, equity and equality, and personnel models fall in this category.
- Systems models deal with interactions among technical models.
- Information system models deal with the flow of information for decision making.

At this level, epidemiological principles are most important to the planning process, because they make it possible (1) to describe the prevalence of disease or disability, as well as the distribution, in the population; (2) to obtain data for planning, implementation, and evaluation; and (3) to identify etiological factors.[8]

> The health needs and demands of a population should be taken into account, and consideration should be given to health promotion and protection in all its aspects: prevention, restoration of impaired health, rehabilitation, and social welfare. Adequate information about the health services required should be collected and evaluated; this would include manpower, investment, equipment, financing, and management.[9]

As emphasized in Chapter 2, community involvement in policy planning is essential in establishing the values and norms of the system. The health planning agency should seek the involvement of all relevant sectors of the community, especially business and civic leaders, residents, and "victims."[10] Unless a total community commitment to health values is attained in this phase, it may be impossible to reach a consensus at a later time. Sigmond suggested the following four steps toward more effective health planning:

1. achieve a consensus
2. identify and fill in gaps in knowledge
3. assist health agencies
4. provide incentives[11]

With this approach, health planners become technical facilitators of the community's decisions.

Finally, at the policy level, forecasting is essential to developing the succeeding levels of planning. Forecasting is the process of modeling or anticipating the likely future. Three broad approaches are possible:

1. *extrapolation of base data to the future.* This can vary from simple straight-line extrapolation based on past history to complex multivariate predictive models that involve causal assumptions, past trends, and indicators.
2. *Delphi or the "expert opinion" forecast.* The essential components of this approach are soliciting the opinions of many experts about future events, averaging their expectations, presenting the results, and repeating the process to refine the forecast. Anonymity of responses is essential to the process.
3. *brainstorming or an open discussion of forecasting.* Members of a group present their opinions on future events and hold discussions to alter or accept specific opinions. As in the Delphi technique, consensus is sought. Because individual responses are public, however, a person with a strong personality or position of authority may dominate the forecast.

Each of these methods has strengths and weaknesses based on the desired results of the forecast. Extrapolation techniques generally require good baseline data and an understanding of causal relationships. The larger data base makes it possible to model future events more precisely and to alter certain variables more selectively so that the sensitivity of the model to changes in the predictive variable can be measured. Delphi techniques and brainstorming are useful when there are few data available to indicate trends or when causal relationships are unclear.

In sum, the policy planning level focuses on futures. Efforts are made to deal with what should be, rather than what is. This level deals with the "invention of anticipations, the design of social systems with preferred dynamic characteristics, the definition of roles for and the creation of institutions, and the feedback interactions between them."[12]

Strategic Planning: What Can Be

Strategic planning deals with "the conception of possible activities, their implications for system structures and system effectiveness, and the creation of instrumentalities. . . . Emphasis is on analysis: system analysis, policy analysis, need analysis, institutional analysis, market analysis."[13] At this point, "the community health planning body converts the general goals, mission, values, or the health aims of the community into specific objectives and criteria for health and health services which the community's operating or delivery systems will be asked to meet."[14]

Bryson consolidated this strategic planning process into eight steps.[15]

1. initiating and agreeing on a strategic planning process
2. identifying the organizational mandates
3. clarifying the organizational mission and values
4. assessing the external environment: opportunities and threats
5. assessing the internal environment: strengths and weaknesses
6. identifying the strategic issues facing an organization
7. formulating strategies to manage the issues
8. establishing an effective organizational vision for the future

These eight steps should lead to actions, results, and evaluation (Fig. 3-1). Bryson also emphasized "that action, results, and evaluative judgments should emerge at each step in the process. In other words, implementation and evaluation should not wait until the end, but should be an integral and ongoing part of the process."[16]

Also at the strategic level, future-oriented goals are established, and the tactical means of achieving these goals are considered. Strategic forecasting deals with the examination of possible activities to carry out the anticipations of society. From that point, specific system structures are established, key result areas are defined, and instrumentalities or means to operationalize institutions are created.

Strategic planning then is the management of processes to reach consensually agreed upon objectives relative to the mission of the organization. The method, in a simplistic sense, requires three continuous actions: (1) environmental scanning; (2) strength, weaknesses, opportunity, and threat (SWOT) analysis; and (3) development of resource allocation strategies that fit the operational (tactical) organization environment. Responsive strategic planning involves all the necessary "actors" in the community; not only do all the community players contribute and receive resources from each other, but also they accept and demonstrate the responsibility of reaching key result measures as defined by the plan.

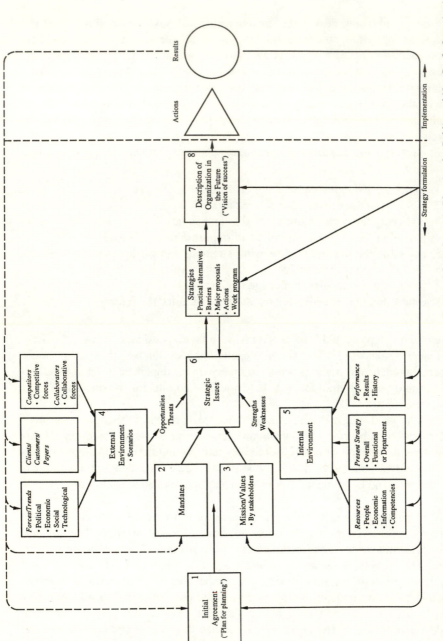

Figure 3-1 Strategic Planning Process for Healthy Public Policy. *Source:* Reprinted from *Strategic Planning for Public and Non-Profit Organizations* by J.M. Bryson, pp. 50–51, with permission of Jossey-Bass, Inc., © 1988.

Strategic plans are usually, but not always, long-term, future-oriented, multi-dimensional, and creative. They focus on identifying specific issues and their resolutions, encouraging divergent thought and, by necessity, accommodating different interests or value groups.

Tactical (Operational) Planning: What Will Be

In the final level of planning, detailed plans are made for carrying out the strategies developed at the second level. At this phase of planning, people are organized to carry out the community's objectives,[17] as "planning can be transmitted into action only by those with operational responsibility for the action."[18] The final outcome is the operation of the system.

For the operational plan to be implemented successfully, it must fit within the operational parameters of the organization. In addition, to achieve any measure of success, there must be responsive evaluation and feedback from all levels. Planning should be seen as a type of closed loop system, such as an electronic circuit, with the evaluation link as the return feedback portion. This part of the system is often neglected or poorly completed, however, which results in a flawed or erroneous measure of the plan's successes. This part of the loop, therefore, requires intensive monitoring—not only to measure the results of the plan accurately, but also to "fine tune" the plan in the face of unforeseen exogenous or endogenous influences.

PLANNING FOR HOLISTIC HEALTH

Each of the three levels of planning deals with specific requirements needed to effect change in society, and, each needs to fit into a holistic health system plan (Fig. 3-2). At present, only the medical care system, the traditional boundary of health care planning, is involved in operational planning (the "will be" aspect). Lifestyle, environment, and biology are still evolving from the strategic level (the "can be" aspect) and the policy level (the "should be" aspect). To achieve holistic health, it is necessary to operationalize all the components (healthy public policy) of holistic health—not only the medical care system—and move to the "will be" level of strategic planning

In developing plans at all three levels, the WHO guidelines for health planning may be useful in developing a holistic approach (healthy public policy).

- Planning should be population-based; that is, the population base or denominator must be appropriate.

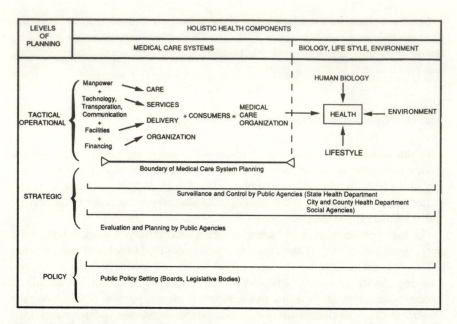

Figure 3-2 Traditional Relationship of Planning Levels to Holistic Health Components. *Source:* Adapted from *Planning for Health: Development and Application of Social Change Theory* by H.L. Blum, p. 278, with permission of Human Sciences Press, © 1974.

- Epidemiology and social sciences are the fundamental health planning components in dealing with the behavior of diseases, individuals, and groups.
- Indicators and proxy measures should be used for attributes and events that are not easy to measure directly.
- Needs, resources, and uses must all be balanced, with attention paid to trade-offs and system dynamics.
- Health is conceived as "the essence of productive life." All sectors of society affect health.
- Other sectors can substitute for the health sector in improving the health status of the population.
- Resources within the health sector can be substituted for otherwise scarce resources; for example, a nurse may provide primary health care.
- Improvement in either productivity or efficiency is of little value if outcomes are not clearly beneficial.
- Effectiveness must be measured in relation to target groups.
- Objective evidence of benefits is necessary in assessing the efficacy either of intervention in treatment or of doing nothing.

- Services must be appropriate to the existing circumstances, adequate, and acceptable.
- What to do is more important than how to do it.
- There must be clear ordering of means and ends.[19]

Finally, planning requires "good judgment, a vast amount of information, a consideration of different points of view, the capacity to think in terms other than the status quo and the ability to develop a deeper frame of understanding."[20]

By applying a community planning model to the concept of wellness in a community, it is possible to illustrate the systems design approach to health planning (Fig. 3-3). The planning paradigm is based on societal values of a high quality of life, an opportunity for a productive life, good education, well-being, health (wellness), clean environment, and appropriate levels of socioeconomic status. The associated norms of literacy, employment, environmental planning, improved well-being, and increased levels of wellness become expectations in the model.

At the policy level, anticipations of wellness, prevention programs, and community- and self-actualization proceed dynamically through appropriate activities toward realization and the achievement of a higher level of quality of life. This holistic design leads to the creation of a community health care system that is not a service system, but a community system based on strength and capacities. In the second phase of planning, strategies that closely parallel the policy phase are developed. For example, anticipations of high-level wellness evolve into such strategies as community exercise, nutritional awareness, coping skills, and stress management programs. At the operational phase of the planning process, running, swimming, cycling, employment opportunities, environmental management, and drug abuse programs are planned to achieve the strategic objectives. These activities incorporate wellness into day-to-day living and pinpoint the need for individual and community responsibility and authority in the management of local health needs.

EVALUATION—ACCOUNTING FOR CHANGE

The second step in holistic health planning is evaluation or accounting for change. Evaluation is the measurable determination of the value or degree of success in achieving specific objectives. The actual process of establishing objectives has several facets, depending on the level of planning and operation. The use of a holistic model that emphasizes the interrelated aspects of environment, lifestyle, human biology, and system of health care delivery requires the design of a system capable of reaching comprehensive goals. Thus, the emphasis should be on a healthy public policy that reflects desired program change.

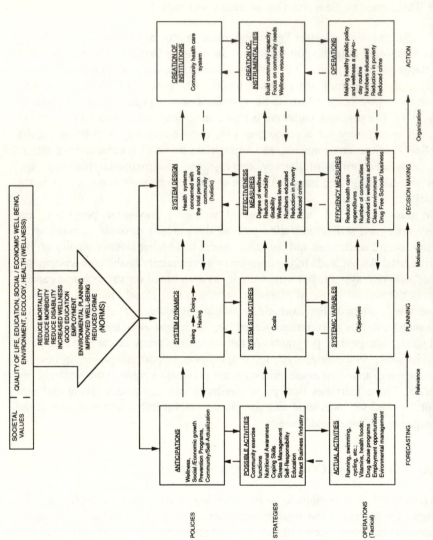

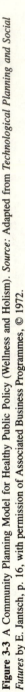

Figure 3-3 A Community Planning Model for Healthy Public Policy (Wellness and Holism). *Source:* Adapted from *Technological Planning and Social Futures* by E. Jantsch, p. 16, with permission of Associated Business Programmes, © 1972.

Establishment of Realistic Objectives

The development of a comprehensive health policy requires environmental scanning, data analysis, and the use of the political process. Data analysis first examines existing conditions, trends, and forecasts to determine community needs. It is essential to establish baseline or benchmark measures, which may be accomplished using these three approaches:

1. If there are no available data on the health status of the population being investigated, collect data for the first year of operation to establish a baseline for the following years.
2. If data are available, develop baseline or benchmark studies to establish past and present levels, making it possible to set realistic objectives for single and multiyear intervals. Essential to this analysis is regional access to timely, accurate, and reliable community-based data.
3. Use experience and intuitive talent.

At this point in data analysis, it is necessary to ask three very critical questions:

1. What kinds of objectives should be included in the health plan?
2. Which issues should be addressed on the strategic level and which on the operational level?
3. How can a realistic level of attainment of objectives be determined?

The answer to the first question is determined by the parameters of the holistic health policy. If the health policy is broad and includes elements of the environment, biology, lifestyle, and system of health care delivery, the objectives should reflect such elements. Both nontraditional and traditional objectives that have a decided impact on changing disease patterns should be identified. A parallel approach would be to identify the disease patterns (specific program problems) for each community—an obvious requirement, but one that is not always met.

There is no absolute test to establish whether an issue is strategic or operational. In fact, many issues fall into a gray area, and the assessment of their strategic importance is a judgment that must be made by top management. To assist managers in making this judgment, it is suggested that the questions in Exhibit 3-1 be applied to each identified issue. Major strategic issues will be characterized by answers that fall predominantly in Columns 2 and 3. Operational issues will tend to be characterized by answers in Columns 1 and 2.

The level of attainment of objectives may be determined by means of value-derived standards of expectations or by means of general, promulgated standards. In addition to baseline or benchmark measures, trends or standards for

Exhibit 3-1 A Litmus Test for Issues

Issues	Operational (1)	(2)	Strategic (3)
1. When will the strategic issue's challenge or opportunity confront you?	Right now	Next year	Two or more years from now
2. How broad an impact will the issue have on your department?	Single unit or division	Several divisions	Entire department
3. How large is your department's financial risk/financial opportunity?	Minor (less than $250,000 or 10% of budget)	Moderate ($250,000 to $1,000,000 or 10 to 25% of budget)	Major ($1,000,000 plus or more than 25% of budget)
4. Will strategies for issue resolution likely require:			
a. Development of new service goals and programs?	No		Yes
b. Significant changes in tax sources or amounts?	No		Yes
c. Significant amendments in federal or state statutes or regulations?	No		Yes
d. Major facility additions or modifications?	No		Yes
e. Significant staff expansion?	No		Yes
5. How apparent is the best approach for issue resolution?	Obvious, ready to implement	Broad parameters, few details	Wide open
6. What is the lowest level of management that can decide how to deal with this issue?	Line staff supervisor	Division head	Department head
7. What are the probable consequences of not addressing this issue?	Inconvenience, inefficiency	Significant service disruption, financial losses	Major long-term service disruption and large cost/revenue setbacks
8. How many other departments are affected by this issue and must be involved in resolution?	None	One to three	Four or more
9. How sensitive or "charged" is the issue relative to community social, political, religious, and cultural values?	Benign	Touchy	Dynamite

specified health status measures must be reviewed, as they may reveal appropriate targets or standards for the attainment of objectives. For example, a reduction in the local infant mortality rate of 20 percent within the next year may be a totally unrealistic objective in light of the fact that the rate has been reduced by only 2 percent per year over the last ten years and is already below the national level. If the infant mortality rate will continue to decrease by 2 percent without any action, the objective of a new program may be a 3 percent decrease. Finally, accounting for rate variations—within certain probability limits—is another way to set realistic objectives. Readjustment of objectives is always feasible in the light of unforeseen issues that may surface to affect a program.

Because of the disparity between the virtually unlimited needs and desires of a community and the scarcity of available resources, the objectives of any health improvement program must be guided by the need to provide the greatest benefit or good at the most equitable cost (social justice). The resources available to communities are likely to decrease further in the 1990s, making it imperative to develop efficient and cost-effective programs.

Types of Evaluation

Evaluation is impossible without goals that are related to the questions of what, how much, who, where, and when, because it assesses health changes in terms of programmatic effects. The results become an input to the continuing process of planning, budgeting, and evaluation. Within the evaluation component are three areas of concern.

1. Fiscal evaluation focuses on and determines cost accountability.
2. Process evaluation determines program activity in terms of (1) the age, sex, race, or other demographic variables in the population receiving the program; (2) the program organization, staffing, and funding; and (3) the program location and timing. Process evaluation is a measure of program efforts or proposed activities, rather than program effects.
3. Outcome evaluation delineates program objectives in terms of effects to determine if health status has changed as a result of the program.

The purpose of evaluation is to answer the practical questions of administrators who want to know whether to continue a program, to extend it to other sites, to modify it, or to end it. Evaluation is more productive when it is a continuous process, with a continuous feedback loop to those administrators, supervisors, and program managers who make decisions. Routine evaluation reports should inform administrators about the effects of policy and program decisions, should alert supervisors to service delivery trends, and should indicate problems that require corrective action. Most management decisions are based on intuition rather than facts; evaluation programs help to determine whether these decisions were appropriate.

The evaluation component is the key to successful planning, but health programs often lack a comprehensive assessment process. Perhaps this reflects a fear that programs will prove inadequate. Indeed, administrators, supervisors, and program managers may well perceive evaluation as a risky process, since it presumes that positions and programs may be reduced as well as increased. Another problem is that most state agencies' information systems are not designed to provide the data needed for effective program evaluation. Sometimes, evaluation is undertaken for inappropriate reasons. Program decision makers may turn to evaluation to delay a decision ("Let's have a study!") or to legitimize a decision already made. In addition, as less tangible performance objectives are addressed and outcome measurement criteria in certain areas become much more difficult to quantify, evaluation problems are compounded.

Too often, program administrators claim success because they completed proposed activities, such as testing or screening a particular number of clients and providing specific hours of therapy (process evaluation), rather than because they improved the health of the people served (outcome evaluation). The introduction of coordinated fiscal, process, and outcome evaluation objectives in an organization will produce the following changes.

- Program planning will be improved as administrators formulate program objectives more precisely, specify plans to achieve objectives, and monitor progress toward accomplishing objectives.

- Management practices will be improved as administrators, supervisors, and health program managers have access to more evaluation and control data to assist them in the planning and direction of their own work, as well as in assessing the work of others.

- Information provided by agency evaluations will allow state and other health agencies to make more timely and relevant reports to the general public and to legislative bodies. This information is becoming more and more critical; legislators are becoming increasingly suspicious of programs that fail to demonstrate concrete accomplishments.

EVALUATION MODEL FOR COMMUNITY HEALTH AGENCIES

The two key components of an evaluation model for community health agencies are (1) monitoring results (fiscal and process evaluation) and (2) assessing change (outcome evaluation).[21] In the context of the planning model previously

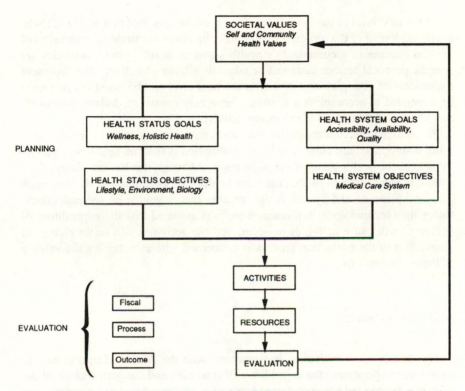

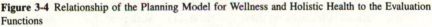

Figure 3-4 Relationship of the Planning Model for Wellness and Holistic Health to the Evaluation Functions

presented (see Fig. 3-3), the evaluation process focuses on the system's relationship to societal values and on the full interdependencies of the system (Fig. 3-4). In this model, social values are used to establish specific health status goals. The goals are broad statements relating to the long-range objectives of the planning model for wellness and holistic health—reduced mortality, morbidity, and disability; increased wellness; good education; employment; environmental planning; and improved well-being.

Within the health system, these goals incorporate major inputs of specific health status and health system objectives. Health status objectives include short-range desired changes in the population's health status, such as a 2 percent reduction in infant mortality or a 30 percent increase in participation in a physical exercise program. The objectives must take into account the population's present health status, be achievable within the specified time frame, and be based on long-term achievement of the desired health status goal (wellness). Health system objectives deal with specific components of the health care system (e.g., accessibility, availability, continuity, quality, and cost).

At the next level of the model, activities must be specified that will lead to the accomplishment of the objectives. Whereas objectives are strategic statements of desired changes in a community's health status or health system, activities are specific practical actions that must be taken to achieve objectives; they represent the process of obtaining objectives. At the next level are the resources that must be expended to accomplish activities. These may consist of dollars, human effort, or any other method of producing activity.

Proceeding upward through the evaluation and planning levels, certain underlying assumptions are clear. The basic assumption is that the health care system influences the health status of the population. Although this has not always been true, it is more likely to be the case if the health care system has evolved through a logical planning and system design process that is guided by societal values, rather than technological brilliance. Too, it is assumed that the expenditure of resources will cause activities to occur, and the activities will cause change to occur. Part of the evaluation process is concerned with ascertaining the validity of these assumptions.

Monitoring Results

The first level of evaluation is concerned with the details of operations. To assess these operations, the expenditure of resources and the performance of activities are subjected to two different kinds of evaluation: fiscal and process.

Fiscal evaluation focuses on these questions: (1) Were resources expended in a planned manner? (2) Did the expenditure of the resources result in the planned activities? (3) Was the expenditure of the resources the most efficient means of ensuring the desired activities? Comparing planned or budgeted expenditures with actual expenditures ensures that resources have been expended for planned activities and not for extraneous purposes; that is, other miscellaneous items have not drawn on resources budgeted to achieve the specified activities. Although one of the easiest methods of fiscal evaluation, it is most often overlooked. In determining whether planned activities occurred as a result of the expenditure of resources, it is important to distinguish activities that would have occurred regardless of the expenditures from those that resulted directly from the expenditures. Further evaluation of such activities will occur at the process level. Finally the actual cost of accomplishing activities and alternative costs are commonly calculated in terms of the cost per unit of activity, for example, the cost per patient served.

Process evaluation deals with activities that are planned to occur. Results are determined by comparing these planned activities with accomplished activities, as in the following:

Actual activities/Planned activities $\times$ 100 = Percentage attainment of activities

Process evaluation is the most frequently conducted evaluation, possibly because of its simplicity. It assumes that the planned activities will result in the achievement of the objectives (which must be separately addressed in outcome evaluation). Not only does process evaluation permit continuous monitoring of results during the duration of a program, thus providing evidence of program operation and a method of program control, but also it can be easily accomplished and, if causal assumptions are correct, can serve as an early indicator of program outcome.

Assessing Change

After program results have been monitored in a fiscal and process evaluation, the next level of evaluation is the assessment of change. Concern at this level focuses on program outcomes and their correlation with the stated objectives. The first step at this level of evaluation is to determine the outcomes desired from a program. From that point, planned accomplishments are compared to actual accomplishments. Program goals at this stage must be specific, a requirement that is not always met. Unless specific goals are established, either explicitly or implicitly, evaluation is impossible; if nothing is planned, there is simply nothing to evaluate.

In determining the program goals, evaluation criteria, and client groups served by the program, the following questions may be helpful:

1. What are the purposes of the program? Why was it (or should it be) adopted?
2. What is to be changed by the program, in both the immediate future and the long run? How would the program manager know if the program was working or not working? What would be accepted as evidence of success?
3. Who are the targets of the program? Is the community as a whole likely to be affected either directly or indirectly? Who else might be affected by the program?
4. What are possible side effects, both immediate and long-run?
5. What would be the likely consequences if the new program were introduced or if an existing program were discontinued? What would be the reaction of citizens in the community? Who would complain? Why would they complain? Who would be glad? Why?[22]

The program objectives and evaluation criteria at this level should be people-oriented. The impact on a community's citizens should be the first concern of any evaluation. Therefore, the evaluation criteria should address the following program characteristics:

1. To what degree does the service meet its intended purposes, such as improving health, reducing crime, or increasing employment?
2. To what degree does the program have unintended adverse or beneficial impacts? For example, does a new industry increase water and air pollution or cause inconvenience to citizens?
3. Is the quantity of the service provided sufficient to meet the needs and desires of citizens? What percent of the eligible "needy" population is actually served?
4. How fast does the program respond to requests for service?
5. Do government employees treat citizens who use the service with courtesy and dignity?
6. How accessible is the service to users?
7. Do citizens who use the service, or who might use the service, view it as satisfactory?
8. How much does the program cost?[23]

More than one objective and one evaluation criterion should be used to evaluate each program. Rarely is a program adequately described with a single objective, and rarely can a single evaluation criterion measure a program impact. Too many objectives and criteria are better than too few. Often it is difficult to determine which objectives or criteria may be important as the evaluation proceeds. Dollar costs should always be included as one criterion, and all resource expenditures should be evaluated fiscally.

Evaluation criteria should not be rejected because of apparent difficulties in measuring them. It is more important to identify the criteria for evaluating a program and then to deal with problems of measurement as the evaluation proceeds.

Weiss proposed the following steps for program evaluations:[24]

- *Formulate program goals.* Goals must be clear, specific, and measurable, and they must address program consequences or outcomes.
- *Choose specific goals to evaluate.* Choices are guided by:
  1. *usability and practicality.* Will the evaluation of a goal prove usable to the community or organization, and is evaluation of the goal possible?
  2. *relative importance.* Is attainment of a goal important enough to a community to make it worth spending valuable resources in an evaluation study?

3. *incompatibilities*. Are the goals to be evaluated compatible with each other, or is the desired outcome of one goal the opposite of that for a second goal?
4. *short-term or long-term goals*. Evaluation of long-term impacts is clearly desired, although there may be an immediate need for evaluation based on short-term results.

● *Establish measurement yardsticks*. What yardstick (standards) will measure successful achievement of a goal? Will a 2 percent reduction in infant mortality be sufficient, or must 10 percent be the goal?

● *Determine unanticipated outcomes*. Unplanned program effects are very likely to occur and may be either negative or positive. Nearly all programs have some negative effects. These should be explicitly identified and, if possible, eliminated. If it is not possible to eliminate them, careful consideration of their negative effects will at least help to put the overall worth of a program into perspective. All unplanned effects are not necessarily bad, however; many desirable unplanned achievements may result from specific programs.

● *Develop indicators of outcomes*. Here several issues arise:
1. *development of measures*. What is the appropriate means of measuring an outcome or indicator of income?
2. *multiple measures*. Several indicators should be measured to gain a better understanding of outcomes. These can then be continued to indicate overall program success.
3. *proximate measures*. When goals are very long range, it is often necessary to use proxy measures to evaluate short-range outcomes with the assumption that the achievement of these short-range goals will result in the achievement of long-range results.
4. *types of measures*. Effects may be measured on several levels:
   (a) *the persons served*. Measurement of changes in patient health status, attitudes, values, and skills must reflect the goals of the organization.
   (b) *agencies*. Assessing the effect of goals that seek to change institutions, for example, makes them more responsive.
   (c) *larger systems*. Some goals seek to change relationships within a network of agencies or an entire community; assessment of such goals must be made at this level.
   (d) *the public*. If the program goals are to change public opinion, public opinion surveys are appropriate.

Exhibit 3-2 presents criteria for selecting the final set of program measures. As a health program management tool, evaluation must demonstrate its worth. It must lead to reduced costs or increased benefits (fiscal evaluation), result in im-

Exhibit 3-2 Criteria for Selecting Final Set of Measures

Importance
Does the measure provide useful and important information on the program that justifies the difficulties in collecting, analyzing, or presenting the data?

Validity
Does the measure address the aspect of concern? Can changes in the value of the measure be interpreted clearly as desirable or undesirable, and can the changes be attributed directly to the program?

Uniqueness
Does the information provided by the measure duplicate information provided by another measure?

Accuracy
Are the likely data sources sufficiently reliable, or are there biases, exaggerations, omissions, or errors that are likely to make the measure inaccurate or misleading?

Timeliness
Can the data be collected and analyzed in time for the decision?

Privacy and Confidentiality
Are there concerns for privacy or confidentiality that would prevent analysts from obtaining the required information?

Costs of Data Collection
Can the resource or cost requirements for data collection be met?

Completeness
Does the final set of measures cover the major aspects of concern?

Source: Reprinted from *Program Analysis for State and Local Governments,* 2nd ed., by Harry Hatry, Louis Blair, Donald Fisk, and Wayne Kimmel, p. 41, with permission of Urban Institute Press, © 1988.

---

proved effectiveness (process evaluation), and be related to changed health status (outcome evaluation). Seldom can one be absolutely positive that a change in health status has been due to a program's effects, but effective evaluation may reduce the degree of uncertainty.

EVALUATION DESIGNS

Figure 3-5 presents five evaluation designs for identifying and quantifying the effects of a program.[25,26] Each design may be applied with limited resources and minimal personnel, or the designs may be used in combination to estimate the net efforts of a program.

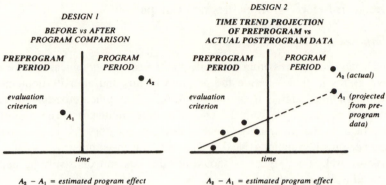

DESIGN 1

BEFORE vs AFTER
PROGRAM COMPARISON

$A_2 - A_1 = $ *estimated program effect*

DESIGN 2

TIME TREND PROJECTION
OF PREPROGRAM vs
ACTUAL POSTPROGRAM DATA

$A_2 - A_1 = $ *estimated program effect*

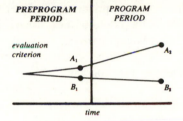

DESIGN 3

COMPARISON WITH OTHER GEOGRAPHICAL AREAS
OR OTHER POPULATION SEGMENTS

geographical area A has a program; geographical area B, the comparison area, does not.
$(A_2 - A_1) - (B_2 - B_1) = $ *estimated program effect (or rate of change might be used rather than absolute amount of change)*

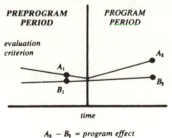

DESIGN 4

CONTROLLED EXPERIMENTATION
COMPARISON OF PREASSIGNED SIMILAR GROUPS
ONLY ONE OF WHICH IS SERVED BY THE PROGRAM

$A_2 - B_2 = $ *program effect*

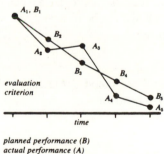

DESIGN 5

PLANNED vs ACTUAL PERFORMANCE

planned performance (B)
actual performance (A)
$(A/B) \times 100 = $ *percent of performance level achieved or percent of objectives targeted*

Figure 3-5 Five Evaluation Designs To Identify and Quantify Program Effects. *Source:* Adapted from *Practical Program Evaluation for State and Local Governments,* 2nd ed., by Harry Hatry, Richard Winnie, and Donald Fisk, p. 27, with Permission of Urban Institute Press, © 1981.

Design 1: Before vs. After Program Comparison

Purpose

Design 1 compares program results in the same geographical area measured at two points in time—before the program begins and after its implementation. Although this design is commonly used, it is often difficult to separate the effects of program activities from the effects of other influences. The design is very practical for the community or public health agency because of time availability and personnel limitations. Next to Design 5, it is the simplest and least expensive type of evaluation. Agencies should use this design extensively in their annual operational plans.

Procedures

1. Identify appropriate goals, objectives, and evaluation criteria.
2. Obtain the values of these criteria at a point before the program begins and after it is implemented.
3. Compare "before" and "after" program data to estimate changes brought about by the program.

Applications

Design 1 is appropriate when the program has a short duration and a narrow scope (e.g., as an intensive health promotion campaign or a physical exercise program). It is also appropriate when conditions are stable over time; that is, the outcome should not be distorted by seasonal changes, such as by immunizations or influenza.

Design 2: Time Trend Projection of Preprogram Data vs. Actual Postprogram Data

Purpose

Design 2 compares actual postprogram data to estimated data from a number of time periods before the program began. Changes are identified as actual differences from earlier projections. In the use of this design, the following should be considered:

- The statistical variations in the data must be accounted for by aggregating time periods, geographical areas, or age groups. Otherwise, projections will be misleading or, possibly, invalid.

- Projections, in addition to being linear ($Y = a + bX$), may also be curvilinear ($Y = ab^x$, $Y = aX^b$).
- Statistical tests of significance can help verify the appropriateness of the projections.
- Added data collection for prior years is required.
- Technical expertise is required for statistical projections.

A health agency can use Design 2 if technical expertise and resources are available for added data collection. If not, Designs 1 or 5 should be followed.

Procedures

1. Identify relevant goals, objectives, and corresponding evaluation criteria.
2. Obtain data on each of the criteria at several time intervals before the program and after implementation.
3. Using statistical methods and the data, make projections to the end of the period covered by the evaluation.
4. Compare actual and projected estimates of numerical changes resulting from the program.
5. Look for other plausible explanations for the changes.

Applications

Design 2 is very useful for health programs that focus on long-term trends in such areas as infant mortality, poverty, illiteracy, major causes of mortality, and hospital needs assessment (e.g., bed needs). The design's projections need not be based only on time trends; they can also be based on changing demographics (e.g., distribution of age, sex, and racial characteristics in urban and rural settings) and disability dysfunctions for special social groups.

Design 3: Comparison with Other Geographical Areas or Population Segments Not Served by the Program

Purpose

Design 3 compares evaluation criteria by means of data from two geographical areas or population groups, one where the program is operating and one where the program is not operating. In order to collect comparable data from the two geographical areas or population groups and to reduce the effects of confounding variables on the program, the segments must be matched as closely as possible. Usual matching criteria are age, sex, race, and sometimes socioeconomic status. One must be careful not to overmatch.

Procedures

1. Identify relevant goals, objectives, and corresponding evaluation criteria.
2. Select similar geographical areas or population groups within the same geographical area where the program is not operating.
3. Obtain data on each of the evaluation criteria of the geographical area or population groups from before implementation of the program to the time of evaluation.
4. Compare the rate and magnitude of change for the geographical areas or population groups.
5. Look for plausible explanations for changes other than the program.

Applications

Design 3 is very useful for the evaluation of state health programs. It should be used in association with Designs 1 and 5 to ensure reliable measures of program efforts, however. Health agencies should concentrate on Designs 1 and 5 and then employ Design 3, using standardized data sources (e.g., infant mortality rates, utilization rates, physician ratios).

Design 4: Controlled Experimentation

Purpose

Design 4 compares preselected, similar groups, some of whom are served and some of whom are not served. The comparison groups must be randomly assigned before program implementation so that they are as similar as possible— except for the program treatment. Because political and ethical problems or pressures may make it difficult to provide a service to one group and not to another, public and community health agencies rarely do this kind of controlled experimentation. Although this design is the best of the five presented, it is also the most difficult and costly.

Procedures

1. Identify relevant goals, objectives, and corresponding evaluation criteria.
2. Select the groups to be compared (control and experimental groups) through a random probability sample.
3. Measure the preprogram performance of each group.
4. Apply the program to the experimental group.
5. Monitor the experiment to see if any actions distort the findings.
6. Measure the postprogram performance of each group.

7. Compare the changes in the evaluation criteria for these groups.
8. Look for plausible explanations for differences between the two groups.

Applications

Design 4 is used typically in the evaluation of clinical research and community medicine programs. It can be used when a program is introduced into one county or area and not into others, which makes it suitable for government programs that can be offered only in limited areas because of limited resources that must be allocated on a priority basis. Under these circumstances, Design 4 is feasible and does not present political or ethical problems.

Design 5: Comparison of Planned vs. Actual Performance

Purpose

Design 5 compares preprogram planned targeted objectives to the actual program performance. Goals or targets must be realistic for the evaluation criteria. Thus, the establishment of targets is likely to become an important issue. The design assumes that the targets that have been set are the best available.

Procedures

1. Identify relevant goals, objectives, and corresponding evaluation criteria.
2. Set specific goals or targets for these criteria for specific time periods.
3. Obtain data on actual performance after the time period (e.g., quarterly).
4. Compare the actual performance to the planned target.
5. Look for plausible explanations for changes in the criteria other than the program.

Applications

Design 5 establishes targets that are the best available indicators of what actual accomplishments should be. This design can be used widely once provisions have been made for the regular collection of the data needed—for example, monthly health program activity reporting—in process evaluation.

BARRIERS TO CHANGE

Planning is designed to bring about change, and evaluation is the science of accounting for change. Planning and evaluation efforts sometimes meet resistance, however. In fact, in some situations, the resistance results in the complete failure of the strategic planning process.

There are four major challenges to the planning process in an organization or community: (1) the human problem, (2) the process problem, (3) the structural problem, and (4) the institutional problem (Table 3-1).[27] Although each is important, the human problem is the most critical to the analysis of community health.

The human problem—the management of attention and commitment—must be viewed from four levels: individuals, groups, organizations, and communities.[28] According to Bryson, individuals have several characteristics that must be taken into account in the strategic planning process.

- Individuals have a limited ability to handle complexity.
- Individuals are highly adaptive and do not recognize gradual change.
- Individuals withdraw, project, and rationalize in crises.
- Individuals lose consciousness and concentration as they gain competence and repeat tasks.
- Commitment increases as individuals take public, binding, and irrevocable actions.[29]

Bryson theorized that individuals can handle only seven or so ideas at a time.[30] Because most strategic planning endeavors involve more than seven ideas, it is imperative that planners limit the key issues so that individuals do not suffer from information overload or stereotype their responses and diagnose the situation incorrectly.[31]

Groups may become barriers to planning or evaluation efforts because they (1) impose strong pressures to conform, (2) try to minimize internal conflict, and

Table 3-1 Barriers to Change in Strategic Planning

Problem	Definition	Issue To Resolve
Human	Management of attention and commitment	Attention of key people must be focused on key issues, decisions, conflicts, and policy preferences at key places in the process and the organizational hierarchy.
Process	Management of strategic ideas into good currency—to sell good ideas	Unconventional wisdom must be focused into conventional wisdom.
Structural	Management of part-whole relations	Internal and external environments must be linked advantageously.
Institutional	Exercise of transformative leadership	Institutional transformation must rely on strong leadership.

Source: Adapted from *Strategic Planning for Public and Nonprofit Organizations* by John M. Bryson, pp. 199–215, with permission of Jossey-Bass, Inc., © 1989.

(3) become homogenous in two to three years.[32] Several organizational barriers must also be resolved for effective planning.

- Strategic planning systems drive out strategic thinking. Repetition and competence can lead to a lack of concentration.

- The average statistical report contains hundreds or even thousands of numbers, which numb most responses. Thus, decisions are based not on data, but on stories that people have individually managed.

- Because of the tendency of specialization to filter options and produce suboptimal behavior, it is necessary to develop settings that facilitate interaction. Retreats, task forces, and seminars bring opposing or specialized narrow views into a wider focus.

- Structure and systems become a substitute for leadership. The key task of leadership is to be creative, view new horizons, suggest strategies and priorities, and embrace healthy public policy—in essence, strategic planning.[33]

Finally, communities have several characteristics that threaten the success of strategic planning. First, because communities are composed of individuals, groups, and organizations, they represent an accumulation of the characteristics and difficulties previously noted. Second, most organizations in a community represent solutions to *old* problems. Third, no organization in any community is likely to contain any important problem. Fourth, in most communities no one person, group, or organization is in charge.[34]

Building strength and capacity in communities has been suggested as the means to empower communities to formulate a healthy public policy via the strategic planning process. Bryson posed a most critical question for communities: "How does one get to a new solution to a new problem when the organizational base is an old solution to an old problem?"[35] He suggested that the answer is to be found in networking; "networks form around new definitions of problems and new solutions in response to those new definitions. New organizations (or reorganizations of old ones) will then institutionalize those new problem definitions and solutions."[36] The solution is the formation of task forces for strategic planning, temporary organizations that address multidimensional problems. Thus, as Bryson noted, "Successful strategic planning for a community is a collective enterprise."[37] By this definition a community must rethink its methods for solving problems.

In health, the service system is a large barrier to strategic planning. Health programs are positioned in communities without reference to the capacity of the community to implement such programs. Thus, new programs are implemented with old solutions; the result is no change. The objective then of community health analysts and planners must be to develop a strategic planning process that promotes changing direction and in which the communities direct the change. A collective process where the ownership is shared is the key to strength and power. This is essential to overcoming the barriers to change and to the successful development of the strategic planning process.

NOTES

1. John P. Van Gigch, *Applied General Systems Theory* (New York: Harper & Row, 1974), 2.

2. Russell L. Ackoff, "Towards a System of System Concepts," *Management Science* 17, no. 11 (July 1971): 661–671.

3. World Health Organization, *International Collaborative Study of Medical Care Utilization, Health Services: Concepts and Information for National Planning and Management* (Geneva: WHO, 1977).

4. Erich Jantsch, *Technological Planning and Social Futures* (London: Associated Business Programmes, 1972), 14.

5. Van Gigch, *Applied General Systems Theory*, 2.

6. N.T. J. Bailey, "Systems Modelling in Health Planning," in *Systems Aspects of Health Planning*, ed. N.T. J. Bailey and M. Thompson (Amsterdam: North Holland Publishing Co., 1975), 9.

7. Ibid.

8. Jan Kostrzewski, "Uses of Epidemiology in the Planning and Evaluation of Health Care Systems," in *Systems Aspects of Health Planning*, ed. N.T. J. Bailey and M. Thompson (Amsterdam: North Holland Publishing Co., 1975), 227–237.

9. Ibid., 233.

10. Henrich L. Blum, *Planning for Health: Development and Application of Social Change Theory* (New York: Human Sciences Press, 1974), 89.

11. Robert M. Sigmond, "Health Planning," in *Dimensions and Determinants of Health Policy*, ed. William L. Kissick, Milbank Memorial Fund Quarterly 46, no. 1, pt. 2 (January 1968): 91–117.

12. Jantsch, *Technological Planning and Social Futures*, 18.

13. Ibid., 19.

14. Blum, *Planning for Health*, 5.

15. John M. Bryson, *Strategic Planning for Public and Non-Profit Organizations* (San Francisco: Jossey-Bass, Inc., 1989), 48.

16. Ibid.

17. Blum, *Planning for Health*, 5.

18. Sigmond, "Health Planning," 95.

19. WHO, *International Collaborative Study*, 108–114.

20. Institute for Health Care Facilities, *View of the Horizons* (Ottawa, Canada: 1988), 39.

21. G.E.A. Dever and Charles M. Plunkett, "Evaluation in Community Health—An Overview," in *A Companion to the Life Sciences*, ed. S.B. Day (New York: Van Nostrand Reinhold, 1979), 93–97.

22. Harry Hatry et al., *Program Analysis for State and Local Governments*, 2nd ed. (Washington, D.C.: The Urban Institute, 1988), 40.

23. Ibid., 32.

24. Carol H. Weiss, *Evaluation Research: Methods of Assessing Program Effectiveness* (Englewood Cliffs, N.J.: Prentice-Hall, Inc., 1972), 24–59.

25. Harry Hatry et al., *Practical Program Evaluation for State and Local Government Officials* (Washington, D.C.: The Urban Institute, 1973), 39–70.

26. S.M. Shortell and W.C. Richardson, "Evaluation Designs," in *Health Program Evaluation* (St. Louis: C.V. Mosby Co., 1978), 38–73.

27. Bryson, *Strategic Planning,* 199–200.

28. Ibid., 200–208.

29. Ibid., 200.

30. Ibid., 201.

31. Ibid.

32. Ibid., 203.

33. Ibid., 204–206.

34. Ibid., 206–208.

35. Ibid., 207.

36. Ibid.

37. Ibid., 208.

Chapter 4

Basic Statistical Measures for Community Health Analysis

Statistics is the means of establishing baseline population characteristics, measuring change, and testing hypotheses. As such, it forms the cornerstone of quantitative evaluation techniques. Above all, it allows inferences to be made to a large population from a small sample through the application of probability concepts and distributional characteristics. Today, statistics is playing an enlarged role in all aspects of community health, including planning and evaluation, as well as in epidemiology and the other health sciences.

DESCRIPTIVE STATISTICS

According to Parsons, "The major emphasis of statistical descriptive techniques is to take a large mass of useful but poorly organized information [health] data and condense it so that the basic characteristics of the data are clearly evident."[1] Descriptive measures establish the characteristics and describe the health status of a population. Several basic concepts must be understood before such analysis is undertaken.

Frequency Distribution

In a simple frequency distribution, all scores ranked from high to low are in one column, and the numbers of individuals or events receiving each score appear as frequencies in the second column. A grouped frequency distribution establishes class intervals of equal width in one column, and the corresponding frequencies are listed in another column. The rules for constructing class intervals in a grouped frequency distribution are as follows:

- In general, there should be between 10 and 20 class intervals, based on the optimal number that will summarize the data efficiently without distorting its shape. Too few intervals compress the data, concealing meaningful changes in its shape; too many stretch out the data, creating unnecessary gaps.
- The width of the class interval is a function of the range of the raw scores and the number of class intervals desired. To illustrate, if the raw score range is $75 - 15 = 60$ and the researcher wants approximately ten class intervals, then $60/10 = 6$. The class interval width should be 6.

As an example, Table 4-1 shows a frequency distribution of live births in a community by age of the mother. The largest number of births occurred in the age group 20–24, the next largest number in age group 25–29, and so on. Raw data do not provide this kind of information. If a graphic technique is desired, class intervals may be marked off on a horizontal axis and frequencies on a vertical axis (Fig. 4-1).

One of the most common frequency distributions is the normal distribution, which forms the basis for statistical inference and hypothesis testing.

Measurement of Distributions

All distributions can be described by measures of central tendency and dispersion.

Measures of Central Tendency. The most commonly used basic measures of central tendency are the arithmetic mean, the median, and the mode. Others, such as the geometric mean and the harmonic mean, are sometimes used, however.

Table 4-1 Frequency Distribution of Live Births by Age of Mother

Age of Mother	Number of Live Births
10–14	607
15–19	18,071
20–24	27,419
25–29	21,246
30–34	8,566
35–39	2,420
40–44	536
45 up	28

Data from *Georgia Vital and Health Statistics,* Division of Physical Health, Georgia Department of Human Resources, 1976, 40.

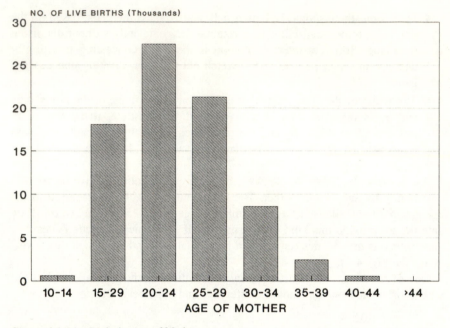

Figure 4-1 Live Births by Age of Mother

The arithmetic mean is often referred to as the simple average. It is computed by summing the values of all observations and dividing by the number of observations. Thus,

$$\overline{X} = \Sigma X / n$$

where $\overline{X}$ = arithmetic mean or average
Σ = Greek letter sigma, indicating the summation
n = the number of values of X
ΣX = sum of the n values of X

For example, given mortality rates of 16.0, 12.0, 14.0, 6.0, 8.0, 9.0, 9.0, 10.0, 11.0, 10.0 for a group of ten census tracts or counties, then

$$\Sigma X = 16.0 + 12.0 + 14.0 + 6.0 + 8.0 + 9.0 + 9.0 +$$
$$10.0 + 11.0 + 10.0 = 105$$
$$n = 10$$
$$\overline{X} = 105/10 = 10.5$$

The value 10.5 is the arithmetic mean of the distribution of mortality rates.

In the normal frequency distribution, the mean is the center of the distribution. In the skewed or nonnormal distribution, the mean is shifted by a large number of low or high observed scores.

The median is the midpoint of a distribution. Like the mean, it represents an average value; but unlike the mean, the median is not influenced by the values of each observation. The median is constructed so that one-half of the observations are above it and one-half are below. Thus, to find the median in the distribution of mortality rates discussed earlier, the observations are ordered from low to high: 6.0, 8.0, 9.0, 9.0, 10.0, 10.0, 11.0, 12.0, 14.0, 16.0. Since there are ten values, the median lies between the fifth and sixth values. In this case, it is equal to 10.

The mode is the most frequently occurring value in a distribution. In the previous example, the mode is 9 or 10, since each appears twice (a bimodal distribution) and no other value appears more than once. In the normal distribution, the mean, median, and mode are all equal.

Isaac had the following suggestions for selecting the appropriate measure of central tendency:[2]

1. Compute the arithmetic mean when any of the following conditions apply:
   a. The greatest reliability is wanted. The mean usually varies less from sample to sample when samples are drawn from the same population.
   b. Other computations, such as finding measures of variability, are to follow.
   c. The distribution is symmetrical about the center, and especially when it is approximately normal.[3]
2. Compute the median when any of the following conditions apply:
   a. Distributions are markedly skewed. This includes the case in which one or more extreme measurements are at one side of the distribution.
   b. We are interested in whether cases fall within the upper or lower halves of the distribution and not particularly in how far from the central point.
   c. An incomplete distribution is given.[4]
3. Compute the mode when any of the following conditions apply:
   a. The quickest estimate of central value is wanted.
   b. A rough estimate of central value will do.
   c. We wish to know the typical case.[5]

Measures of Dispersion

Although measures of central tendency provide some indication of the average value of a distribution, they provide no information about the distribution of values around this average. Values may be clustered closely around the mean, in which case the mean is an effective representation of the distribution, or values may be scattered over a broad range, in which case the mean is less representative. The range, standard deviation, and coefficient of variation are three measures of dispersion in a distribution.

The range is the simplest measure of dispersion to compute. It is computed by subtracting the lowest value from the highest value in the distribution. It is thus based only on the extreme values of the distribution. The standard deviation, the most important measure of dispersion about the mean, forms the basis for most statistical analysis. The coefficient of variation is useful when two populations with differing means are compared. This measure of dispersion adjusts the standard deviation for the mean value and is computed as follows:

$$CV = \bar{S}/X$$

where CV = coefficient of variation
       S = standard deviation
       $\bar{X}$ = mean

The coefficient of variation is often expressed as a percentage by multiplying the computed value by 100.

THE SIGNIFICANCE OF RATES: DESCRIBING COMMUNITIES

The epidemiological approach to the determination of community health problems rests on the comparison of mortality and morbidity rates in the population of concern to some other standard or target rate. The identification of a problem has meaning only in relation to some standard. A standard, then, refers to the value associated with a particular indicator (criterion) that is acceptable to the decision makers. For example, an infant mortality rate of 20 per 1,000 has marginal meaning by itself. It must be compared with an infant mortality rate in another geographical area or another time period or with some arbitrarily set standard or target value.

When comparing rates, it is necessary to determine the degree of difference or deviation from the standard that is significant. Significance is based on three factors: the variability of rates, the significance of the difference between two rates, and the significance of excess deaths.

Variability of Rates

An observed mortality or morbidity rate is only an estimate of the true rate and, as is the case with any estimate, is subject to chance variation. As Kleinman pointed out, the number of deaths in an area varies by chance, depending on the size of the population and the probability of death—the true mortality rate.[6] As the size of the population increases, the chance component becomes less important, and the observed mortality rate becomes a better estimate of the true rate. For example, the observed death rate in an area where there are few deaths may be very different from the true rate. Consequently, the variability of rates must be assessed. This can be done easily through basic statistical measures.

Standard Deviation

As noted earlier, the standard deviation is the most important measure of dispersion about the mean value of a distribution and forms the basis for most statistical analysis. It consists of the square root of the sum of the squared deviations of each value from the mean, divided by the number of observations, or

$$S = \sqrt{[\sum_{i=1}^{n}(X_1 - \overline{X})^2] / n}$$

where
$$S = \text{standard deviation}$$
$$(X_1 - \overline{X})^2 = \text{the mean value X from the value of } X_1 \text{ then squared}$$
$$n = \text{number of observations}$$

One unique property of the standard deviation in the normal distribution is that 68 percent of the observed values fall within one standard deviation on either side of the mean, 95 percent within two standard deviations, and 99 percent within three standard deviations. This property has important consequences for testing hypotheses and significant levels through statistical analysis.

Sample Mean

Because every value in the population cannot be measured, the true mean is estimated from some smaller number of measurements. Thus, when a population mean or some other population parameter is to be determined, the true population mean or parameter is estimated from a small sample of the total population. If all possible samples of a given size were taken from the same population, the result would be a distribution of sample means with the shape of a normal distribution.

Regardless of the shape of the population distribution, the distribution of the sample means is approximately normal. This is expressed in the central limit theorem, which states that, for almost all populations, the sampling distribution of the means will be distributed about normally, given a sufficient sample size. This theorem allows inferences to be drawn about population means and mortality rates from information extracted from samples in time or space.

Like a population distribution, a distribution of sample means involves a variance. The variance of the sample means is equal to the variance calculated from a sample, divided by the size of the sample used to calculate the variance:

$$S_{\bar{x}}^2 = S^2 / n$$

The square root of the variance of the sample mean is called the standard error of the mean:

$$S_{\bar{x}} = \sqrt{S^2 / n} = S \sqrt{(n)}$$

where $S_{\bar{x}}$ = standard error of the mean
$\quad S$ = standard deviation
$\quad n$ = number of observations

The standard error of the mean is the statistic that permits statements to be made regarding population estimates of the true mean with specified levels of confidence. Similarly, the standard error of a rate is the standard deviation of the (theoretical) sampling distribution of the rate.

Levels of Confidence

The standard error is used to estimate the range within which the true population lies; this range is called the confidence interval.

It is always necessary to construct a confidence interval when presenting data derived from a sample of a population or when presenting rates for a population. Such calculations are often based on relatively low numbers of values, and the width of the confidence interval will take this into account. If few values are used, the confidence interval will be quite wide. With a great many values, however, the confidence interval is narrower, indicating that the estimates are more accurate.

The probability that the true population rate is contained within the confidence interval is called the degree of confidence. The value most commonly used for the degree of confidence is .95, or 95 percent. This indicates that users of the data can be 95 percent confident that the true rate lies within the calculated confidence interval. In other words, there is a 95 percent probability that the confidence interval includes the true rate and a 5 percent probability that it does not. When a 5 percent chance of error is not acceptable, a 99 percent confidence interval is commonly used.

Confidence Intervals for a Population Rate. The calculation of the confidence interval is based on the assumption that the distribution of the observed rates approximates the standard normal curve. There are three primary methods for the construction of confidence intervals.

Method 1: A rate that has been computed for a population at a given time can be considered a sample estimate of the true rate or a sample in time or space, thereby allowing confidence interval estimations to be used. An estimate of the true rate reflects the true rate plus random error. To construct a confidence interval for the rate, the following formula is used:[7]

95 percent confidence limits:

$$\text{Upper limit} = 1,000/n[d + 1.96 \sqrt{(d)}]$$
$$\text{Lower limit} = 1,000/n[d - 1.96 \sqrt{(d)}]$$

where d = number of deaths upon which rate is based
n = denominator of rate (i.e., the target population)

The step-by-step procedure for calculating the 95 percent confidence interval is shown in Exhibit 4-1. For the 99 percent confidence interval, 1.96 ($\pm$ 2 standard deviations based on the normal curve) is replaced with 2.58 ($\pm$ 3 standard deviations based on the normal curve). If the rate is greater than 100 per 1,000, $\sqrt{(d)}$ is replaced by $\sqrt{d[1 - (d/n)]}$. If the rate is of some base other than 1,000 (10,000 or 100,000), this base is exchanged for 1,000. An application of this procedure for calculating 95 percent confidence intervals using Method 1 is illustrated in Exhibit 4-2. The calculated confidence interval indicates that we are 95% confident that the true death rate is between 6.46 and 8.88 per 1,000.

Method 2: A 95 percent confidence interval for more than 30 observations can also be derived from the following formula:

$$CI = p \pm 1.96 \sqrt{[(p \times q)/n]}$$

where CI = confidence interval
p = the rate
$q = (1 - p)$
n = the population for the rate

To calculate the confidence interval:

1. Divide the rate (p) by 1,000 to put it on a per person basis.
2. Multiply the rate (p) by 1 minus the rate (q): $p \times q$.
3. Divide the product of $p \times q$ by the population for the rate (n): $(p \times q)/n$.
4. Find the square root for the preceding quotient: $\sqrt{[(p \times q)/n]}$.
5. Multiply the preceding square root by 1.96: $1.96 \times \sqrt{[(p \times q)/n]}$. Multiply the product by the number used to get the rate to a per person basis.
6. To find the two specified confidence limits, add the preceding product to the rate for the high limit and subtract the product from the rate for the low limit. Thus, the confidence interval = rate $\pm 1.96 \sqrt{[(p \times q)/n]}$.

Exhibit 4-1 Calculating a Confidence Interval for a Population Rate

1. Find the square root of d.	$\sqrt{d}$
2. Multiply the square root of d by 1.96	$1.96 \times \sqrt{d}$
3a. For the upper limit, add d to $1.96\sqrt{d}$.	$d + 1.96\sqrt{d}$
b. For the lower limit, subtract $1.96\sqrt{d}$ from d.	$d - 1.96\sqrt{d}$
4. Divide 1,000 by n.	$1{,}000 / n$

5a. Multiply the quotient in #4 ($1{,}000 / n$) by the sum in #3a ($d + 1.96\sqrt{d}$) to get the upper limit.
  b. Multiply the quotient in #4 ($1{,}000 / n$) by the difference in #3b to get the lower limit.

Exhibit 4-2 Method 1 for Calculating 95 Percent Confidence Interval for a Population Rate

In DeKalb County, Georgia, there were 155 deaths of white males aged 45 to 54 years. A total of 20,201 white males lived in the county. The death rate was 7.67 per 1,000:

$$\left(\frac{155}{20{,}201} \times 1{,}000\right)$$

The 95 percent confidence interval is

$$CI = \frac{1{,}000}{n} [d \pm 1.96\sqrt{d}]$$

1. $\sqrt{155} = 12.450$

2. $12.45 \times 1.96 = 24.402$

3. a. $155 + 24.402 = 179.402$ (+ for high limit)
  b. $155 - 24.402 = 130.598$ (− for low limit)

4. $1{,}000 / 20{,}201 = .0495$

5. a. $.0495 \times 179.402 = 8.88$
  b. $.0495 \times 130.598 = 6.46$

$$CI = 6.46 \text{ to } 8.88 \ (95\%)$$

The procedure for calculating 95 percent confidence intervals by means of Method 2 is illustrated in Exhibit 4-3.

Method 3: The third and simplest method to calculate the confidence interval approximates the standard error of the rate. The standard error (*SE*) of a rate can be calculated easily:

$$SE = \frac{r}{\sqrt{d}}$$

where r = rate
    d = observed number of deaths (upon which the rate is based)

Exhibit 4-3 Method 2 for Calculating a 95 Percent Confidence Interval for a Population Rate

---

Using the data for DeKalb County (see Exhibit 4-2), the 95 percent confidence interval for the death rate among white males aged 45 to 54 is

$$CI = p \pm 1.96\sqrt{[(p \times q)n]}$$

1. $7.67 / 1,000 = .00767$

2. $.00767 \times .99233 = .0076111$ (.99233 is obtained by subtracting .00767 from 1.00, as defined for q)

3. $.0076111 / 20,201 = .0000003$

4. $\sqrt{.0000003} = .0006138$

5. $1.96 \times .0006138 = .001203 \times 1,000 = 1.20$ (multiplying by 1,000 returns the rate to a per 1,000 population basis)

6. $7.67 + 1.20 = 8.87$ (high limit)
   $7.67 - 1.20 = 6.47$ (low limit)

$$CI = 6.47 \text{ to } 8.87$$

The 95 percent confidence interval is constructed using the following formula:

$$CI_{(95\%)} = \text{rate} \pm (1.96 \times SE)$$

The 99 percent confidence interval would simply be

$$CI_{(99\%)} = \text{rate} \pm (2.58 \times SE)$$

A step-by-step procedure to calculate the 95 percent confidence interval is as follows:

1. Find the square root of d: $\sqrt{d}$.
2. Calculate the standard error (SE): divide the rate (r) by the square root of d: ($\sqrt{d}$).
3. Multiply the SE by 1.96.
4. Add the preceding product to the rate for the high limit, and subtract it for the low limit.

This procedure is illustrated in Exhibit 4-4.

The three methods described can be used to assess the variability of any rates or ratios, including the standardized mortality ratio and birth rates. Method 3 uses an approximation of the standard error of a rate, but it is the simplest and easiest to calculate and is more than adequate for use in community health planning. Using Method 3, the standard error of a standardized mortality ratio is

Exhibit 4-4 Method 3 for Calculating a 95 Percent Confidence Interval for a Population Rate

---

Using the data from Exhibit 4-2:

1. $\sqrt{155} = 12.45$

3. $SE = 7.67 / 12.45 = .616$

3. $1.96 \times .616 = 1.21$

4. $7.67 + 1.21 = 8.88$ (high limit)
   $7.67 - 1.21 = 6.46$ (low limit)

$$CI = 6.46 \text{ to } 8.88$$

$$SE = \frac{SMR}{\sqrt{d}}$$

where d = number of observed deaths

The standard error of a birth rate (r) is:

$$SE = \frac{r}{\sqrt{b}}$$

where b = number of births

Confidence Intervals for Mortality Indexes. Mortality index values may require the estimation of confidence intervals. Therefore, confidence intervals can be constructed for adjusted mortality indexes by means of the general formula:[8]

$$I \pm 1.96 \, SE_I$$

where I = mortality index
   1.96 = standard deviation for 95 percent confidence interval
   SE_I = standard error of the index

Before applying this formula it is necessary to calculate the standard error of the index being used. For example, the formulas used to calculate the standard error for three mortality indexes are:

1. Standardized Mortality Ratio[9]

$$SE_{SMR} = \sqrt{(d)}/[(1/1,000)(\Sigma M_a p_a)]$$

where d = number of deaths
   M_a = standard age-race-sex–specific rates per 1,000
   p_a = area population in age-race-sex group a
   Σ = sum over all age-sex-race groups

2. Comparative Mortality Figure[10]

$$SE_{CMF} = \sqrt{\{\Sigma\ 1{,}000m_a/p_a\ (P_a/P)^2\}}/\Sigma\ (M_a)\ (P_a/P)$$

where $m_a = d_a/p_a \times 1{,}000$ (area's age-specific death rate per 1,000)

p_a = area population in age group a

P_a = standard population in age group a

P = total standard population = ΣP_a

M_a = standard age-specific death rates

3. Years-of-Life-Lost (YLL) Index[11]

$$SE_{YLL} = \sqrt{\Sigma d_a\ (70 - y_a)^2/1}/1{,}000\ \{\Sigma M_a p_a\ (70 - y_a)\}$$

where d_a = deaths in each age group a

M_a = standard age-specific death rates

p_a = area population in age group a

y_a = the midpoint of each age interval a

If the years-of-life-lost index for DeKalb County, Georgia, is .851 (based on the data in Table 4-2), and since the formula for the years-of-life-lost index extends only to age 70, we will use the age group 55–64 as the last one in the computation. Therefore,

For $d_a\ (70 - y_a)^2$:

$$
\begin{aligned}
64(69.5)^2 &= 64(4{,}830.25) & &= 309{,}136 \\
12(67)^2 &= 12(4{,}489) & &= 53{,}868 \\
13(60)^2 &= 13(3{,}600) & &= 46{,}800 \\
31(50)^2 &= 31(2{,}500) & &= 77{,}500 \\
41(40)^2 &= 41(1{,}600) & &= 65{,}600 \\
68(30)^2 &= 68(900) & &= 61{,}200 \\
155(20)^2 &= 155(400) & &= 62{,}000 \\
235(10)^2 &= 235(100) & &= \underline{23{,}500} \\
& & \Sigma d_a\ (70 - y_a)^2 &= 699{,}604 \\
& & \sqrt{\Sigma\ d_a\ (70 - y_a)^2} &= 836.42
\end{aligned}
$$

For $1/1{,}000\ M_a p_a\ (70 - y_a)$

$$
\begin{aligned}
70.26(69.5) &= 4{,}883.07 \\
10.64(67) &= 712.88 \\
18.18(60) &= 1{,}090.8 \\
49.82(50) &= 2{,}491.0 \\
48.47(40) &= 1.938.8 \\
83.33(30) &= 2{,}499.9 \\
178.37(20) &= 3{,}567.4 \\
245.15(10) &= \underline{2{,}451.5} \\
\Sigma\ M_a p_a\ (70 - Y_a) &= 19{,}635.4
\end{aligned}
$$

Table 4-2 Years-of-Life-Lost Data

a (Age Group)	p_a (Population)	d_a (Deaths)	y_a (Midpoint)	m_a (Mortality Rate/ 1,000)	$M_a p_a$* (Expected Deaths)
<1	3,325	64	.5	19.25	70.26
1–4	12,669	12	3	.95	10.64
5–14	38,883	13	10	.34	18.18
15–24	29,136	31	20	1.06	49.82
25–34	27,383	41	30	1.50	48.47
35–44	24,223	68	40	2.81	83.33
45–54	20,201	155	50	7.67	178.37
55–64	11,128	235	60	21.12	245.15
65+	7,103	520	75	73.21	235.74
Total	174,051	1,139			

*M_a is the U.S. age-specific death rate.

Source: Reprinted from *Statistical Notes for Health Planners,* February 1977, p. 9, National Center for Health Statistics, U.S. DHHS.

Since

$$SE_{YLL} = \sqrt{\Sigma \; d_a \; (70 \; - \; y_a)^2/1}/1{,}000 \; \{\Sigma \; M_a p_a \; (70 \; - \; y_a)\}$$

Therefore

$$SE_{YLL} = \sqrt{699{,}604}/19{,}635.4 = 836.423/19{,}635.4 = .0426$$

Given the standard error for YLL as .0426, the 95 percent confidence interval is

$$I \pm 1.96 \; (SE_{YLL}) = .851 \pm 1.96 \; (.0426)$$
$$= .851 \pm .083$$
$$= (.934, .768)$$

Thus, 95 percent of the time, the years-of-life-lost index for DeKalb County will be between .768 and .934.

In health planning, the years-of-life-lost index appears to be the most useful of the three statistics that have been discussed. The data needed to compute the index and the confidence intervals are readily available. In addition, this index may be used to compare different areas, although a slightly modified formula is required when the ratio of the index values is used. Finally, the index need not be based on total values or all ages, but may be used for portions of the age range (e.g., groups 15–44).

Significance of Difference between Two Rates

When comparing an observed rate with an arbitrarily set standard, goal, or target value, the confidence interval for the observed rate provides the significance of the difference. If the standard is included in the confidence interval of the observed rate, there is no significant difference at the level of confidence chosen. The situation is somewhat more complex, however, when comparing rates of two different areas or of two different times for the same area. This requires a direct extension of the concept of a confidence interval. The objective is to determine whether a difference between the rates is significant or whether it is caused solely by random effects. Different methods must be used, depending on whether the rates are independent.

When Rates Are Independent

Two rates are independent when they do not include any of the same observations or events (e.g., births, deaths) in their numerator. Thus, rates from overlapping time periods or areas are not independent. For example, rates from a county and the state that the county is in are not independent; rates from two different counties are independent.

To determine whether there is a significant difference between two independent rates, the confidence interval for the ratio between the two rates or the difference between the two independent rates is used.[12] The ratio is defined as

$$R = r_1/r_2$$

where R = ratio

r_1 = rate for area 1 or period 1

r_2 = rate for area 2 or period 2

The 95 percent confidence interval for the ratio (R) is defined as

$$R \pm 1.96 \, R \, \sqrt{(1/d_1) + (1/d_2)}$$

where d_1 = number of events for area 1 or period 1 (i.e., the rate numerator)

d_2 = number of events for area 2 or period 2

To establish a significant difference, it must be determined whether the confidence interval contains the figure one. If it does not, it can be stated that the two rates are significantly different. If the interval does contain the figure one, it cannot be concluded that there is a significant difference. Kleinman provided the example:[13]

Years	Number of Infant Deaths	Number of Live Births	Infant Mortality Rate per 1,000 Live Births
1961–1965	200	5,000	40
1966–1970	100	4,000	25

$$R = 40/25 = 1.6$$

The 95 percent confidence interval is

$$1.96R \sqrt{(1/d_1) + (1/d_2)} = 1.96(1.6)\sqrt{(1/200) + (1/100)}$$
$$= 1.96(1.6)(.1225) = .384$$
$$1.6 + .384 = 1.984 \text{ (upper limit)}$$
$$1.6 - .384 = 1.216 \text{ (lower limit)}$$
$$CI_{(95\%)} = 1.216 \text{ to } 1.984$$

Thus, the infant mortality rate for 1961 to 1965 can be said, with 95 percent confidence, to be from 1.22 to 1.98 times the rate for 1966 to 1970. Because the interval does not contain one, there is a statistically significant difference in the area's infant mortality rate between the two time periods. If the interval did contain one, there would not be a statistically significant difference.

An alternate method of computing the 95 percent confidence interval for the ratio between two rates is to use the confidence intervals for each rate. If the confidence limit (CL) is defined as the value that is added to and subtracted from the rate to give the confidence interval, the formula is

$$CL = 1.96 \times SE = 1.96 \times (r/\sqrt{d})$$

where SE = standard error (See Method 3 for calculating a confidence interval.)

The confidence interval for the ratio R then is

$$CI = R \pm R \sqrt{\{[(CL_1/r_1)^2] + [(CL_2/r_2)^2]\}}$$

where CL_1 = confidence level for rate 1
CL_2 = confidence level for rate 2
r_1, r_2 = rates for periods 1 and 2, respectively

In the previous example

$$CL_1 = 1.96 \times (40/\sqrt{200}) = 1.96 \times 2.828 = 5.54$$
$$CL_2 = 1.96 \times (25/\sqrt{100}) = 1.96 \times 2.5 \quad = 4.9$$

and

$$CL = R \pm R \sqrt{(CL_1/r_1)^2 + (CL_2/r_2)^2}$$
$$= 1.6 \pm 1.6 \sqrt{(5.54/40)^2 + (4.9/25)^2}$$
$$= 1.6 \pm 1.6(.240) = 1.6 \pm .384$$
$$\text{Upper limit} = 1.6 + .384 = 1.984$$
$$\text{Lower limit} = 1.6 - .384 = 1.216$$
$$CI = 1.216 \text{ to } 1.984$$

This confidence interval does not include one, which indicates that the two rates are significantly different at the 95 percent confidence interval.

These two formulas for the construction of the confidence interval for the ratio between two independent rates are valid only when the rate in the denominator (r_2) is based on 100 or more events; moreover, (r_1) must be greater than (r_2) so that the resulting ratio will always be greater than or equal to 1.

An alternative way of testing the difference between two independent rates is to construct a confidence interval directly for the difference rather than for the ratio. The confidence interval for the difference between two independent rates $(D = r_1 - r_2)$ is given by

$$D \pm \sqrt{CL_1^2 + CL_2^2}$$

where D = difference between the two rates

CL_1, CL_2 = confidence limits for rates 1 and 2

The confidence limit (CL) then is the value that is added to and subtracted from the rate to construct the confidence interval of the rate:

$$CL = 1.96 \times SE = 1.96 \times (r/\sqrt{d})$$

where d = number of events

In this case, if the interval includes 0, it cannot be concluded that the difference between the two rates is significant. In the previous example,

$$D = r_1 - r_2 = 40 - 25 = 15$$
$$CL_1 = 5.54 \qquad CL_2 = 4.9$$
$$CI = D \pm \sqrt{CL_1^2 + CL_2^2}$$
$$= 15 \pm \sqrt{5.54^2 + 4.9^2}$$
$$= 15 \pm 7.4$$
$$\text{Upper limit} = 15 + 7.4 = 22.4$$
$$\text{Lower limit} = 15 - 7.4 = 7.6$$
$$CI = 7.6 \text{ to } 22.4$$

The 95 percent confidence interval for the difference between the two rates ranges from 7.6 to 22.4. Since this interval does not include 0, there is 95 percent confidence that the difference between the two rates is significant. Kleinman presented the following example:[14]

	Santa Cruz, California	DeKalb County, Georgia
Population (n), white males, 45–54	6,051	20,201
Number of deaths (d)	63	155
Death rate per 1,000	10.41	7.67

The confidence limits (95 percent) are as follows:

$$\text{Santa Cruz: } CL_1 = 1.96 \times (10.41/\sqrt{63}) = \pm\, 2.57$$
$$\text{DeKalb: } \quad CL_2 = 1.96 \times (7.67/\sqrt{155}) = \pm\, 1.21$$

The confidence interval for the difference between the two rates is

$$D = 10.41 - 7.67 = 2.74$$
$$CI = D \pm \sqrt{(CL_1^2 + CL_2^2)}$$
$$= 2.74 \pm \sqrt{(2.57)^2 + 1.21^2)}$$
$$= 2.74 \pm \sqrt{8.0690}$$
$$= 2.74 \pm 2.84$$
$$CI = -.10 \text{ to } 5.58$$

Because the interval does include 0, it can be concluded that the rates for the two counties are not significantly different.

When Rates Are Not Independent

When comparing an observed rate to a standard rate that may not be independent, a slightly more complex formula is needed:[15]

$$\mu = (r - s)\,\sqrt{n/s - s^2}$$

where r = the observed rate or rate to be compared
s = the standard rate (e.g., in the state, region, nation)
n = the denominator (population on which the rate is based)

The formula is calculated as follows:

1. Square the standard rate s. Change all rates to a per person basis by dividing by the rate's denominator.
2. Subtract the square of s from s: $s - s^2$.
3. Divide the denominator on which the rate is based, n, by the difference of $s - s^2$: $n/(s-s^2)$.
4. Find the square root of the quotient from the last step: $\sqrt{n/s - s^2}$.
5. Subtract the standard rate s from the observed rate, r: $r - s$.
6. Multiply the square root in the fourth step by the difference in the fifth step: $\mu = (r - s)\sqrt{n/s - s^2}$.

If μ exceeds 1.96, it can be concluded that the rate differs significantly at the 95 percent confidence level from the standard rate to which it is compared. If it exceeds 2.58, it is significantly different at the 99 percent level. If for example, a county has a population of 16,400 persons and a death rate of 20.9 per 1,000, the objective may be to find out whether the county rate is significantly different from the state rate of 16.8 per 1,000:

Observed rate, r = 20.9 per 1,000

Standard rate, s = 16.8 per 1,000

Population (denominator n on which the rate is based) = 16,400

1. $(.0168)^2 = .0168 \times .0168 = .000282$
2. $.0168 - .000282 = .016518$
3. $16,400/.016518 = 992856.27$
4. $\sqrt{992856.27} = 996.42173$
5. $.0209 - .0168 = .0041$
6. $.0041 \times 996.42173 = 4.09 \ (\mu)$

Since the value of 4.09 (μ) is greater than 2.58, it can be concluded that the difference between the rates is significant at the 99 percent confidence level. In other words, there is 99 percent confidence that the county death rate is higher than the state death rate.

When rates are based on a very low number of events (e.g., births, deaths, cases), the actual number of events is used instead of the rate:

$$\mu = (o - e)/\sqrt{e}$$

where o = the observed number(s) to be compared

e = the standard number (e.g., state, region, nation)

This formula is calculated as follows:

1. Find the square root of the standard number e: $\sqrt{e}$.
2. Subtract the standard number e from the observed number o: $o - e$.
3. Divide the difference between the observed and standard numbers (Step 2) by the square root of e: $(o - e)/\sqrt{e}$.

Thus, to determine whether a county infant mortality rate is significantly higher than the state infant mortality rate,

$$\mu = (o - e)/\sqrt{e}$$

where o = 20.2 per 1,000 (65 deaths)

e = 17.5 per 1,000 (117 deaths)

Thus

$$\sqrt{117} = 10.81$$
$$65 - 117 = -52$$
$$-52/10.81 = -4.81$$

Since the value -4.81 in absolute terms (that is, without considering the sign) is greater than 2.58, it can be concluded that the two rates are significantly different at the 99 percent confidence level.

Reasons for Differences in Rates

Statistical differences are not the only reasons for rate variations. Weir noted several others.[16]

- Physicians, coroners, and their assistants in different locations may complete death certificates in different ways.
- Although such classification is a highly standardized process done by well-trained and experienced technicians, there may be differences in the way that health departments' nosologists determine the underlying cause of death and assign a code to it.
- Data entry clerks may make different types of coding errors, although this seems less   likely in view of data-processing patterns.

- Differences may result from program errors or from decisions, such as excluding death records that lack age, sex, and/or county data.
- Geographical areas may differ in the proportional distribution of residents at each year of age during the time period.
- The Census Bureau's undercount percentages among health service areas and between sexes may be different.

Significance of "Excess Deaths"

A problem may also be defined by an excess of morbidity or mortality. In an analysis of "excess deaths," for example, there are two major steps. Initially, it must be determined whether there is a difference between the number of deaths expected and the number that actually occurred (observed). If so, it must be determined whether the excess deaths result merely from chance or are actually significant statistically. This analysis requires the following data on both the population being investigated and the standard population:

- demographic data categorized by age, sex, race, occupation, or other specifics
- mortality data categorized by cause of death, either in actual number observed or in death rates

If death rates are available for the selected standard population, the expected number of deaths can be derived for the population being investigated.

Determining the Number of Expected Deaths

Each of the following two methodologies is statistically valid for health problem analysis and should produce the same results. The selection of one methodology over the other, therefore, depends solely on the availability of data and personal preference.

Using the Actual Number of Deaths. The expected number of deaths can be calculated using the following formula:

$$E = P_1/P_2 \times D$$

where E = expected deaths
P_1 = population being investigated
P_2 = standard population
D = actual deaths in standard population

The ratio, P_1/P_2, should be age-sex-race–specific. If the subject is deaths among white men aged 55 to 64, both P_1 and P_2 should refer to the number of white men of these ages; on the other hand, if deaths among the overall population are being studied, P_1 and P_2 should refer to the total population.

For example, in Massachusetts between 1969 and 1973 there were 52 deaths from fires and flames among men aged 60 to 64. There were 113,128 men of this age in the state; 4,055 in the city being investigated. Assuming that the risk of dying in a fire was the same in the city as in the state as a whole, the expected number of deaths in the city was calculated as follows:

$$E = \frac{P_1}{P_2} \times D = \frac{4,055}{113,128} \times 52 = 1.9 \text{ deaths}$$

Thus, 1.9 (rounded to 2) is the expected number of such deaths in the city among men aged 60 to 64. There were three actual deaths because of fires and flames in the city being investigated, a difference of one death.

Using Death Rates. If, instead of the actual number of deaths, death rates are available for the standard population, the expected number of deaths is given by

$$E = P_1 \times M_2$$

where P_1 = population being investigated

M_2 = specific death rate in the standard population

Since $M_2 = \dfrac{D}{P_2}$, it can be seen this is algebraically equivalent to the previous method.

Testing the Significance of Results

Once the difference between the expected and the observed (actual) deaths has been determined, a statistical test must be applied to determine whether the difference has any significance. If so, a greater than expected number of deaths is not likely to be the result of chance alone; however, there is always a possibility that a certain number of events in 100 could have occurred solely on the basis of chance.

The significance of a difference may be tested by means of standardized mortality ratios (SMRs), which are developed and tested using the standard error and confidence intervals, or the chi square "goodness-of-fit" test. Although each of these methods is statistically sound for this purpose, health analysts with limited statistical backgrounds generally find the standardized mortality ratio easier to use. It requires more subjective judgment in interpreting the results, but the chi square test is more complex and may require some statistical expertise.

Standardized Mortality Ratio. The standardized mortality ratio (SMR) is calculated as follows:

$$SMR = \frac{\text{Observed deaths}}{\text{Expected deaths}} \times 100$$

A ratio of 100 indicates that the observed number of deaths equals the expected number of deaths. A ratio of 130 indicates that there were 30 percent more deaths than expected; a ratio of 90 indicates 10 percent fewer deaths than expected.

The next step is to calculate the confidence interval of the standardized mortality ratio. Using Method 3 for the calculation of a 95 percent interval (see Exhibit 4-4), the 95 percent confidence interval of a standardized mortality ratio is obtained by

$$CI = SMR \pm (1.96 \times SE)$$

where $SE = \dfrac{SMR}{\sqrt{d}}$

d = number of observed deaths

Data on observed and expected deaths in a county, as compared to a state, are presented in Table 4-3.

The confidence interval of a standardized mortality ratio is interpreted as follows:

- If the lower confidence limit is below 100 and the upper limit is above 100, there is no significant difference between the number of observed and the number of expected deaths.
- If the lower confidence limit is above 100, the number of observed deaths is significantly higher than expected, and it is unlikely that the excess is merely a chance occurrence.
- If the upper confidence limit is below 100, the number of observed deaths is significantly fewer than expected.
- If a confidence interval is quite wide, regardless of what the limits are, more data are required or the data should be grouped before any conclusions can

Table 4-3 Observed and Expected Deaths from Heart Disease for County A, by Age Group, 1970–1974

Age Group	Observed Deaths	Expected Deaths
20–29	16	16
30–39	18	20
40–49	22	18
50–59	51	56
60–69	55	72
70–79	62	64
80–89	22	28
90+	14	15
Totals	260	289

$$SMR = \frac{260}{289} \times 100 = 89.97$$

$$SE = \frac{SMR}{\sqrt{d}} = \frac{89.97}{\sqrt{260}} = 5.58$$

$$CI_{(95\%)} = 89.97 \pm (1.96 \times 5.58)$$

Upper limit = 89.97 + 10.94 = 100.91

Lower limit = 89.97 − 10.94 = 79.03

$$CI = 79 \text{ to } 101$$

be reached. Although no clear-cut rules specify what constitutes a "wide" range, a range of 50 or more is excessive.

In the preceding example (see Table 4-3), it is somewhat difficult to decide whether the result is significant, since the upper confidence limit is barely above 100. It can be concluded that the standardized mortality ratio seems moderately, although not significantly, low at the 95 percent confidence level.

Chi Square Test. The chi square or "goodness-of-fit" test makes it possible to compare an observed frequency with an expected frequency distribution. The formula for chi square is

$$\chi^2 = \Sigma \frac{(O - E)^2}{E}$$

where χ^2 = chi square

Σ = sum across all groups

O = observed deaths

E = expected deaths

Table 4-4 presents the calculation of chi square for the data presented in Table 4-3. The computed chi square value of 6.97 is compared with a tabular value

Table 4-4 Calculation of Chi Square for Observed and Expected Deaths from Heart Disease for County A, 1970–1974

Age Group	Observed Deaths	Expected Deaths	$\dfrac{(O - E)^2}{E}$
20–29	16	16	0.00
30–39	18	20	0.20
40–49	22	18	0.89
50–59	51	56	0.45
60–69	55	72	4.01
70–79	62	64	0.06
80–89	22	28	1.29
90+	14	15	0.07
Totals	260	289	6.97

$$\chi^2 = 0 + .20 + .89 + .45 + 4.01 + .06 + 1.29 + .07$$
$$\chi^2 = 6.97$$

of chi square with $(k - r)$ degrees of freedom, where k equals the number of categories that can be calculated $(O - E)^2/E$ (that is, the number of age groups in this example), and r equals the number of restrictions (quantities) that were determined from observed data and used in calculating the expected frequencies.[17]

In most cases in which the expected frequencies are determined by using the chi square test (or the standardized mortality ratio), the only observed quantity involved in calculating the expected frequencies is the population (P_1). Under these circumstances, the degree of freedom is $(k - 1)$. In the example in Table 4-4, there are no restrictions, as the expected frequencies were not calculated from observed data.

There are eight degrees of freedom (eight age groups). The value of chi square for eight degrees of freedom at the 95 percent level is 15.507. If the calculated value (6.97) is less than the tabular value, as is the case here, then it can be said that there is no significant difference between the observed and the expected deaths. If the calculated value were greater than the tabular value, the difference would be significant.

Testing for Significance: Small and Large Samples

A test of differences between hypothetical population parameters and estimates derived from samples requires a direct extension of the concept of a confidence interval. Health analysts are interested most often in comparing rates of two different areas or of two different times for the same area to determine if a difference between the rates is significant or if the difference is due solely to random effects. There are several commonly used methods to test such differences in health data.

Testing the Difference between Two Means for Large Samples (n>30)

In order to determine whether two mean values were derived from two samples drawn from the same population or drawn from two populations, a health analyst uses the Z test. Z is the value of the standard normal deviation, corresponding to a standard deviation on a standard normal distribution (95 percent of values with ± 1.96 standard deviation). Values are obtained from a table of Z values available in most statistics texts. The formula is

$$Z = (\overline{X}_1 - \overline{X}_2) / \sqrt{(S_{x_1}^2 / n_{x_1}) + (S_{x_2}^2 / n_{x_2})}$$

where $\overline{X}_1$ = mean from sample 1

$\overline{X}_2$ = mean from sample 2

$S_{x_1}^2$ = variance from sample 1

$S_{x_2}^2$ = variance from sample 2

n_{x_1} = number of observations in sample 1

n_{x_2} = number of observations in sample 2

A critical value (μ) is selected from a table for the normal distribution. Three commonly used values are

μ	90%	95%	99%
Z	1.65	1.96	2.33

For example, if the average number of miles jogged per month by 50 persons from Atlanta is 69.5 miles, with a standard deviation of 2.5 miles, and the average number of miles jogged by 60 people from a second city is 70.1 miles, with a standard deviation of 2.3 miles, the significance of the difference can be tested by the following formula:[18]

$$Z = \frac{70.1 - 69.5}{\sqrt{[(5.29)/(60)] + [(6.25)/(50)]}} = 1.29$$

Thus it can be concluded that the joggers in the two cities are not significantly different in their habits at the 90 percent level.

Testing the Difference between Two Means for Small Samples (n<30)

When sample sizes are small, the distribution of the sampling statistic is more closely approximated by the t distribution than by the Z test. The formulas are:[19]

$$t = |\overline{X} - \overline{Y}| / S\sqrt{[(1) / (n_x)] + [(1) / (n_y)]}$$

$$\text{and } S = \Sigma(X_1 - \overline{X})^2 + \Sigma(Y_1 - \overline{Y})^2 / n_x + n_y - 2$$

where S = pooled estimate of the standard deviation

$\overline{X}$ = mean of first sample

$\overline{Y}$ = mean of second sample

n_x = number of observations in first sample

n_y = number of observations in second sample

$\Sigma(\overline{X}_1 - \overline{X})^2$ = sum of the squared deviation of the first sample observations from $\overline{X}$

$\Sigma(Y_1 - \overline{Y})^2$ = sum of the squared deviation of the second sample observations from $\overline{Y}$

The critical value, found in a table of the t distribution, is dependent on the number of values in the sample. The t table is entered at the desired level of significance and degrees of freedom. Degrees of freedom in this case are equal to the sum of the sample sizes less 2 ($n_x + n_y - 2$). For example, if one group of children was instructed to take multivitamins and another group to take vitamin C in order to find out whether vitamin C is important to the prevention of colds, the significance of vitamin usage can be determined by means of the t test:

	Multivitamin Group	*Vitamin C Group*
Number of observations	$n_x = 10$	$n_y = 10$
Average number of colds in a year	$\overline{X} = 25.5$	$\overline{Y} = 22.0$

Sum of Squared Deviation $\Sigma(X_1 - \overline{X})^2 = 168.5$ $\Sigma(Y_1 - \overline{Y})^2 = 178.0$

$$S = \sqrt{[(168.5 + 178.0)/10 + 10 - 2)]} = \sqrt{19.25} = 4.39$$

$$t = (25.5 - 22.0) / 4.39\sqrt{[(1 / 10) + (1 / 10)]} = 3.5 / 1.96 = 1.786$$

The t value for a 95 percent significance level at (10 + 10 − 2) 18 degrees of freedom with a one-tail test is 1.72. Since 1.786 is more than 1.72, it can be concluded that the mean for the group using multivitamins is significantly higher than the mean for the group using vitamin C. Potentially, therefore, vitamin C is a preventive measure for the common cold.

Testing for the Difference between Two Sample Variances: The F Test

Once the variances have been computed from two samples, any significant difference between the two can be computed by means of the F test. The value of F is calculated by dividing the variance of the first sample by the variance of the second:

$$F = S_1^2/S_2^2$$

Normally, the larger of the two variances is placed in the numerator so that the values of F will exceed 1. In fact, if the two variances are exactly equal, the value of F will equal 1. The F test for significance indicates whether, given the sample sizes, the computed F value is significantly larger than 1, showing that the two variances are unequal.

For example, to test for the difference between the sample variance of group A, nonsmokers who can run 2 miles ($n = 40$, $S_1^2 = 8.4$), and the sample variance of group B, smokers of two packs per day who can run 2 miles ($n = 30$, $S_2^2 = 4.5$), the calculation is

$$F = 8.4 / 4.5 = 1.867$$

A table of F at the 95 percent confidence level, for 39 ($n - 1$) degrees of freedom in the numerator and 29 ($n - 1$) in the denominator, produces a critical value of $F = 1.64$. Because the calculated F value of 1.867 exceeds the critical value, the two variances are significantly different. Alternatively, there is a significant difference in the variances of smokers and nonsmokers who can run 2 miles.

Testing for the Difference between a Sample Variance and a Population Variance: The Chi Square Test

In order to determine if a calculated sample variance is significantly different from a known population variance, the chi square test is used. As in the F test, the chi square value is calculated as the ratio between two variances, but this time the sample variance is divided by the population variance:

$$\chi^2 = (n - 1)S^2 / \sigma^2$$

where S^2 = sample variance
σ^2 = population variance

The analysis proceeds as for the F test, except that the critical value from the table of chi square is used to determine the degrees of freedom from the sample ($n - 1$).

A HEALTH PLANNER'S CHECKLIST FOR STATISTICAL TESTING

The following checklist is helpful for health planners who are carrying out statistical testing.

- Formulate the problem.
- State the assumptions about the population(s) and the sampling procedures. (Rates can be assumed to be samples in time and space.) Usually, it is assumed that
  1. the data approximate a normal distribution with a population mean (μ) and a population standard deviation (σ)
  2. S (sample standard deviation) is an unbiased estimate of σ (population standard deviation)
  3. X (sample mean) is an unbiased estimate of μ (population mean)
  4. the samples are random and the observations independent

When the rates are not independent,

- set the null hypothesis (H_0) in such a way that the planner expects to reject it. In this way, the probability of a Type I error can be calculated and controlled. The null hypothesis usually states that there is no significant relationship or difference between the rates.
- formulate an alternative (H_1) hypothesis that can be accepted on rejection of the null hypothesis.
- obtain the sampling distribution. Given the assumptions and the characteristics of the data, select the appropriate sampling distribution in which to associate probabilities with outcomes.
- select the level of significance or the probability of making a Type I error. Specify n, the sample size or number of observations.
- define the critical region. Determine which values of the statistic indicate rejection of the null hypothesis (rejection region) and which indicate acceptance of the hypothesis. Do so on the basis of the type of sampling distribution at a specified level of significance, whether the critical region is to include one or both tails of the sampling distribution.
- compute the test statistic from the observed data.
- make the decision.
  1. Compare the test statistic for that sampling distribution with the values of the critical region.
  2. Accept or reject the null hypothesis, depending on whether the value obtained is inside or outside the critical region.
  3. Specify the level of significance (confidence) of this decision.
  4. Evaluate the specific problem as originally formulated.
- review statistical testing procedures to ensure that (1) small or large samples, (2) means or variances (Fig. 4-2), and (3) confidence levels between rates are being taken into account.

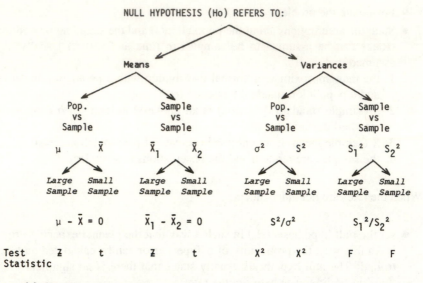

Figure 4-2 Checklist in Statistical Testing

ADDITIONAL STATISTICAL TECHNIQUES

The application of statistics is rapidly growing in importance as practitioners become more proficient, as the demands for reliable information collected in a cost-efficient manner increase, and as statistical techniques improve. The number of techniques being applied to health analysis often seems unlimited. It is important to remember, however, that the more powerful the technique, the greater the opportunity for misapplication or misunderstanding.

Correlations

Analysts may examine the degree of association between variables by means of correlation techniques, which are provided for different levels of measurement (Table 4-5).

The ultimate concern of health planners is the identification of cause-and-effect relationships. Because such relationships are always correlated, there is a strong tendency to reverse the process and infer a cause-and-effect status between two or more correlated variables. Correlation does not imply causation, however; two variables may be correlated with a third variable.

In its simplest form, a correlation coefficient is a number indicating the extent to which variations in one variable coincide with variations in another.[20] A perfect

Table 4-5 Appropriate Correlational Techniques for Different Forms of Variables

Technique	Symbol	Variable 1*	Variable 2*	Remarks
Product-moment correlation	r	Continuous	Continuous	The most stable technique
Rank difference correlation	p	Ranks	Ranks	Often used instead of product-moment when number of cases is under 30
Kendall's tau	τ	Ranks	Ranks	Preferable to rho for numbers under 10
Biserial correlation	r_{bis}	Artificial dichotomy	Continuous	Sometimes exceeds 1—has a larger standard error than r—commonly used in item analysis
Widespread biserial correlation	r_{wbis}	Widespread artificial dichotomy	Continuous	Used when you are especially interested in persons at the extremes of the dichotomized variable
Point-biserial	r_{pbis}	True dichotomy	Continuous	Yields a lower correlation than r and much lower than r_{bis}
Tetrachoric correlation	r_t	Artificial dichotomy	Artificial dichotomy	Used when both variables can be split at critical points
Phi coefficient	ϕ	True dichotomy	True dichotomy	Used in calculating interitem correlations on multiple choice or two choice items
Contingency coefficient	C	Two or more categories	Two or more categories	Comparable to r_t under certain conditions—closely related to chi square

*In these columns, a *continuous* variable is one representing an underlying continuum tending to be normally distributed. Examples include such variables as height, weight, and ability or achievement as measured by standardized tests. *Artificial dichotomies* can be constructed by arbitrarily dividing continuous variables into two groups, usually about the center of the data. Examples include such classifications as achiever-nonachiever, above average–below average, pass-fail, and warm-cold on an attitude scale. *True dichotomies* involve relatively clear-cut (though not necessarily absolute) differences, allowing the data to be categorized into two groups. Examples include such dichotomies as male-female, living-dead, teacher-nonteacher, dropout-nondropout, and smoker-nonsmoker. Other variables that can be treated as if they were true dichotomies for the purpose of computing (for example, computing a point-biserial correlation coefficient) include color blind–noncolor blind, alcoholic-nonalcoholic, and right-wrong responses with respect to a particular test item in item analysis. The distributions underlying true dichotomies, if not absolute differences, tend to be bimodal and/or relatively discontinuous.

Source: Reprinted from *Handbook in Research and Evaluation* by S. Isaac, pp. 126–127, with permission of Edits Publishers, © 1971.

positive correlation (1.0) means that changes in one variable are, without exception, accompanied by equivalent changes in the *same* direction in the other variable. No correlation (0.0) means that changes in one variable have no relationship or are only randomly related to changes in the other variable. A perfect negative correlation (-1.0) means that changes in one variable are, without exception, accompanied by equivalent changes in the *opposite* direction in the other variable. A correlation coefficient requires two sets of measurements on the same groups of individuals or on matched pairs of individuals.

The correlation coefficient, r, does not represent a percentage of the determinants that two variables have in common unless it is squared and becomes an estimate of variance called the coefficient of determination (r^2). Multiplying the coefficient of determination by 100 indicates the percentage of variance held in common by the two variables, X and Y. It answers the question, How much of the variance in Y is accounted for, associated with, or determined by the variance in X?

The standard assumption underlying most correlation coefficients is that the relationship between the two variables is linear; as one variable increases or decreases, so does the other. The simplest procedure for detecting nonlinear trends in correlation data is to construct a scatter diagram and inspect the shape of the plots for bends and curves.

A major weakness of the correlation method is that it encourages the adoption of a "shotgun" approach to research, in which all available data are used indiscriminately. In such cases, the results are extremely difficult to interpret and generally useless. Moreover, the reliability of a correlation coefficient varies directly with the sample size. Problems involving more than two variables—as in partial correlation, multiple correlation, and factor analysis—require advanced treatments of correlation methodology.

Regression

The statistical technique that specifies the relationship between one dependent variable and a set of one or more independent variables is regression. In simple linear regression, a value for Y, the dependent variable, in relation to the value of X, the independent or predictor variable, is estimated. The estimating equation takes this form:

$$Y = a + bX$$

where a = a constant equal to the Y intercept
  b = the estimated regression weight equal to the slope of the regression line

The a and b coefficients both represent estimates of true regression coefficients and, thus, are measured with error. Like the sample mean, they have a distribution that can be used to develop confidence levels. The regression coefficients are estimated through the solution of a set of normal equations. If more than one set of predictor variables is involved, matrix algebra techniques are used to solve for the regression coefficients.

Regression is one of the most frequently used techniques in the statistical analysis of large data sets. Major violations of the assumptions that are made in a regression analysis can cause misleading results, however, and specialized regression techniques have been developed to deal with such occurrences. Particular attention must be paid to the error variances of the dependent variable and to intercorrelations within the set of independent variables.

STATISTICAL SIGNIFICANCE VS. PRACTICAL SIGNIFICANCE

Although statistical significance provides evidence of differences, characteristics, or associations, it does not provide proof because it is based on several assumptions. Statistical significance deals with probabilities based on repeated sampling from a population. For any one sample, the true probability is either 0.0 or 1.0; either the sample statistic is a reliable estimate of the true population parameter, or it is not.

Statistical significance testing focuses on the probability of making an error (or the probability of being correct), given the results obtained. Thus, a 95 percent confidence level (or a 5 percent error level) means that 95 times out of 100 a value will fall within two standard errors of the true mean; 5 times out of 100, a value will exceed two standard errors. If a value exceeds the established critical level and falls outside the range of likely values, two things are possible. Either the true mean is different from the one hypothesized (rejection of a false null hypothesis), or the sample value falls in the 5 percent region only by chance (rejection of a true null hypothesis).

Although the confidence level (often referred to as α) indicates the probability that a value will exceed the critical region by chance, it does not indicate the probability that the true statistic is actually different from the hypothesized statistic. The latter is the β probability, which involves the ability to detect a false null hypothesis. Although the computation of the β probability is much more difficult than the computation of the α probability, once the desired α level and the sample size are set, the β level is fixed. Because the β level value is usually unknown and is often very small, it is impossible to conclude that it is true, even when a null hypothesis is not rejected. Rather, it is said that the results are inconclusive or, more commonly, that the null hypothesis has not been rejected. Any decision maker must consider the consequences of an error on a test of significance— either rejecting a true null hypothesis or failing to reject a false null hypothesis.

Only someone who is familiar with the hypothesis being tested or with the program being evaluated can assess the practical significance of a difference. A statistically significant difference may be so small that it is meaningless in terms of programmatic impact, especially when large samples or rates based upon large populations are involved. As statistical significance is a function of both sample size and the variation in the population, it is quite possible that any differences in a large sample will be significant. Thus, consideration must be given to the real impact of a statistically significant difference on the program or population being tested.

A problem for the administrator then is the difference between statistical and practical significance. Indexes in health services may always be significantly different in a statistical sense, because the data involve large populations. The health professional must decide whether the differences are of significant magnitude to justify action, such as revising a program.

NOTES

1. Robert Parsons, *Statistical Analysis: A Decision Making Approach* (New York: Harper & Row, 1974), 7.

2. Stephen Isaac, *Handbook in Research and Evaluation* (San Diego: Edits Publishers), 116–148.

3. Ibid., 117.

4. Ibid.

5. Ibid.

6. Joel C. Kleinman, "Infant Mortality," *Statistical Notes for Health Planners,* vol. 2 (Washington, D.C.: National Center for Health Statistics, July 1976), 4.

7. Joel C. Kleinman, "Mortality," *Statistical Notes for Health Planners,* vol. 3 (Washington, D.C.: National Center for Health Statistics, February 1977), 6.

8. Ibid., 16.

9. Kleinman, "Infant Mortality," 12.

10. Kleinman, "Mortality," 14.

11. Ibid.

12. Kleinman, "Infant Mortality," 11.

13. Ibid.

14. Kleinman, "Mortality," 7.

15. D.E. Drew and E. Keeler, "Algorithms for Health Planners," *Hypertension* 6 (U.S. DHEW, HRA, R-221516, Santa Monica, Calif.: HEW: The Rand Corporation, August 1977), 63.

16. William M. Weir, "Confidence Level Estimation To Help Data Users Evaluate Differences in Health Related Rates." Paper presented at the Third Data Use Conference, Phoenix, November 14–16, 1978, iii, 27–53.

17. Drew and Keeler, "Algorithms," 64.

18. J. Virgil Peavy and William W. Dyal, *Analytical Statistics: Statistical Methods—Testing for Significance* (Atlanta: Centers for Disease Control, 1981), 1.

19. Peavy and Dyal, *Analytical Statistics,* 11.

20. Adapted from Isaac, *Handbook,* 148–151.

Simple Math—Always on Your Mind

RATES, CASES, POPULATION, AND CONSTANTS

Health planners often need to know values related to the interrelationships of rates, cases, populations, and constants. It is not unusual, for example, for a health planner to need to know how many cases are represented by a rate. The number of cases based on a rate can be determined by the following procedure:

$$\text{Rate} = \frac{\text{Cases}}{\text{Population}} \times k \text{ (constant)}$$

where k may be 100, 1,000, 10,000, 100,000

Multiply both sides by population:

$$\text{Population} \times \text{Rate} = \text{Population} \times \frac{\text{Cases}}{\text{Population}} \times k$$

Then cancel:

$$\text{Population} \times \text{Rate} = \cancel{\text{Population}} \frac{\text{Cases}}{\cancel{\text{Population}}} \times k$$

$$\text{Population} \times \text{Rate} = \text{Cases} \times k$$

Divide both sides by k:

$$\frac{\text{Population} \times \text{Rate}}{k} = \frac{\text{Cases} \times k}{k}$$

Then cancel:

$$\frac{\text{Population} \times \text{Rate}}{k} = \frac{\text{Cases} \times \cancel{k}}{\cancel{k}}$$

$$\frac{\text{Population} \times \text{Rate}}{k} = \text{Cases}$$

If the infant mortality rate is 40 per 1,000 live births and the number of births is 5,000, the number of infant deaths can be determined:

$$\frac{\text{Population} \times \text{Rate}}{k} = \text{Cases}$$

$$\frac{5,000 \times 40}{1,000} = 200 \text{ (infant deaths)}$$

Therefore, the rate of 40/1,000 live births represents 200 infant deaths (cases).

To determine the population on which a rate is based, the following procedure is used:

$$\text{Rate} = \frac{\text{Cases}}{\text{Population}} \times k$$

Multiply both sides by population:

$$\text{Population} \times \text{Rate} = \text{Population} \times \frac{\text{Cases}}{\text{Population}} \times k$$

Then cancel:

$$\text{Population} \times \text{Rate} = \cancel{\text{Population}} \times \frac{\text{Cases}}{\cancel{\text{Population}}} \times k$$

$$\text{Population} \times \text{Rate} = \text{Cases} \times k$$

Divide both sides by rate:

$$\frac{\text{Population} \times \text{Rate}}{\text{Rate}} = \frac{\text{Cases} \times k}{\text{Rate}}$$

Then cancel:

$$\frac{\text{Population} \times \cancel{\text{Rate}}}{\cancel{\text{Rate}}} = \frac{\text{Cases} \times k}{\text{Rate}}$$

$$\text{Population} = \frac{\text{Cases} \times k}{\text{Rate}}$$

Using the earlier infant mortality example and the following formulas,

$$\text{Population} = \frac{\text{Cases}}{\text{Rate}} \times k$$

$$\text{Population} = \frac{200 \times 1,000}{40}$$

$$\text{Population} = 5000$$

These simple formulas are important in community health analysis. Rates are certainly critical to the determination of the variation in health status; however, numbers (i.e., cases and population) are critical to the allocation of resources. Knowing these simple calculations makes it unnecessary to turn to the original documents, which are not always readily available.

PERCENTAGES

One of the most frequently, but often inappropriately, used calculations in community and public health is the determination of percentages. Three basic types of percentage problems are expressed in the following questions:

1. An infant mortality rate of 20 (a community rate) is what percentage of 11.2 (a state rate)?
2. 30 teenagers die as a result of homicides and they represent 20 percent of all teenage deaths in the community, how many deaths are there?
3. If an objective is to reduce the number of cases by 30 percent and the number of cases is 126, what is the number of cases that must be prevented to meet the objective?

These problems may be restated as follows:

1. 20 is what percentage of 11.2?
2. 30 is 20 percent of what number?
3. What number is 30 percent of 126?

To solve question 1, set up a blank proportion and fill in the spaces:[1]

$$\frac{?}{?} = \frac{?}{?}$$

Because the unknown, x, is a percentage, it is put over 100:

$$\frac{x}{100} = \frac{?}{?}$$

$$\frac{x}{100} = \frac{20}{11.2}$$

$$11.2x = 20 \times 100$$

$$11.2x = 2,000$$

$$x = \frac{2,000}{11.2}$$

$$x = 178.6 \text{ percent}$$

The infant mortality rate of 20.0/1,000 live births is 178.6 percent of the state rate of 11.2/1,000 live births. This calculation is identical to that for a standardized mortality ratio in which 20.0/1,000 live births is the observed rate and therefore

$$SMR = \frac{O}{E} \times 100$$

where O = observed
E = expected

$$SMR = \frac{20}{11.2} \times 100$$

$$= 178.6 \text{ percent}$$

The community infant mortality rate of 20.0 is 78.6 percent greater than the expected rate of 11.2.

Solving questions 2 and 3 involves the same steps, but excludes the SMR calculations. Therefore, to determine how many teenage deaths occurred in a community if 30 teenage homicide deaths are 20 percent of them,

$$\frac{?}{?} = \frac{?}{?}$$

$$\frac{20}{100} = \frac{?}{?}$$

$$\frac{20}{100} = \frac{?}{x}$$

$$\frac{20}{100} = \frac{30}{x}$$

$$20x = 3,000$$

$$x = 150$$

There were 150 teenage deaths.

To reduce the number of cases by 30 percent if the total number of cases is 126 or, simply, to determine what number is 30 percent of 126,

$$\frac{?}{?} = \frac{?}{?}$$

$$\frac{30}{100} = \frac{?}{?}$$

$$\frac{30}{100} = \frac{?}{126}$$

$$\frac{30}{100} = \frac{x}{126}$$

$$100x = 30 \times 126$$

$$100x = 3,780$$

$$x = \frac{3,780}{100}$$

$$x = 37.8$$

Therefore, in order to meet the objective of reducing the cases by 30 percent, the number of cases should be reduced by 37.8, rounded to 38.

PERCENTAGE CHANGE

The calculation of percentage change (increase or decrease) is probably the most used—and misused—statistic in community and public health analysis. The need for such a calculation generally arises in connection with the percentage change in a mortality or morbidity rate between two time periods. For example, what was the percentage change in the family planning objective over the past five years? What is the percentage change in population over the last three years for the age group over age 65?

To calculate the percentage change, the following formula is used:[2]

$$\frac{\text{Change}}{\text{Starting point}} \times 100 = \text{Percentage change}$$

If, in 1985, there were 2,486 people aged 65 and over in a rural county and, in 1990, there were 3,215, the percentage change between 1985 and 1990 is calculated as follows:

$$\text{Change} = 3215 - 2486 = 726$$

$$\frac{\text{Change}}{\text{Starting point}} = \frac{726}{2486} = .292 \times 100 = 29.2 \text{ percent}$$

If the mortality rate for this group was 869 per 100,000 in 1985, and 792 per 100,000 in 1990, the percentage change in mortality for this group is calculated as follows:

$$\frac{\text{Change}}{\text{Starting point}} \times 100 = \% \text{ change}$$

$$\text{Change} = 869 - 792 = 77$$

$$\frac{77}{869} \times 100 = 8.9 \text{ percent}$$

The percentage change formula is also used for other types of problems. For example, the national objective for infant mortality in the year 2000 is 7 per 1,000 live births. In 1990, the infant mortality rate for a state is 12.5 per 1,000 live births, representing 1,325 infant deaths for the year. If the birth rate remains constant and the number of infant deaths do not increase, the number of infant deaths that must be prevented for this state to meet the national objective is calculated as follows:

$$\frac{1325}{12.5} = \frac{x}{7.0}$$

$$12.5x = 1325 \times 7.0$$

$$12.5x = 9275$$

$$x = \frac{9275}{12.5}$$

$$x = 742$$

Thus, the state needs to reduce the number of infant deaths from 1,325 to 742 by the year 2000 to reach a rate of 7 per 1,000 live births (the national standard). Using the percentage approach,

$$\text{Change} = 12.5 - 7.0 = 5.5$$

$$\frac{\text{Change}}{\text{Starting point}} = \frac{5.5}{12.5} = .44 \times 100 = 44 \text{ percent}$$

To reduce the infant mortality rate by 44 percent (i.e., achieve the national standard of 7.0), it is necessary to prevent 44 percent of 1,325 infant deaths:

$$\frac{44}{100} = \frac{x}{1325}$$

$$100x = 44 \times 1325$$

$$100x = 58300$$

$$x = \frac{58300}{100}$$

$$x = 583$$

These simple calculations are both easy and important to understand. Their application to the problems encountered in community health analysis will enhance the ability of analysts to put forth some very basic presentations to policy and decision makers.

NOTES

1. Jerry Bobrow, *Math Review for Standardized Tests* (Lincoln, Nebr.: Cliff Notes, Inc.), 52–59.
2. Ibid., 59–60.

Chapter 5

Basic Epidemiological Methods

The science of epidemiology has its roots in the study and control of infectious diseases. Today, as discussed earlier, emphasis has shifted from infectious disease to chronic disease and to social disease epidemiology. Yet, even with the change in emphasis, many concepts of infectious disease epidemiology continue to be useful in the analysis of current and future epidemiological and community health status investigations.

DESCRIPTIVE EPIDEMIOLOGY

As the "study of the amount and distribution of disease within a population by person, place, and time,"[1] descriptive epidemiology seeks to answer three basic questions regarding disease:[2] (1) Who is affected (person)? (2) Where do the cases occur (place)? and (3) When do the cases occur (time)? Friedman pointed out that descriptive epidemiological studies are of fundamental importance in that they can (1) indicate what types of persons are most likely to be affected by a disease, where the disease will occur, and when; (2) assist in planning health facilities; (3) provide clues, questions, or hypotheses as to disease etiology for further study; and (4) determine the health status of a population in a geographical area.[3]

Who Is Affected by the Disease?

To determine who is affected by a disease, it is necessary to look at such factors as age, sex, racial or ethnic origin, socioeconomic status, lifestyle, occupation, parental age, birth order, and family size. Community epidemiological studies focus primarily on groups, rather than on specific individuals. Thus, rates become a natural tool in the study of the persons whom a disease affects.

114

Age

The personal attribute most strongly related to disease occurrence is age; in fact, age is usually included in studies of other personal attributes. One method of examining the age characteristics of a disease is to analyze age-specific death rates. As shown in Table 5-1, adjusted, crude, and age-specific death rates per 100,000 population for white and black males and females are high at infancy, but decline rapidly. The rates increase gradually after age 10 and exponentially after age 40. Chronic diseases, specifically lung cancer, often show a dramatic relationship to age (Fig. 5-1).

The disease pyramid is an alternate method of examining diseases by age, as well as by sex and race (Fig. 5-2). It provides an immediate visual analysis of disease mortality by age, sex, and race, indicating at a glance the dominance of a specific age, sex, or race for the selected disease. Target groups may then be identified, depending on the specificity of the age groups studied. For example, an inverted pyramid indicates that the disease occurs primarily in the older age groups, whereas a pyramid that bulges to the left of the central axis at midpoint indicates a disease, such as cirrhosis of the liver that occurs predominantly in middle-aged men. The pyramid, however, does not give the absolute risk of dying by age, sex, and race because the values are not weighted according to the distribution of population for each age, sex, and race grouping.

Table 5-1 Death Rates for All Causes According to Sex, Race, and Age: United States, 1986

Ages	1986 Rates Per 100,000 Population				
	Total	White Male	Black Male	White Female	Black Female
All ages, age adjusted	541.7	679.8	1,026.9	387.7	588.2
All ages, crude	873.2	954.4	987.7	840.7	733.9
Under 1 year	1,032.1	976.6	2,181.7	759.1	1,731.1
1–4 years	52.0	52.2	90.0	40.7	76.5
5–14 years	26.0	29.9	42.0	18.6	26.9
15–24 years	102.3	145.9	190.5	50.4	64.3
25–34 years	132.1	168.8	385.6	60.4	146.5
35–44 years	212.9	248.4	675.9	121.3	290.2
45–54 years	504.8	592.2	1,266.5	330.3	654.6
55–64 years	1,255.1	1,573.1	2,545.5	853.3	1,469.8
65–74 years	2,801.4	3,634.8	4,789.9	2,031.8	2,892.3
75–84 years	6,348.2	8,341.7	9,290.8	5,108.7	6,148.8
85 years +	15,398.9	18,576.1	15,488.1	14,502.9	12,510.3

Source: Reprinted from *Health United States*, p. 61, U.S. DHHS, Public Health Service, 1988.

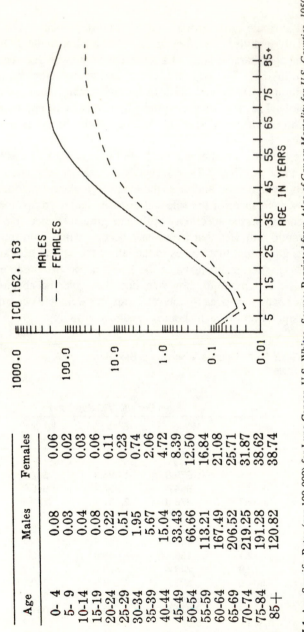

Age	Males	Females
0- 4	0.08	0.06
5- 9	0.03	0.02
10-14	0.04	0.03
15-19	0.08	0.06
20-24	0.22	0.11
25-29	0.51	0.23
30-34	1.95	0.74
35-39	5.67	2.06
40-44	15.04	4.72
45-49	33.43	8.39
50-54	66.66	12.50
55-59	113.21	16.84
60-64	167.49	21.08
65-69	206.52	25.71
70-74	219.25	31.87
75-84	191.28	38.62
85+	120.82	38.74

Figure 5-1 Age-Specific Rates (per 100,000) for Lung Cancer, U.S. Whites. *Source:* Reprinted from *Atlas of Cancer Mortality for U.S. Counties, 1950–1969,* by T.J. Mason, et al., p. 81, U.S. DHHS Pub. No. NIH 15–780.

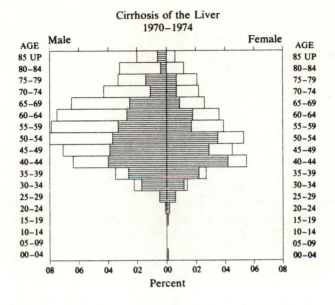

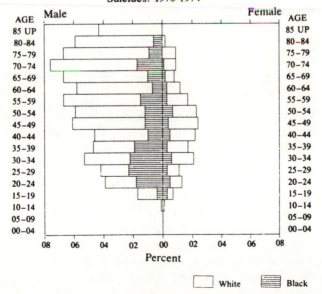

Figure 5-2 Disease Pyramids. *Source:* Reprinted from *Health Services Research and Statistics*, Division of Physical Health, Georgia Department of Human Resources, pp. 116, 121, and 137, 1976.

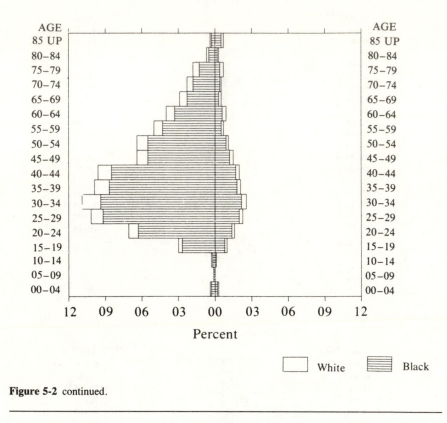

Figure 5-2 continued.

Studies by age may be done as current analysis or as cohort analysis. Current analysis examines the relationship between age and, in some instances, sex and race to death or disease at one point in time (see Table 5-1, Fig. 5-1, and Fig. 5-2). In contrast, a cohort analysis examines the relationship between age and death or disease in successive birth cohorts (persons born during a specified time). In Figure 5-3, for example, a cohort method has been used to plot suicide rates for males and females in the 15–24 age group. Each bar indicates the rate in a single cohort. Instead of displaying the data cross-sectionally, cohort analysis shows the relationship between death (or disease) and age through time. The graph depicts a major difference in male and female suicide rates. Additionally, it shows that the suicide rate for the 1951–1960 cohort increased dramatically over that of the 1941–1950 cohort.

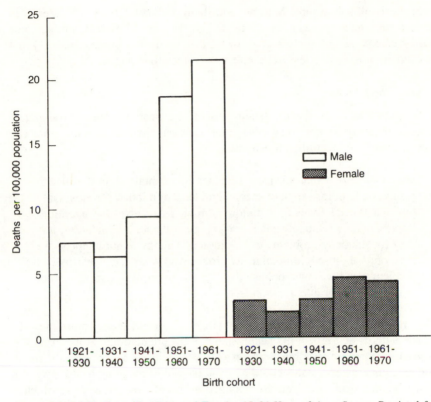

Figure 5-3 Suicide Rates for Males and Females 15–24 Years of Age. *Source:* Reprinted from *Health, United States, 1987,* p. 19, U.S. DHHS, Pub. No. 88–1232, 1988.

Sex

The differential mortality experience of males and females is evident in both Table 5-1 and Figure 5-1. For nearly all forms of cancer, the number of male deaths exceeds the number of female deaths. The ratio of male to female deaths for age-adjusted cancer rates varies from more than three to one to less than one to one.[4] Particularly significant is the fact that the ratio of male deaths to female deaths exceeds three to one for four forms of cancer—larynx, esophagus, tongue, and lung. Lung cancer has been related specifically to the greater incidence of smoking by men. Current evidence suggests, however, that this ratio will decrease as more women begin to feel the effects of long-term smoking. Although mortality rates are generally higher in males, morbidity rates are usually higher in females.[5] For females, both reported morbidity and physician visits are higher in all age groups. Mausner and Bahn postulated that these differences between men and women may be related to the possibility that women seek medical care at an earlier stage of a disease than do men or to the possibility that the cited diseases have a less lethal effect on women than on men.[6]

Race or Ethnic Group

The examination of specific health statistics, especially those pertaining to ethnic or minority groups, may raise more questions than the investigations can answer. Therefore, according to Haynes,

> We should insist that adequate statistics be maintained so that health planners do not lose sight of special problems of minority groups. Only by such special focus will minority problems receive due attention. Representing a relatively small percentage of the total population, it is easy for minority problems to be ignored. This must not happen. We must oppose those within minority groups who wish to conceal special problems, and we must oppose those of the majority group who want to ignore these problems.[7]

To provide adequate health care for all citizens, a health agency must know the disease patterns that reflect the health status of the population that it serves. Because socioeconomic standing has been associated with some diseases, the socioeconomic patterns of a state should be most helpful in planning health services. Socioeconomic data, however, are obtained primarily through census, which is taken only every ten years. For this reason, mortality and, increasingly, morbidity statistics are employed to depict areas of relative need. To plan adequately for the minority population, the health planner should consider racial differences in mortality and morbidity rates.

Compared to whites, blacks have a higher death rate at every age group, except that of 85 and over (see Table 5-1). Death rates for heart disease, cerebrovascular accidents, homicide, and accidental deaths are all higher among blacks.[8] Whites have higher death rates for arteriosclerotic heart disease, suicide, and leukemia. Whites and blacks also have different rates for several forms of cancer; for example, black women have a higher incidence of cervical cancer than do white women, whereas white women have a higher incidence of breast cancer than do black females.[9]

Socioeconomic Status

Although some diseases are related to race or ethnic background, most differences in the incidence of disease may be accounted for by differences in socioeconomic status and environments. In an analysis by socioeconomic status, age-adjusted death rates are usually compared on the basis of income, occupation, education, or on some combination of indicators. For example, one study related the ten leading causes of death in Georgia to standardized measures of socioeconomic status, median education, median income, and occupation (Table 5-2).[10] Based on Spearman's rank-order correlation, seven of the ten causes of death

Table 5-2 Spearman's Rank-Order Correlation Coefficients of Mean Mortality Rates with Combined Socioeconomic Status, Median Education, Median Income, and Occupation, Georgia, 1969–1972

Mortality Categories	Combined Socioeconomic Status		Median Education		Median Income		Occupation	
	"r" Value	Significance	"r" Value	Significance	"r" Value	Significance	"r" Value	Significance
Total mortality	−.62	.001	−.50	.001	−.72	.001	−.25	.001
Other accidents	−.36	.001	−.32	.001	−.45	.001	−.15	.05
Motor vehicle accidents	−.32	.001	−.35	.001	−.29	.001	−.23	.01
Infant mortality	−.27	.001	−.17	.05	−.33	.001	−.16	.05
Ischemic heart disease	.21	.01	.24	.01	.13	NS	.18	.05
Influenza and pneumonia	−.18	.05	−.19	.05	−.21	.01	−.04	NS
Cancer of the trachea, bronchus, and lung	.18	.05	.16	.05	.09	NS	.21	.01
Cerebrovascular disease	−.17	.05	−.11	NS	−.24	.01	−.04	NS
Homicide	−.15	.05	−.09	NS	−.23	.01	−.02	NS
Acute myocardial infarction	−.14	NS	−.10	NS	−.14	NS	−.16	.05
Other forms of heart disease	.01	NS	.006	NS	−.007	NS	−.04	NS

Note: NS = not significant.

Source: Reprinted from "Socioeconomic Analysis of the Disease Patterns of the 70s," *Health Services Research and Statistics,* Division of Physical Health, Georgia Department of Human Resources, August 1977, p. 10.

showed significant inverse relationships to increasing socioeconomic status. Two (ischemic heart disease and cancer of the trachea, bronchus, and lung) showed significant direct relationships, indicating that the incidence of death from these causes increases as socioeconomic status increases.

The relationship of occupation to disease has been studied intensively in recent years. Occupational exposure to asbestos has been related to mesothelioma, as well as to lung and gastrointestinal cancer;[11] free silica exposure, to pulmonary fibrosis;[12] and other chemical agents and toxic substances, to various forms of morbidity and mortality. Other studies, such as that by Cobb and Rose on air traffic controllers,[13] have shown an increased incidence of hypertension, peptic ulcer, and diabetes to be associated with certain occupations.

Several investigators have examined the relationship between socioeconomic status and cancer (Table 5-3). In many instances, a positive association has been shown between socioeconomic status and cancer survival. As Freeman pointed out, these differences most often reflect the level of poverty in a population group, not race; "poverty acts through the prison of culture (race)."[14] Specifically, Freeman noted, "Poverty is a proxy for other elements of living, including lack of education, unemployment, substandard housing, poor nutrition, risk promoting lifestyle and behavior and diminished access to health care."[15]

In the American Cancer Society special report about socioeconomic disparities,[16] it was noted that controlling for socioeconomic status greatly reduces (and sometimes nearly eliminates) the apparent mortality and incidence differences between ethnic groups. This suggests that ethnic differences in cancer are largely secondary to socioeconomic factors and associated processes. Furthermore, there are consistent excesses of cancer mortality overall and cancer mortality of many specific sites for patients of low socioeconomic status, compared to those of high socioeconomic status. The overall five-year survival rate of the poor in the United States, regardless of race, is estimated to be 10 to 15 percent lower than that of the middle-class and the affluent.

Lifestyle Characteristics

Tables from the government report, *Health, United States, 1987*[17] and *Health, United States, 1988*[18] illustrate lifestyle characteristics, such as self-assessment of health, limitation of activity caused by chronic conditions, smoking, and use of alcohol or drugs. Such lifestyle data make it possible to approach health problems holistically. For example, Table 5-4 indicates the consumption of alcohol by persons 18 years of age and over in relation to sex, race, family income, marital status, and education. A profile can be developed of the problem drinker who imbibes 0.551 ounces or more of alcohol per day. A heavy drinker may be characterized as a single white male with a family income of $15,000 or more and with either high school or some college education. Such a profile may serve

Table 5-3 Summary of Multiple-Site Studies of Survival Differences between Different Socioeconomic Groups and between Blacks and Whites

Reference	Survival	Socioeconomic Status Indicator	Time Period	Population	Observed Association between Socioeconomic Status and Survival
Berg et al., 1977	Five-year, adjusted and relative	Hospital type (private, clinic-pay, indigent)	1940–1969	University of Iowa Hospitals Tumor Registry	Positive, adjusted for stage
Haenszel and Chiazze, 1965	Five-year, relative	Census (family income)	1947–1948	Chicago, Pittsburgh, Dallas	No association
Linden, 1969	Five-year, relative	Hospital type (private, public)	1942–1956	California Tumor Registry	Positive, adjusted for stage
Lipworth et al., 1970	Three-year, relative	Census (family income)	1960–1962	Connecticut	Positive, adjusted for stage and type of hospital
Lipworth et al., 1972	Less than one year	Hospital type (private, public)	1964–1966	Boston hospitals	Positive, adjusted for stage and treatment
Axtell et al., 1975	Five-year, relative	Black/White	1955–1964	NCI—End Results Group	Positive (white survival rate higher), stage-adjusted
Axtell and Myers, 1978	Five-year, relative	Black/White	1960–1973	NCI—End Results Group and SEER	Positive (white survival rate higher), stage-adjusted
Page and Kuntz, 1980	Five-year, relative	Black/White	1958–1963	VA hospitals	No association (except for bladder cancer), stage-adjusted
Young et al., 1984	Five-year, relative	Black/White	1973–1979	NCI—SEER	Positive

Note: Table is adapted from American Cancer Society Special Report on Cancer in the Economically Disadvantaged.
Rates are adjusted for sex and age.

Source: Data from *CA—A Cancer Journal for Physicians*, Vol. 39, No. 5, pp. 276–277, American Cancer Society, Inc., 1989.

Table 5-4 Consumption of Alcohol by Persons 18 Years of Age and Over, According to Selected Characteristics: United States, January 1975 (Data are Based on Household Interviews of a Sample of the Civilian Noninstitutionalized Population.)

				Drinking Level			
		Abstainers or Less Than 1 Drink per Year	Infrequent Drinkers (1–6 Drinks per Year)	Drinkers, Average Daily Consumption of Absolute Alcohol			
Characteristic	All Levels			0.100 oz. or less	0.101– 0.200 oz.	0.201– 0.500 oz.	0.501 oz. or more
			Percent Distribution				
Total	100	34	10	21	7	11	16
Sex							
Male	100	25	8	18	7	14	25
Female	100	43	11	25	6	8	7
Race							
White	100	33	10	22	7	11	16
Black	100	47	10	19	3	7	9
Family Income							
Less than $5,500	100	53	10	16	3	5	11
$5,000–$9,999	100	39	11	15	4	11	16
$10,000–$14,999	100	28	10	25	9	12	15
$15,000 or more	100	16	8	27	10	16	21
Marital Status							
Single	100	19	11	22	8	13	28
Married	100	33	9	22	8	11	15
Separated, divorced, or widowed	100	51	11	19	2	6	9
Education							
Less than high school graduate	100	50	9	16	3	6	13
High school graduate	100	27	10	23	8	13	18
Some college	100	22	13	26	8	12	18
College graduate	100	21	6	28	11	16	16

Source: U.S. Department of Health and Human Services, *Health United States, 1976–77,* Pub. No. (HRA) 77-1232, Table 41, p. 197. Calculated from tables in M. Rappeport, P. Labaw, and J. Williams, *The Public Evaluates the NIAAA Public Education Campaign, A Study for the U.S. Department of Health, Education, and Welfare,* Vols. I and II. Princeton. Opinion Research Corporation, July 1975.

two purposes. First, it may become the basis for experimental designs in epidemiological studies. Second, it provides a market segmentation that can be used for health education and health promotion programs. Alternatively, health promotion programs may use such information to target and market primary prevention activities.

Other Person-Related Attributes

There are several other personal attributes that should not be overlooked in epidemiological studies. Religious groups may have different rates of morbidity and mortality, for example, as studies have shown that Amish women have a lower rate of cervical cancer morbidity than do other groups[19] and many studies have shown lower morbidity and mortality rates among Mormons. Marital status also has been shown to have an impact on some causes of death; the age-adjusted mortality rate was found to be lower in both married men and married women than in single, widowed, or divorced groups.[20]

Studies on the birth order and the race of the mother have demonstrated considerable variation in neonatal, postneonatal, and infant mortality (Table 5-5). The higher the birth order, the higher the infant mortality rate. In addition, studies that have focused on the age of the mother and birth order have shown a direct relationship between these factors and infant mortality rates. Older women and high birth order produce high infant mortality rates.[21] It is quite apparent that first and second births have the lowest risk of infant deaths. Thus, birth order is a significant personal characteristic to be investigated in the descriptive phase of a community epidemiological study.

Where Does the Disease Occur?

The search for a geographical pattern of disease occurrence involves mapping disease patterns and making comparisons between geographical areas in tables, graphs, and charts. The objectives are to suggest possible relationships between location and disease for further study and to lay the basis for the planning of specific programs for attacking problem areas.

The most important step in analysis by place is choosing the proper scale. The level of analysis must be specific enough to determine geographical variations of the phenomenon being studied. A second aspect of the analysis relates to the particular disease being studied. If the disease has a very low incidence, however, it is often necessary to use a large scale of analysis and to plot the location of occurrences. Most community-specific analyses deal with diseases of relatively widespread incidence and prevalence. Consequently, the choice of scale depends on the basis of the need for data.

A classic example of an analysis of epidemiology by place is Snow's study of cholera in London in 1848–1854.[22] Snow mapped the exact location of the cholera deaths that occurred during a ten-day period in 1848 (Fig. 5-4). As a result of this visual analysis, Snow noted that the deaths were clustered around the Broad Street pump, from which residents received their water supply. After removal of the pump handle, no new cholera cases were reported.[23] This fact, together with

Table 5-5 Infant Mortality Rates by Birth Order and Race, Georgia, 1980–1984

| | Infant Mortality Rates* | | | | |
| | Neonatal | | Postneonatal | | Infant |
Birth Order	White	Black	White	Black	All Races
Single Births					
First birth	6.1	12.4	2.3	4.8	11.0
Second birth	5.4	11.8	2.8	6.1	11.2
Third birth	5.3	9.5	3.3	8.1	12.1
Fourth birth	7.7	10.3	4.1	7.5	14.8
Fifth birth	6.4	13.6	6.7	9.2	18.8
Sixth birth	9.0	16.3	3.0	6.8	19.3
Seventh or more	7.4	14.8	10.3	11.8	24.3
Multiple Births					
Twins or more	48.2	85.8	8.7	12.3	74.2
Total	6.9	13.8	2.9	6.6	13.6

*Rates per 1,000 live births.

Source: Reprinted from Vital Records, Georgia Infant Death Fact File, Department of Physical Health, Georgia Department of Human Resources, p. 154, 1988.

Snow's earlier work, suggested that cholera was transmitted by contaminated water. By determining the relationship between location and disease, Snow discovered the etiological factors of the disease.

Place-related studies make it possible to compare mortality and morbidity rates in different areas. Age-adjusted rates are compiled and then either plotted or mapped for the areas under consideration. In a study in Georgia, for example, investigators mapped several of the leading causes of death by county (Fig. 5-5).[24] Similar analyses may be done on enumeration districts or census tracts, depending on the purpose of the study. Probably one of the largest place-related studies of disease was conducted by the U.S. Environmental Protection Agency;[25] cancer rates were mapped by cause, by county, and, in some cases, by state economic area for the entire United States.

Urban and rural differences in disease patterns may also occur. As shown in Table 5-6, for example, rates for several chronic conditions vary according to metropolitan or nonmetropolitan residence. Nonmetropolitan areas have higher rates for the majority of conditions, although metropolitan areas have higher rates for some of the digestive conditions. Examination of cause-specific death rates showed that lung cancer deaths were higher in urban areas, whereas stomach cancer rates were higher in rural areas.[26]

Information about the geographic pattern of disease occurrence should be re-

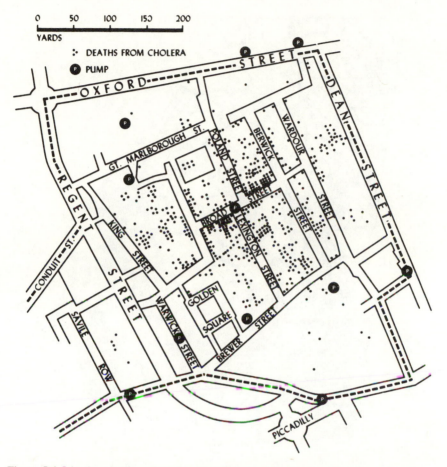

Figure 5-4 John Snow's Map of Cholera Deaths in the Soho District of London, 1848. *Source:* Adapted from *Health Care Delivery: Spatial Perspectives* by G. Shannon and G.E.A. Dever, p. 3, McGraw-Hill Book Company, 1974, and from *Some Aspects of Medical Geography* by L.D. Stamp, p. 16, Oxford University Press, 1964.

lated to differences in environment, socioeconomic status, and lifestyle. The analysis of disease patterns by place can then

- demonstrate high- and low-risk areas for specific diseases
- provide a "community diagnosis" for further investigation by health officials
- provide a basis for determining the health status of the population
- provide a reliable method of presenting data to concerned groups
- serve as an aid in establishing priorities for allocation of resources
- serve as an aid in developing policy for community health and social programs

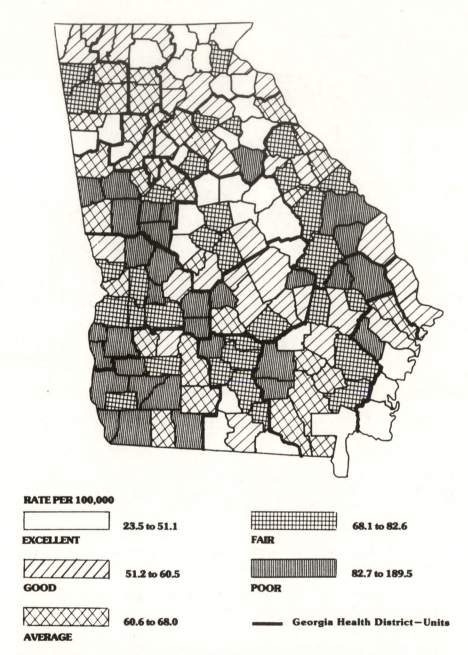

RATE PER 100,000

☐ 23.5 to 51.1	▦ 68.1 to 82.6
EXCELLENT	**FAIR**
▨ 51.2 to 60.5	▮ 82.7 to 189.5
GOOD	**POOR**
▩ 60.6 to 68.0	▬ **Georgia Health District—Units**
AVERAGE	

Figure 5-5 Cerebrovascular Disease, 1980–1984, Age-Sex Adjusted Death Rates Per 100,000. *Source:* Reprinted from *Disease Patterns of the 80's,* Division of Physical Health, Georgia Department of Human Resources, p. 110, 1987.

Table 5-6 Selected Reported Chronic Conditions for Metro and Nonmetro Areas, 1985

Type of Chronic Condition*	Number of Conditions per 1,000 Persons	
	Metro	Nonmetro
Selected Skin and Musculoskeletal Conditions		
Arthritis	119.7	158.1
Gout, including gouty arthritis	8.8	12.7
Intervertebral disc disorders	16.4	20.5
Bone spur or tendinitis, unspecified	8.9	9.0
Disorders of bone or cartilage	4.8	6.3
Trouble with bunions	11.1	11.7
Bursitis, unclassified	20.1	22.6
Sebaceous skin cyst	7.4	7.8
Trouble with acne	18.4	21.9
Psoriasis	8.3	8.2
Dermatitis	38.9	39.3
Trouble with dry (itching) skin, unclassified	16.6	19.4
Trouble with ingrown nails	20.8	31.3
Trouble with corns and calluses	21.7	23.2
Impairments		
Visual impairment	34.3	43.0
Color blindness	10.3	12.2
Cataracts	22.5	32.9
Glaucoma	7.9	8.8
Hearing impairment	86.0	106.4
Tinnitus	26.1	28.4
Speech impairment	9.3	12.5
Absence of extremities (excludes tips of fingers or toes only)	6.2	7.7
Paralysis of extremities, complete or partial	5.6	7.3
Deformity or orthopedic impairment	108.8	125.2
Back	61.0	66.2
Upper extremities	11.4	17.7
Lower extremities	45.7	54.0
Selected Digestive Conditions		
Ulcer	18.3	24.6
Hernia of abdominal cavity	18.2	28.1
Gastritis or duodenitis	11.9	15.8
Frequent indigestion	22.1	32.0
Enteritis or colitis	10.4	15.7
Spastic colon	6.7	6.5
Diverticula of intestines	8.5	8.3
Frequent constipation	15.3	19.2

*Chronic condition: a condition is considered chronic if the respondent indicates it was first noticed more than three months before the reference date of the interview or if it is a type of condition that ordinarily has a duration of more than three months.

continues

Table 5-6 continued

Source: In Health Services Research Special Issue: A Rural Health Service Research Agenda,by Norton, C.H., and McManus, M.A. Background Tables on Demographic Characteristics, Health Status, and Health Services Utilization. Vol. 23, No. 6. Feb. 1989, p. 739–740. Data from National Center for Health Statistics, *Vital and Health Statistics.* Current Estimates from the National Health Interview Survey, United States, 1985. Series 10, No. 160. Hyattsville, MD: NCHS, September 1986, Tables 61 and 66.

When Does the Disease Occur?

The relationship between diseases and units of time varies with the particular disease under study. Hours are significant when studying an outbreak of food poisoning; days may be significant when studying cases of respiratory illness in a boys' camp. Occupational exposure to hazardous substances may not be evident until years or even decades later. Indeed, many chronic diseases are characterized by long latency periods and an indefinite time of onset.

In examining diseases, particularly chronic diseases, over time, analysts commonly look at the changes in mortality rates. Two major kinds of changes may be observed: secular trends (i.e., changes that take place over a long period of time) and cyclical trends (i.e., recurring patterns of disease over periods of time).

Secular Trends

Figure 5-6 shows the trend of the leading causes of cancer mortality for males and females in the United States for the period 1930 to 1986. The age-adjusted death rates from cancer of the lung for males and females and cancer of the liver for males increased, while death rates from cancer of the stomach for both males and females and colon and rectum for females decreased.

In some cases, a secular trend reflects historical events. Adult per capita consumption of cigarettes in the United States, for example, increased from 1900–1950, leveled off between 1960 and 1965, and then decreased as a result of the first report of the Surgeon General on smoking (Fig. 5-7). When changes in a line graph can be accounted for in this way, the secular trend approach is highly recommended.

Some rates need to be seasonally adjusted. Figure 5-8 shows the seasonally adjusted fertility rate for 1985–1989. A moving average smooths out most random variations that occur within individual time periods; this effect can be seen in a comparison of the line of the moving average with the line showing the monthly data. In some instances, the kind of data desired may require the use of a moving average to portray secular trends accurately.

**AGE-ADJUSTED CANCER DEATH RATES* FOR
SELECTED SITES, FEMALES, UNITED STATES, 1930-1986**

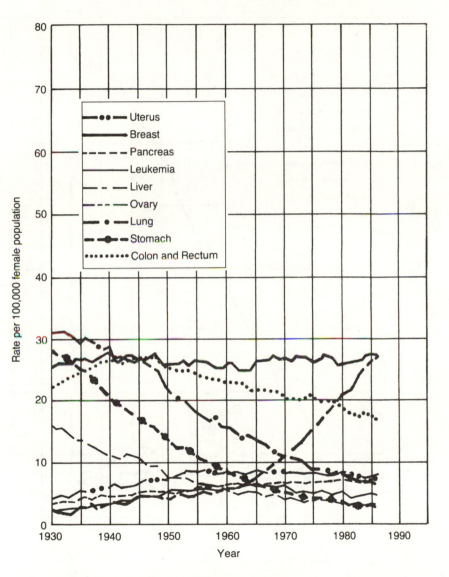

*Adjusted to the age distribution of the 1970 US Census Population.

Figure 5-6 Secular Trends in Cancer Mortality. *Source:* Reprinted from *CA—A Cancer Journal for Clinicians,* Vol. 40, No. 1, p. 16–17, with permission of American Cancer Society, Inc., © 1990. Data from U.S. National Center for Health Statistics and U.S. Bureau of the Census.

**AGE-ADJUSTED CANCER DEATH RATES* FOR
SELECTED SITES, MALES, UNITED STATES, 1930-1986**

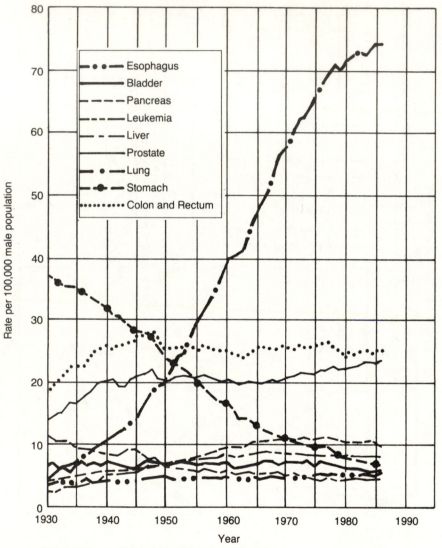

*Adjusted to the age distribution of the 1970 US Census Population.

Figure 5-6 continued

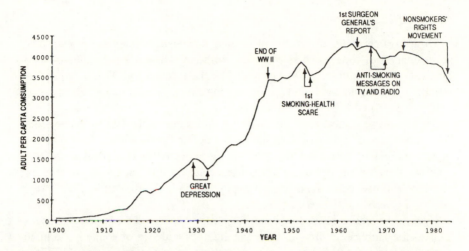

Figure 5-7 Adult Per Capita Consumption of Cigarettes in the United States, 1900–1985. *Source:* Kenneth E. Warner, *Selling Smoke* (Washington, D.C.: American Public Health Association, 1986), p. 22; *Prevention Report,* Jan 89, p. 5, Reported Per Capita Consumption by Year, U.S. 1900–1985.

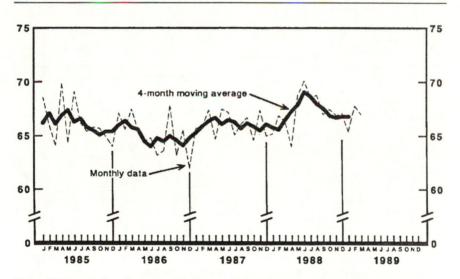

Figure 5-8 Seasonally Adjusted Fertility Rates per 1,000 Women Aged 15–44: United States, 1985–1989. *Source:* Reprinted from *Monthly Vital Statistics Report,* Vol. 38, No. 3, p. 2, U.S. DHHS, 1989.

Cyclical Trends

To determine cyclical patterns of disease occurrence, rates are plotted for a short interval of time, such as one year. Some of the best known depictions of cyclical trends are in the graphs provided by the Centers for Disease Control on monthly pneumonia and influenza deaths (Fig. 5-9). These graphs indicate when epidemic levels of a disease are reached.

An epidemic, a short-term fluctuation in a disease cycle, has been defined as "the occurrence of a disease in members of a defined population clearly in excess of the number of cases usually or normally expected in that population."[27] In contrast, the endemic occurrence of a disease has been defined as the regular and continuous presence of the disease in a population in a defined place and over a period of time.[28]

Cyclical trends in disease or death rates may be related to seasonal changes, such as the increase in drownings or the greater incidence of some of the infectious diseases transmitted by insects in summer. Such trends may be observed

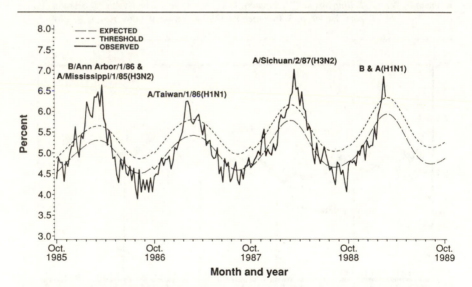

*Reported to CDC from 121 cities. P&I deaths include all deaths for which pneumonia is listed as a primary or underlying cause or for which influenza is listed on the death certificate. The predominant virus type is shown above the peak of mortality for each epidemic season. The epidemic threshold for each influenza season was estimated at 1.645 standard deviations above the values projected on the basis of a periodic regression model applied to observed P&I deaths for the previous 5-year period but excluding the observations during influenza outbreaks.

Figure 5-9 Cyclical Trends Illustrated by Pneumonia and Influenza (P&I) Deaths as a Percentage of Total Deaths* in the United States, October 1985–February 11, 1989. *Source:* Reprinted from *MMWR,* Vol. 30, No. 7, p. 115, U.S. DHHS, 1989.

over long periods of time (e.g., the two- to three-year cycle of influenza Type A epidemics or in the four- to six-year cycle of influenza Type B epidemics) or over short periods (e.g., the weekly cycle of motor vehicle deaths, which peak on weekends).

Epidemics, it should be emphasized, are not limited to infectious diseases. In fact, the major chronic diseases—heart disease, cancer, and stroke—are at epidemic levels, and the really universal epidemics are obesity, poor nutrition, inactivity, stress, poverty, illiteracy, and unemployment.

ORGANIZATION OF COMMUNITY HEALTH DATA

When organizing descriptive epidemiological data to present the characteristics of person, place, and time, health agencies must deal with voluminous amounts of data generated from many statistical systems. They must present such data effectively so that consumers, program directors, and decision makers can make informed judgments and decisions about program direction, support, planning, and evaluation. Using the various modes of data presentation (tables, graphs, and charts), an agency must provide a product that is an effective and efficient communication device.

Organizing data in graphic form has several advantages:

- Graphic forms make it easy for both the layperson and the statistician to read data.
- Graphics have popular appeal and convey information quickly. Readers often skip lengthy tables or texts; graphics are forceful and attractive as learning devices.
- Results shown in graphic form are remembered easily. Visual impressions are more revealing, convincing, and lasting than are those from sets of figures or words.
- Patterns and trends are easy to identify and interpret in graphic form.

Like any method or technique, however, organizing data in graphic form also has disadvantages:

- The use of graphic forms entails a loss of information and, thus, a loss of precision in the information presented.
- The input data for graphics must be carefully scaled geographically and statistically in order to avoid oversimplification.
- In hand-drawn graphics, errors and changes can be very costly, although the use of computer graphics is helping to eliminate this problem.

Moroney stated well the need for graphics in organizing community health data:

> Cold figures are uninspiring to most people. Diagrams help us to see the pattern and shape of any complex situation. Just as a map gives us a bird's-eye view of a wide stretch of country, so diagrams help us to visualize the whole meaning of a numerical complex at a single glance. Give me an undigested heap of figures and I cannot see the woods for the trees. Give me a diagram and I am positively encouraged to forget detail until I have a real grasp of the overall picture. Diagrams register a meaningful impression almost before we think.[29]

The selection of the method for organizing and presenting health data depends on several factors:

- the purpose of the presentation: oriented toward policy making, toward management, or toward the consumer
- the type of data summary required: by person, place, or time
- the type of data message involved: counts, frequencies, rates, ratios, proportions
- the type of presentation to be made: slides, transparencies, flip charts
- the individual who is to use the data: health planner, epidemiologist, or statistician

Tables

Quantitative data are usually organized in tabular form. In many instances, a table is all that is needed. Tables do have limitations, however; the basic limitation stems from the fact that the difficulty of determining patterns and trends in the data hinders interpretation.

Although there are no specific rules for the construction of tables, the following general standards are more or less accepted:

- Tables should be as simple and as self-explanatory as possible. Titles, rows, columns, and totals should be marked clearly and concisely; the units of data measurement should be provided; and codes, abbreviations, and symbols should be explained in footnotes.
- The title should indicate what (person or thing), when (time), and where (place).
- The source of reproduced data should be given in a footnote.

- The layout should be well spaced.
- To enhance clarity, not more than three variables should be displayed. Indeed, small tables are often preferred to a single large table.

Tables have several advantages. First, they can display numbers extremely well. Second, the numbers in a tabular design may be expressed in various ways (e.g., absolutes, rates, ratios, percentages, or correlation coefficients). Third, if absolute numbers are used, the data can be used for allocation of resources. Finally, graphs and charts can be prepared as natural outgrowths of tabular data.

Graphs

One of the oldest forms of graphic presentation, a graph is a method of organizing quantitative data by a coordinate system of x and y points. Examples of graphs are arithmetic, semilogarithmic, and logarithmic line graphs; histograms; and frequency polygons.

Line Graphs

A line graph not only shows maximum and minimum values, but also indicates directional change, thereby demonstrating trends. A line graph may permit analysts to project or predict rates and percentages by extrapolating the trend line. On a multiple line graph, changes in one quantity can be related to changes in another.

Data plotted on a line graph can reflect point or period information. Point data, which refer to a particular point in time, are seldom used in summarizing health data. Period data, however, refer to a period of time; such period data as annual mortality rates, average annual occupancy rates, and the annual percentage of the gross national product expended on health care are frequently used by health planners.

Guidelines for effective line graphs include the following:[30]

- The simplest graphs are the most effective. The number of lines and symbols in a single graph should be limited to those that the eye can easily follow.
- Every graph should be self-explanatory.
- The title may be placed at either the top or the bottom of the graph.
- When more then one variable is shown on a graph, each should be clearly differentiated by means of legends or keys.
- Coordinate lines should be lighter than the data lines of the graph itself.

- Usually, frequency is represented on the vertical scale; method of classification, on the horizontal scale.
- On an arithmetic scale, equal increments must represent equal numerical units.
- Scale divisions and their units should be indicated clearly.
- For comparative purposes, the zero point should be shown on the y axis.

Arithmetic Line Graphs. Although an arithmetic line graph is generally constructed on paper with equal intervals on the vertical (*y*) axis and the horizontal (*x*) axis, there are some situations in which intervals may be uneven. When a time period displayed on the horizontal axis is related to mortality rates on the vertical axis, for example, a scale break may be needed in the vertical axis to clarify the appropriate interpretation (Fig. 5-10). Such a scale break can be used only in an arithmetic line graph. On an arithmetic line graph, an arithmetic progression will yield a straight line.

Semilogarithmic and Logarithmic Line Graphs. While arithmetic line graphs illustrate absolute magnitudes, both semilogarithmic and logarithmic line graphs illustrate proportional rates of change and relationships between two or more variables with significant differences (Fig. 5-11). On a semilogarithmic line graph, logarithmic units are measured on the vertical axis, and arithmetic units are measured on the horizontal axis; on a logarithmic line graph, logarithmic values are measured on both the vertical and the horizontal axes. Logarithmic

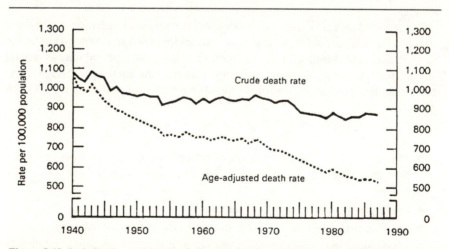

Figure 5-10 Scale Break on a Line Graph Illustrated by Crude and Age-Adjusted Death Rates in the United States, 1940–1987. *Source:* Reprinted from *Monthly Vital Statistics Report,* Vol. 38, No. 5, p. 2, U.S. DHHS, 1989.

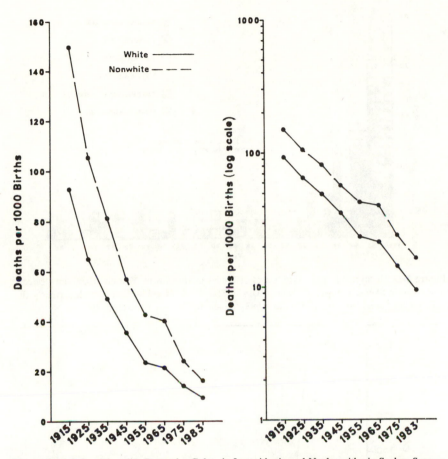

Figure 5-11 Infant Mortality Rates, by Color, in Logarithmic and Nonlogarithmic Scales. *Source:* A. Donabedian, et al. Medical Care Chartbook, 8th Edition, Health Administration Press, Ann Arbor, MI, 1986, p. 24. Data from National Center for Health Statistics. Vital statistics of the United States, 1979. Vol II-Mortality, Part A. Hyattsville, MD: NCHS, 1984; DHHS Publ. No. (PHS)84–1101: Section 2, p. 1; National Center for Health Statistics. Annual summary of births, deaths, marriages and divorces: United States, 1981. Hyattsville, MD: NCHS, 1984 Sept. 21: Table 7, p. 16. (Monthly vital statistics report: Vol 33; No. 7).

scales can have one or more cycles and do not have to start at zero. For instance, the scale can begin with 0.1, 1.0, 10.0, 100.0, or 1,000.0—with the larger number always ten times greater than the smaller number. A geometric progression is shown on a logarithmic line graph by a straight line; equal increases or decreases represent equal percentage changes, and equal slopes reflect equal rate of change.

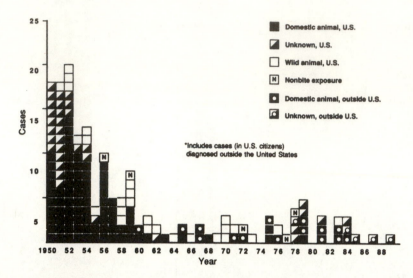

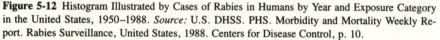

Figure 5-12 Histogram Illustrated by Cases of Rabies in Humans by Year and Exposure Category in the United States, 1950–1988. *Source:* U.S. DHSS. PHS. Morbidity and Mortality Weekly Report. Rabies Surveillance, United States, 1988. Centers for Disease Control, p. 10.

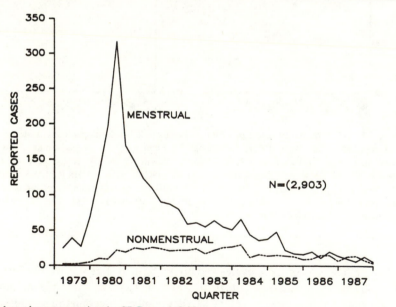

*Includes only cases meeting the CDC case definition.

Figure 5-13 Frequency Polygon Illustrated by Toxic-Shock Syndrome—By Quarter in the United States, 1979–1987*. *Source:* Reprinted from *MMWR*, Vol. 36, No. 54, p. 42, U.S. DHHS.

Histograms and Frequency Polygons

Both the histogram and the frequency polygon are special forms of graphics that are portrayed on two quantitative scales, a vertical and a horizontal. Data on a variable are usually converted into class intervals on the horizontal axis, and the frequency of the variable is plotted on the vertical axis. The vertical and horizontal axes should reflect interval or ratio measurements, such as the distribution of dentists by age groups.

A histogram is a graph of frequency distributions on arithmetic paper. Although it resembles a bar chart in appearance, a histogram shows frequencies on both axes (Fig. 5-12). Because the height of each column is compared, there should be no scale break in the histogram. A histogram must satisfy two conditions: (1) the width of each rectangle must represent the width of the corresponding group, and (2) the area of each rectangle must represent the frequency of the corresponding group. Thus, the area under the histogram (the sum of the area of all rectangles) represents the total frequency.

A frequency polygon is constructed from a histogram. Plotting class interval midpoints of the histogram reveals a trend line (Fig. 5-13). Because it permits a clearer, more concise comparison of two or more sets of data, the frequency polygon is preferred to the histogram.

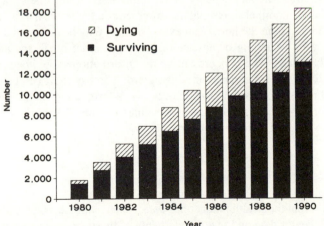

Estimated cumulative number of surviving and dying infants with spina bifida born since 1980, by outcome and year — United States, 1980–1990

Figure 5-14 Two-Dimensional Bar Chart. *Source:* Reprinted from *MMWR*, Vol. 38, No. 15, p. 265, U.S. DHHS, 1989.

Quality of Life and Youth Mortality, Ages 10–19, Georgia, 1978–1987

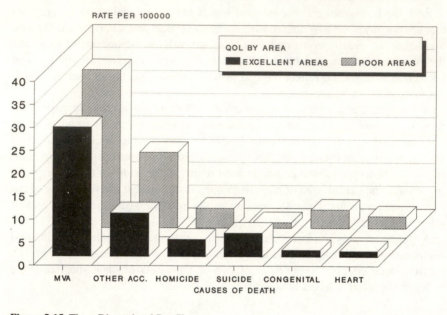

Figure 5-15 Three-Dimensional Bar Chart.

Charts

The bar chart is the most widely used of all charts. It is a one-scale chart that portrays data of nominal or ordinal measurement on the vertical axis. No quantitative scale is used on the horizontal axis. The bars may be arranged horizontally or vertically in ascending or descending order. A scale break should never be used on a bar chart. The bars presenting the information should be separated by spaces to avoid the appearance of a histogram. The bar chart can take the form of a two-dimensional bar chart (Figure 5-14), a three-dimensional multiple bar chart (Figure 5-15), or a component bar chart (Figure 5-16). Figure 5-17 is a special type of chart called a pie chart.

Selection of Organizational Method

Assuming that the health planner has constructed summary tables of important community health data and that the elements of these tables require illustration, Table 5-7 will help the planner to select the most appropriate graphic. Each question in the guide should be answered yes or no. The last column gives appropriate directions either to a follow-up question or to the suggested method.

Adolescent Mortality by Cause, Georgia, 1977–1986

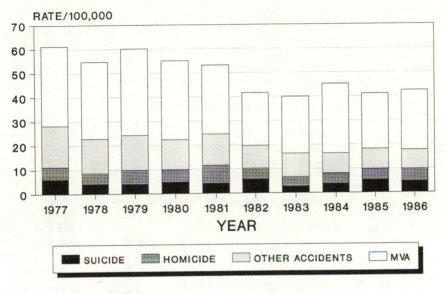

Figure 5-16 Component Bar Chart.

Percent of Total Deaths, Selected Causes, Georgia, 1980–84

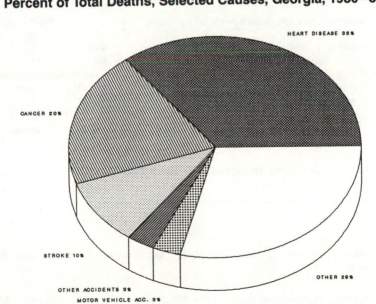

Figure 5-17 Pie chart.

Table 5-7 Guide for Selecting a Method To Illustrate Community Epidemiological Data

Question No.	Question	Answer	Go to Number Indicated or Use Method Shown
1	Data to be illustrated are either continuous or time series	Yes	5
2	If comparisons are to be made among magnitudes of:		
	a. Component parts of a total, then		Bar Chart
	b. Different categories of things, people, conditions, etc., then		Bar Chart
	c. Things, conditions, etc., in different places, then		3
3	Places to be compared are readily identifiable on a map	Yes	4
		No	Bar Chart
4	Specific site of occurrence is important	Yes	Dot Map
		No	Area Map
5	Data are time series	Yes	6
		No	7
6	Data are cases of disease in an outbreak	Yes	7
		No	9
7	Not more than two sets of data are to be compared (e.g., males and females, cases and deaths)	Yes	Histogram or Frequency Polygon
		No	8
8	More than two sets of data are to be compared		Frequency Polygon
9	Intent is to show *variation* in frequency of one or more items	Yes	10
		No	11
10	Range from minimum to maximum values to be illustrated does not exceed two orders of magnitude	Yes	Arithmetic Line Graph
		No	11
11	Either the intent is to show rates of change in one or more items, or the range of values to be illustrated exceeds two orders of magnitude		Semilogarithmic Line Graph

Source: Adapted from *Methods for Organizing Epidemiological Data,* pp. 33–36, CDC, U.S, DHHS, 1977.

NOTES

1. Judith S. Mausner and Anita K. Bahn, *Epidemiology: An Introductory Text* (Philadelphia: W.B. Saunders Co., 1974), 43.

2. Ibid.

3. Gary D. Friedman, *Primer of Epidemiology* (New York: McGraw-Hill Book Co., 1974), 52–53.

4. Abraham M. Lilienfeld, *Foundations of Epidemiology* (New York: Oxford University Press, 1976), 96.

5. Mausner and Bahn, *Epidemiology,* 47.

6. Ibid., 48–49.

7. Alfred M. Haynes, "Minorities and Health Statistics," *Urban Health* (June 1975): 14.

8. Department of Health and Human Services, Public Health Service, *Health, United States, 1988,* Pub. no. (PHS) 89-1232 (Washington, D.C., March 1989), 66–75.

9. Ibid.

10. Health Services Research and Statistics, Division of Physical Health, *Socioeconomic Analysis of the Disease Patterns of the '70s* (Atlanta: Georgia Department of Human Resources, August 1977), 51.

11. I.J. Selikoff et al., "Asbestos Exposure, Smoking, and Neoplasia," *Journal of the American Medical Association* 204 (1968).

12. V.M. Trasko, "Silicosis, A Continuing Problem," *Public Health Reports* 73 (1958).

13. S. Cobb and R.M. Rose, "Hypertension, Peptic Ulcer, and Diabetes in Air Traffic Controllers," *Journal of the American Medical Association* 224 (1973).

14. H.P. Freeman, "Cancer in the Socioeconomically Disadvantaged," CA: *Cancer Journal for Clinicians* 39, (September/October 1989): 280.

15. Ibid., 285.

16. Ibid., 281–282.

17. Department of Health and Human Services, Public Health Service, *Health, United States, 1987,* Pub. no. (PHS) 88-1232 (Washington, D.C., March 1988), 91–95.

18. Department of Health and Human Services, *Health, United States, 1988,* 92–99.

19. H.E. Cross, E.F. Kennel, and A.M. Lilienfeld, "Cancer of the Cervix in the Amish Population," *Cancer* 21 (1968).

20. John P. Fox, Carrie E. Hall, and Lila R. Elveback, *Epidemiology: Man and Disease* (London: Collier MacMillan, 1970), 202.

21. *Missouri Monthly Vital Statistics* (Columbia, Mo.: Center for Health Statistics, Division of Health, 1975), 3.

22. Gary Shannon and G.E. Alan Dever, *Health Care Delivery: Spatial Perspectives* (New York: McGraw-Hill Book Co., 1974), 141.

23. L.D. Stamp, *Some Aspects of Medical Geography* (New York: Oxford University Press, 1964), 103.

24. Georgia DHR, DPH. Center for Health Statistics. *Georgia: Disease Patterns of the 80's with Epidemiological Profiles* (January 1987), 217.

25. W.B. Riggan et al., *U.S. Cancer Mortality Rates and Trends, 1950–1979,* vol. 4 (Washington, D.C.: U.S. Environmental Protection Agency, September 1987), 363.

26. Ibid., 154, 62.

27. Friedman, *Primer of Epidemiology,* 67.

28. Fox, Hall, and Elveback, *Epidemiology,* 240.

29. M.J. Moroney, *Facts from Figures* (Baltimore: Penguin Books, 1963), 20.

30. U.S. Department of Health, Education, and Welfare, Public Health Service, *Methods for Organizing Epidemiological Data* (Atlanta: Centers for Disease Control, February 1977), 9.

REFERENCES

Axtell, I.M., M.H. Myers, and E.M. Shambaugh. 1975. *Treatment and survival patterns for black and white cancer patients diagnosed 1955 through 1964.* DHEW Pub. No. (NIH) 75-712, 1–41. Washington, D.C.: U.S. Department of Health, Education and Welfare.

Axtell, I.M., and M.H. Myers. 1978. Contrasts in survival of black and white cancer patients, 1960–1975. *J. Natl. Cancer Inst.* 60:1209–14.

Berg, J.W., R. Ross, and L.B. Latourette. 1977. Economic status and survival of cancer patients. *Cancer* 39:467–77.

Haenszel, W., and L. Chiazze, Jr. 1965. Survival experience of cancer patients enumerated in morbidity surveys. *J. Natl. Cancer Inst.* 34:85–101.

Linden, G. 1969. The influence of social class in the survival of cancer patients. *J. Natl. Cancer Inst.* 59:267–74.

Lipworth, L., B. Bennett, and P. Parker. 1972. Prognosis of nonprivate cancer patients. *J. Natl. Cancer Inst.* 48:11–16.

Page, W.F., and A.J. Kuntz. 1980. Racial and socioeconomic factors in cancer survival: A comparison of Veterans Administration results with selected studies. *Cancer* 45:1029–40.

Young, J.L. Jr., L.G. Ries, and E.S. Pollack. 1984. Cancer patient survival among ethnic groups in the United States. *J. Natl. Cancer Inst.* 73:341–52.

Chapter 6

Basic Demographics: Methods and Issues

Demography, the study of human populations, is a scientific discipline closely related to epidemiology. It is the study of the size, composition, distribution, density, growth, and other characteristics of the population, as well as of the causes and consequences of changes in those factors.[1] Demographic data are almost always prerequisites for basic community health analysis, since demographic trends directly influence health and disease patterns. Accompanying any demographic trend is a public and health policy implication reflective of a healthy public policy. Thus, a basic understanding of demographic principles and techniques is required for community health analysis.

TOOLS OF DEMOGRAPHIC MEASUREMENT

Demographic analysis focuses on population statics and dynamics.[2] Population statics describe the size, geographical distribution, and composition of a population at a fixed point in time. Population dynamics covers population change and components of change. The principal tools of demographic measurement are crude counts, rates, ratios, proportions, cohort measures, and point and period measures.

Population Statics

Studying the geographical distribution of the population is similar to determining the place component of health and disease patterns. The person characteristics used by demographers to describe the population composition are age, sex, race, marital status, and socioeconomic status.

Age and Sex Composition

A population's age and sex composition at any point in time is dependent on the dynamics or changes that took place earlier through births, deaths, and migration. Because both age and sex influence disease patterns and utilization of health services, the analysis of the age-sex composition of the population of interest is a fundamental prerequisite of health planning and management.

Median Age. The age at which half the population is older and half is younger—the median age—is an indicator of the age composition of a population. The median age of the U.S. population in 1987 was 32.1 years. In contrast, the median age in Syria was 15 in 1975, and that in the German Democratic Republic was reported to be 37 in 1980.[3]

Age-Dependency Ratio. The ratio of persons in the "dependent" ages (under 15 and over 64) to those in the economically productive ages (15–64) is the age-dependency ratio. It is usually expressed as the number of persons in the dependent ages for every 100 persons in the productive ages:

$$\text{Age-dependency ratio} = \frac{\text{Population under 15} + \text{Population over 64}}{\text{Population aged 15–64}} \times 100$$

The age-dependency ratio indicates (with questionable validity) the economic burden that the productive portion of a population must carry; the higher the ratio, the heavier the burden. The U.S. age-dependency ratio projected for 1990 is 51.6:100, meaning that there are likely to be 51.6 persons in the dependent ages for every 100 persons in the working ages. Less developed areas with rapidly growing populations usually have a greater burden of dependency. For example, in 1980, the ratio in Turkey was 78:100; in 1976, the ratio in Syria was 114:100.[4,5] The dependency burden has been suggested as one factor that affects health, social patterns, consumption, and labor force quality.[6]

The age-dependency ratio can be subdivided into old age dependency (the ratio of those over 64 to those 15–64) and child dependency (the ratio of those under 15 to those 15–64). This is portrayed graphically in Figure 6-1 for Kenya and Switzerland.

Sex Ratio. The sex composition of a given population is usually expressed as the number of males per 100 females. The sex ratio at birth in any population is approximately 106 males per 100 females. Because of different mortality and migration patterns, however, this ratio subsequently varies among places and age groups. The ratio can be particularly useful in analyzing small areas, as the variations in sex distribution may be more significant in these areas.

Population Pyramids. The best way to illustrate age and sex composition graphically is the population pyramid, which shows the numbers or proportions

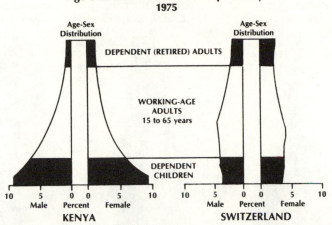

Figure 6-1 Age-Dependency Ratios in Kenya and Switzerland. *Source:* Reprinted from Population Crisis Committee, Population Growth and Economic Development, Population No. 14, Feb. 1985, p. 5, with permission of Population Crisis Committee, © 1985. Data from RAPID II, The Futures Group.

of males and females in each age group and is a vivid picture of a population's composition. The age-sex composition of a population tends to fall into one of three general profiles (Figure 6-2).[7] Expansive populations have larger numbers of people in the younger age groups, with each age cohort larger than the one born before it. Constrictive populations have smaller numbers of people in the younger age groups. Stationary populations have roughly equal numbers in almost all age groups, until the numbers gradually decrease at the older levels.

Because the most important influence on the shape of the population pyramid is the fertility rate (Fig. 6-3), the age-sex population pyramid also reveals the changing nature of population growth. The larger the number of children for each parent, the broader the base of the pyramid (and the younger the median age). Mortality has a somewhat less simple effect on the age distribution. Contrary to what might be assumed, lower mortality rates actually produce a slightly younger age distribution, as differences in mortality rates among populations are much more likely to result from variances in the mortality rates for younger age groups (mostly infants and children).[8]

Pyramids provide a demographic window for a community, giving health analysts a general sense of the social and economic structure of an area. Figure 6-4 shows ten different age-sex pyramids, each representing a different demographic and socioeconomic situation. The Liberty County pyramid is typical of a military base (predominantly young male); Clarke County has a college town (large num-

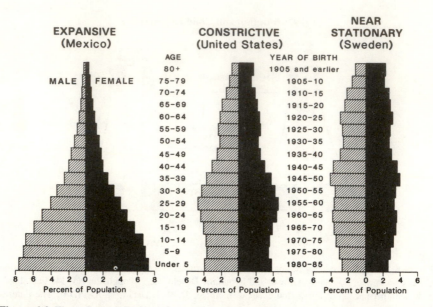

Figure 6-2 Three General Profiles of Age Composition, Based on 1985 Estimates. *Source:* Reprinted from *Population Handbook, International Edition* by A. Haupt and T. Kane, p. 24, with permission of Population Reference Bureau, © 1980.

bers in the 20–24 age group); Stewart County is a very poor county, with the old and young remaining while those in the economically productive ages have left; Gwinnett County and Columbia County look full and fat, representing young, socioeconomically advanced, suburban counties that are growing very fast; and Fannin County is an older county where many retirees are making their home. Clearly, the age-sex pyramid is a very useful tool for determining an area's age-sex and socioeconomic character and for comparing the area to others.

Other Variables To Describe Population Composition

Other demographic variables commonly used to describe the composition of a population include race, socioeconomic status, marital history, and other family-related characteristics. Just as sex ratios are expressed as the number of males per 100 females, race ratios are usually expressed as the number of whites per 100 blacks. Income, occupation, and education data indicate socioeconomic status; these variables can be used individually or combined into a socioeconomic index. Marital history refers to the number of times a person has married, when each marriage occurred, and when and how each previous marriage ended. Age at first marriage can be a good demographic and social indicator. The mean (av-

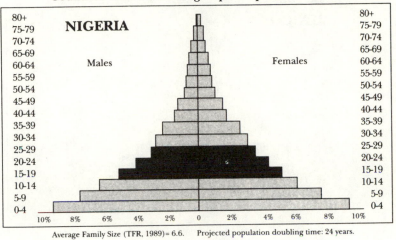

**Characteristic Age Structure for
Countries With Continuing Rapid Population Growth**

Average Family Size (TFR, 1989)= 6.6.   Projected population doubling time: 24 years.

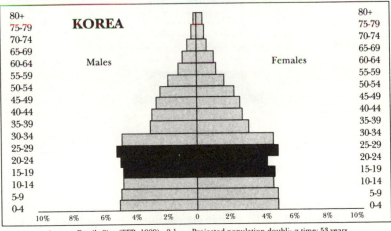

**Characteristic Age Structure for
Countries with Dramatic Fertility Declines Beginning in the 1960s**

Average Family Size (TFR, 1989)= 2.1.   Projected population doubling time: 53 years.

Figure 6-3 Age Structures in Relation to Fertility Rates. *Source:* Reprinted from *Population Pressures Abroad and Immigration Pressures at Home,* p. 17, with permission of Population Crisis Committee, © 1989. Data from United Nations, *Demographic Indicators of Countries.*

Characteristic Age Structure for
Countries with Modest and Recent Fertility Decline

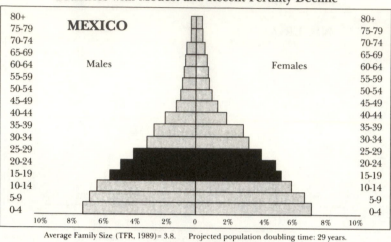

Average Family Size (TFR, 1989) = 3.8.   Projected population doubling time: 29 years.

Characteristic Age Structure for
Countries with Dramatic Fertility Declines Beginning in the 1940s

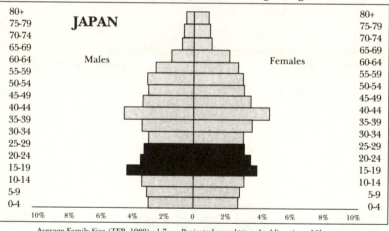

Average Family Size (TFR, 1989) = 1.7.   Projected population doubling time: 141 years.

Figure 6-3 continued

---

erage) size of household[9] and the mean size of family,[10] as well as the number of children of dependent ages, are also used as demographic indicators.

Population Distribution

The patterns of settlement and dispersal of population within a county or other area indicate the distribution of the population.[11] The main descriptive concepts

AGE-SEX PYRAMIDS FOR SELECT COUNTIES, GEORGIA, 1980

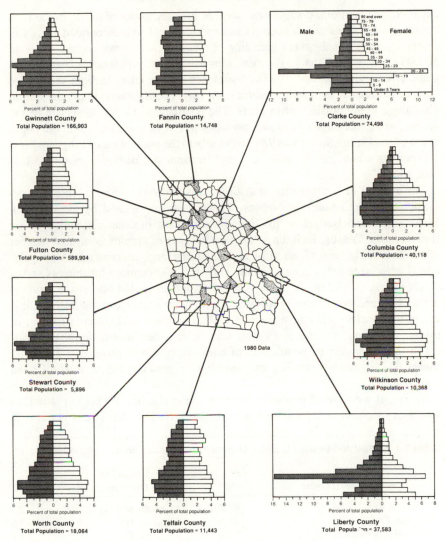

Figure 6-4 Age-Sex Pyramids for Select Counties in Georgia, 1980. *Source:* Reprinted from *The Atlas of Georgia,* by T.W. Hodler and H.A. Schretter, p. 205, with permission of Institute of Community and Area Development, The University of Georgia at Athens, © 1986.

are urban versus rural, metropolitan status, population density, and population size.

There is surprisingly little agreement on the definition of the term *urban.* Different authors offer different definitions based on any one or combination of the following criteria: population size, density, concentration, structure, types of occupation, sociocultural distinctions, ways of life, and states of mind. In the U.S. census, urban areas are defined as incorporated and unincorporated places of 2,500 or more inhabitants, including the contiguous areas around cities of 50,000 or more. In Canada, the minimum size is 1,000 inhabitants, with a population density of at least 1,000 persons per square mile. In both the United States and Canada, as in most countries, the rural population is simply the residuals—those living outside urban areas. The population in urban areas can be expressed as a percentage of the total population. For example, in 1989, the population of the United States was 74 percent urban; the population of Singapore was 100 percent urban, and the populations of Burundi and Bhutan were only 5 percent urban.[12]

The concept of metropolitan statistical areas (MSAs) is used often in the description of population distributions. These areas are defined by the Office of Management and Budget on the basis of a long list of criteria supplied by the Bureau of the Census, including size, density, type of employment, and number of commuters. In general, an MSA is defined as a large concentration of population (i.e., a large urban area), usually with 100,000 or more inhabitants and at least one city of 50,000 or more. Administrative areas that border the city and are socially and economically integrated with it are included in the MSA.[13] It is useful to calculate whether a particular MSA or other local area is gaining or losing population, because this simple statistic provides information that is critical to the expansion or contraction of community health programs. Table 6-1 shows the ten fastest growing and ten slowest growing MSAs in the United States.

The usual measure of population density is the number of people per unit of land area (population per square mile or kilometer). This measure is not always

Table 6-1 Fastest and Slowest Growing Metropolitan Statistical Areas: 1980–1986

10 MSAs with Greatest Gains	%	10 MSAs with Greatest Losses	%
1 Naples, FL	41.2	1 Duluth, MN-WI	−8.7
2 Ocala, FL	39.6	2 Elmira, NY	−7.3
3 Fort Myers-Cape Coral, FL	36.0	3 Peoria, IL	−7.0
3 Fort Pierce, FL	36.0	4 Waterloo-Cedar Falls, IA	−6.9
5 Amarillo, TX	35.3	5 Muncie, IN	−6.0
6 Anchorage, AK	34.7	6 Beaver County, PA	−5.5
6 Midland, TX	34.7	6 Parkersburg-	
8 Melbourne-Titusville-Palm Bay, FL	32.3	Marietta, WV-OH	−5.5
9 West Palm Beach-Boca Raton-	31.0	8 Wheeling, WV-OH	−5.4
Del Ray Beach, FL		9 Cumberland, MD-WV	−5.2
10 McAllen-Edinburg-Mission, TX	29.1	10 Buffalo, NY	−5.0

Source: Reprinted from *Interchange: Where is Metropolitan U.S.?*, Vol. 16, No. 4, with permission of Population Reference Bureau, Inc., © 1987.

satisfactory, however, because it is based on the assumption that the population is dispersed evenly over the entire area considered.[14] In places where the inhabitants are concentrated in a small portion of an area, the population density is very low, even though the people live in high-density areas. Consequently, other measures of population density have been used, such as the percentage of the population in multifamily dwellings and the population per square mile for urban areas only.[15]

The main advantage of using the crude size of the population in analyzing distributions is that a classification by multiple size categories can be established instead of the dichotomous urban-rural or MSA–non-MSA classifications. Population distribution, therefore, can be examined on a continuum of urbanization.

Interaction among Variables

Some demographic variables may interact with each other in such a way that a composite analysis yields results that are different from those obtained in a study of the components alone.[16] In other words, the relationship between one demographic variable and health, disease, or utilization may depend in part on another demographic variable. For example, an analysis of the utilization of health services may show no difference among age or income groups. A composite analysis by age and income may show that utilization is higher among both older age–lower income groups and younger age–higher income groups. This finding would indicate that utilization is related not to age and income separately, but to the composite age-income variable. Data to perform such a composite analysis are not always available, but, when possible, it is always wise to check for interaction among variables.

Population Dynamics

In addition to the description of population composition (i.e., population statics), demography is concerned with the changes in the composition of a population over time (i.e., population dynamics). Population change involves three components: births, deaths (see Chapter 4), and migration.

Natality

The term *natality* refers to the role of births in population change. Although some authors use the term *fertility* in this same broad sense, most restrict their use of this term to actual birth performance,[17] that is, to the number and tempo of births that actually occur in a population.[18]

Although this was not always the case, measures of natality, fertility, and births have come to refer only to live births. Stillbirths, fetal deaths, and abortions are not included in these statistics.

Crude Birth Rate. The most common measure of natality is the crude birth rate (CBR). It is simply the number of births in a year per 1,000 midyear population (the population as of July 1):

$$CBR = \frac{\text{Number of births}}{\text{Total midyear population}} \times 1,000$$

The crude birth rate is a valid measure of the number of babies a population is producing in a given year. It is not very useful for temporal or spatial comparisons, however, because it does not eliminate the impact of differential population structures.[19] In other words, it does not reveal much about the reproductive experience or about the intensity or tempo of births, because it does not account for the age-sex composition of the population.

General Fertility Rate. Because it relates the number of births to the population at risk of giving birth, that is, the female population aged 15–44, the general fertility rate (GFR) is a more refined measure than the crude birth rate.[20] The general fertility rate is defined as the number of live births per 1,000 women aged 15–44:

$$GFR = \frac{\text{Total births}}{\text{Females aged 15–44}} \times 1,000$$

The total number of births, regardless of the age of the mother, is used in the numerator.[21] Unlike the crude birth rate, the general fertility rate can be used for comparison purposes, as it takes into account the age and sex composition of the population involved.

The current situation in the United States illustrates the difference between these two rates. Although the crude birth rate has been increasing in recent years, the general fertility rate has remained constant. There are more babies born—not because women are having more babies, however, but because more women are having babies; the women who were born during the Baby Boom after World War II are now in their reproductive years.

Age-Specific Fertility Rate. Health analysts use age-specific fertility rates for the comparison of different populations over time and for the detection of differences in fertility behavior at different ages. An age-specific fertility rate (ASFR) is defined as the number of live births to women in an age group in one year per 1,000 women in that age group (at midyear):[22]

$$ASFR\ (15\text{--}19) = \frac{\text{Live births to women aged 15--19 in the year}}{\text{Midyear population of women aged 15--19}}$$

Calculation of the age-specific rates for every five-year age group between 15 and 49 gives a complete picture of the fertility differences, which can be valuable for planning purposes.

A standardized fertility rate can be calculated by means of the same methods (direct or indirect adjustment) used to standardize mortality rates (see Chapter 4). It indicates how many births per 1,000 women there would be in the population of interest if its age and sex composition was the same as that of a standard (arbitrarily chosen) population. Fertility rates can also be adjusted (standardized) for other demographic variables, such as marital status, race, urban-rural residence, and duration of marriage.

Some authors refer to specific and standardized fertility rates as specific and standardized birth rates.[23,24] The use of the term *fertility* seems more appropriate, however, since the denominators are always limited to the female population at risk of childbearing while the denominator of the crude birth rate is the total population. Furthermore, the general fertility rate is in fact a weighted average of these age-specific rates.

Total Fertility Rate. A hypothetical measure (a synthetic estimate) of the average number of children that would be born alive to a woman during her lifetime if she were to pass through all her childbearing years conforming to the age-specific fertility rates of a given year is the total fertility rate (TFR).[25] This measure is one of the most important fertility measures, because it indicates as nearly as possible how many children women are having. Unlike the general fertility rate, the total fertility rate is adjusted for the age and sex composition of the population. It is actually a summary measure of the age-specific fertility rates over all ages of the childbearing period:

$$TFR = \frac{5\left(\sum\limits_{a=15\text{--}19}^{a=45\text{--}49} fa\right)}{1,000}$$

where fa = An age-specific fertility rate per 1,000

In the formula, 5 is used because each group encompasses five years. Thus, the total fertility rate is calculated as follows:

Age group	Age-specific fertility rate per 1,000 women
15–19	17.3
20–24	95.8
25–29	143.9
30–34	74.3
35–39	20.8
40–44	3.0
45–49	0.2
	$\Sigma fa = 355.3$

$$TFR = \frac{5 \times \Sigma fa}{1,000}$$

$$TFR = \frac{5 \times 355.3}{1,000} \times 1.777$$

where TFR = Total fertility rate
Σ = Summation
fa = Age-specific fertility
Σfa = Sum of all age-specific fertility rates

A total fertility rate of 1.78 means that, if the age-specific fertility rates were to continue, women on the average would have 1.78 children during their child-bearing years.

The total fertility rate is extremely useful in a comparison of the fertility rates in two or more areas. For example, in 1973, the general fertility rate was 60.9 per 1,000 women in the United States and 60.1 in Canada.[26] Age-specific fertility rates show that fertility is really higher in the United States only at ages under 25, whereas in Canada it is higher for all age groups over 25. Furthermore, the total fertility rates, which take into account the age and sex composition of the population, are essentially identical (1.896 in the United States and 1.890 in Canada). Thus, it can be concluded that, in 1973, women in the United States had their children at earlier ages than did women in Canada; over their lifetime, however, women in both countries have the same number. The difference in the general fertility rate was caused by the fertility calendar, not by real differences in total fertility.

The gap between the total fertility rate of the developed nations and that of the developing nations narrowed since 1950 (Table 6-2). The rate is lowest in western Europe and highest in sub-Saharan Africa. These variations are indicative of the disease cycles (i.e., infectious, chronic, or social transformation). This information is most important to a community health analyst or administrator who is thinking of providing new programs, expanding old programs, or intensifying

Table 6-2 Total Fertility Rate per Woman

	1950	1960	1970	1980	1985
World	4.9	4.9	4.4	3.6	3.4
Developed	2.8	2.7	2.2	2.0	2.0
Developing	5.9	5.9	5.3	4.1	3.8
North America	3.5	3.4	2.0	2.0	2.0
Latin America	5.9	6.0	5.1	4.2	3.9
Western Europe	2.5	2.7	2.1	1.8	1.8
Eastern Europe and USSR	2.9	2.5	2.4	2.3	2.3
Middle East	6.6	6.6	6.2	5.6	5.1
South Asia	6.4	6.4	5.8	4.8	4.2
Far East	5.5	5.2	4.5	2.9	2.6
Oceania	3.7	3.8	3.0	2.6	2.5
Africa	6.4	6.5	6.4	6.3	6.1
Sub-Saharan	6.4	6.5	6.6	6.6	6.6
Other Africa	6.3	6.3	5.8	5.5	5.7

Source: Adapted from *Women: A World Survey* by R.L. Sivard, p. 38, with permission of World Priorities, © 1985.

efforts to develop community capacity. The demographic trend becomes critical to the needs for and success of such endeavors.

Together with the age-specific fertility rates, the total fertility rates remain the most useful fertility measures for community health analysts. Like mortality rates (see Chapter 4) these rates can be made specific for any population subgroups (Table 6-3). Additionally, variations in fertility rates are strongly associated with economic progress. Low fertility is generally related to strong economic progress. (The United States and Canada are good examples.) Countries now experiencing fertility rate declines generally have a strong economy. A moderate to high fertility rate—an average family size of four to five children— suggests the potential strength of a developing economy or a fair economy. A high fertility rate generally reflects an extremely poor economic outlook. The average family size is six or more children, which remains stable; high infant mortality rates are common. This pattern frequently occurs in Third World countries or developing countries.

Migration

The geographical or spatial movement of population in changing a usual residence from one clearly defined geographical unit to another is migration.[27] Demographers usually distinguish between international and internal migration. International migration refers to moves between countries and is designated as emigration from the nation left and as immigration to the receiving nation.[28] Internal migration refers to movements between different areas within a country.

Table 6-3 General Fertility Rates and Total Fertility Rates, U.S., 1980: Selected Characteristics

Characteristics	General Fertility Rate per 1,000 Women	Total Fertility Rate per 1,000 Women
Total, 18–44 years old	71.1	2.059
Age		
18–24 years old	96.6	2.023
25–29 years old	114.8	2.022
30–34 years old	60.0	2.150
Race		
White	68.5	2.036
Black	84.0	2.227
Spanish origin*	106.6	2.363
Marital Status		
Currently married†	95.0	2.187
Widowed, divorced, and separated	27.5	2.035
Single	28.4	1.807
Years of School Completed		
Not a high-school graduate	91.9	2.427
High school, 4 years	71.5	2.018
College, 1 to 3 years	58.4	2.018
College, 4 years	65.9	1.857
College, 5 or more years	52.1	1.765
Labor Force Status		
In labor force	40.9	1.901
Employed	37.4	1.882
Unemployed	75.0	2.053
Not in labor force	130.1	2.370
Family Income		
Under $5,000	94.3	2.190
$5,000–$9,999	86.8	2.071
$10,000–$14,999	83.9	2.099
$15,000–$19,999	77.1	2.048
$20,000–$24,999	69.8	2.015
$25,000 and over	48.5	2.014
Region of Residence		
Northeast	62.4	2.061
North Central	70.8	2.122
South	71.7	1.984
West	80.2	2.098

*Persons of Spanish origin may be of any race.
†Except separated women.

Source: Adapted from *American Demographics,* Vol. 4, No. 1, p. 27, with permission of American Demographics, Inc., © 1982.

The terms *in-migration* and *out-migration* may be used instead of immigration and emigration, respectively. In the United States and Canada, interstate (inter-provincial) migration and intrastate (intraprovincial) migration may also be dealt with separately.

The immigration (or in-migration) rate is the number of immigrants (in-migrants) arriving at a destination per 1,000 population at that destination in a given year:[29]

$$\text{Immigration rate} = \frac{\text{Number of immigrants in a year}}{\text{Total midyear population at destination}} \times 1{,}000$$

Similarly, the emigration (out-migration) rate is the number of emigrants who depart an area of origin per 1,000 population at that area of origin in a given year:

$$\text{Emigration rate} = \frac{\text{Number of emigrants in a year}}{\text{Total midyear population at area of origin}} \times 1{,}000$$

Immigration and emigration are more precisely referred to as gross immigration and gross emigration, as the balance of the two for a given area during a given time (usually a year) is called net immigration or net emigration, depending on which is larger.[30] The net migration rate shows the net effect of immigration and emigration on an area's population, expressed as an increase ($+$) or a decrease ($-$) per 1,000 population of the area in a given year:[31]

$$\text{Net migration rate} = \frac{\text{Number of immigrants} - \text{Number of emigrants}}{\text{Total midyear population}} \times 1{,}000$$

For example, in 1976, the United States had a net migration rate of $+1.7$ per 1,000 population—a net increase of 1.7 persons per 1,000 population.

Temporary Migration

It is a relatively easy task to count individuals and project population counts for people who are permanently settled or who migrate for new opportunities. It is a more difficult task to estimate temporary populations—those who spend only a month, six months, or a few days in an area. For instance, the number of migrant workers, farm and seasonal workers, and the homeless is sizable, and they need housing, health care, transportation, education, protection and most other goods and services. Therefore, it is essential in many areas to attempt to count these temporary migrants. Smith suggested two ways to estimate a temporary population: directly, by using census statistics and surveys, and indirectly, by contacting local agencies and programs for changes in utilization.[32] The number of poorer temporary residents may be estimated by contacting migrant camps, homeless shelters, motels, trailer parks, and campgrounds; the number of wealthier temporary residents, by examining the number of electric/water customers, enrollment in adult education, and traffic counts. The task of making these counts is complex, but it is necessary if appropriate services are to be in appropriate places at appropriate times.

Measures of Population Change

The relationship among the three components of population change—births, deaths, and migration—and population change over time can be expressed by the balancing equation:[33]

$$P_2 = P_1 + (B - D) + (I - E)$$

where P_2 = Population at the later date

P_1 = Population at the earlier date

B = Births

D = Deaths between the two dates

I = Immigration or in-migration

E = Emigration or out-migration between the two dates

The difference between the number of births and the number of deaths is the natural increase (NI). The rate of natural increase is the rate at which a population is increasing (or decreasing) in a given year because of a surplus (or deficit) of births over (or under) deaths, expressed as a percentage of the base population:[34]

$$\text{Rate of natural increase} = \frac{\text{Births} - \text{Deaths}}{\text{Total midyear population}} \times 100$$

or

$$\text{Rate of natural increase} = \frac{\text{Birth rate} - \text{Death rate}}{10}$$

The rate of natural increase in the United States in 1989 was 0.7 percent.[35]

The growth rate is the rate at which a population is increasing (or decreasing) in a given year because of a natural increase and net migration, expressed as a percentage of the base population:

$$\text{Growth rate} = \frac{(B - D) + (I - E)}{\text{Total midyear population}} \times 100$$

or

$$\text{Growth rate} = \text{Rate of natural increase} + \text{Net migration rate}$$

The growth rate, which takes into account all the components of population change (i.e., births, deaths, and migration), should not be confused with the rate of natural increase, which involves only births and deaths, nor with the birth rate, which involves only births.

Another common way of measuring population change is to calculate the intercensus change (*IC*), which is simply the difference between the population indicated in a previous census (P_1) and a subsequent census (P_2) of the same area:

$$IC = P_2 - P_1$$

The intercensus change in percentage (*IC%*) can be used to compare the growth of different populations:

$$IC\% = \frac{P_2 - P_1}{P_1} \times 100$$

These rates related to population dynamics are important to community health analysts. The increased need for services, the marketing of new ones, expansion into a new location, and the demand for care in institutions are dependent on the changing nature of population characteristics. Further, the application of these concepts to preventive medicine in a changing population structure requires a knowledge of the lifestyles and environment of the existing structure. The use of the techniques that have been discussed should enhance the development of a healthy public policy for migrating populations.

POPULATION ESTIMATES

In most countries, the most reliable and complete source of information on population composition is the national census. The population is changing constantly, however, so population data quickly become out of date. For this reason, demographers have developed several methods and techniques for estimating intercensus and postcensus (current) populations. These methods and techniques are valuable to health planners, because valid estimates of population are of special importance for an epidemiological approach to community health analysis.

Techniques for estimating population fall into two broad categories (Exhibit 6-1): demographic and statistical. Demographic techniques use data on any or all of the components of population change (i.e., births, deaths, migration). Statistical techniques, on the other hand, rely on predictors of population change, even though they may not be directly related to the three components of population change.[36]

Exhibit 6-1 Methods for Estimating Population

Demographic Methods	_Statistical Methods_
Component Methods	Ratio-Correlation Methods
Housing Unit Methods	Censal Ratio Methods
Composite Methods	Extrapolation of Past Growth
Death Rate Method (ASDR)*	Sample Surveys

*ASDR = Age-Specific Death Rate.

Source: Adapted from _American Demographics,_ Vol. 4, No. 4, p. 3, with permission of American Demographics, Inc., © 1982.

Demographic Methods

Component Method

Because component methods deal with the three components of population change separately, the estimating formula is exactly the same as that previously referred to as the balancing equation:

$$P_2 = P_1 + (B - D) + (I - E)$$

The population is estimated by adding the numbers resulting from natural increase and net immigration for the period since the last census to the latest census count. When data are available, this is without doubt the easiest way of estimating population.

It is not usually difficult to obtain data on births and deaths from vital statistics reports, but net migration data may not be so readily available. Sometimes it is necessary to assume that the net migration rate for the years since the last census is the same as that reported in the last census or to extrapolate from past trends. If net migration data are not available from the last census, they can be estimated by using figures from the two previous censuses (P_2 and P_1) and from vital statistics:

$$(I - E) = P_2 - P_1 - (B - D)$$

Housing Unit Method

In the housing unit method, the first step is to determine the number of housing units that have been added and the number lost through demolition. These data are usually available from municipal records of building permits. Next, the vacancy rate is determined, usually from the last census or again from municipal building authorities. Finally, data on the average household size and on the number of households at the last census date are assembled from census data. The estimating formula is as follows:[37]

$$P_2 = [HH\ Census + ((NHH - DHH) \times OR)] \times AHS$$

where P_2 = Population estimate

   HH = Number of household units at last census date

   NHH = Number of new housing units

   DHH = Number of household units lost through demolition

   OR = Occupancy rate (1 − vacancy rate)

   AHS = Average household size

Composite Method

In some cases, analysts use a composite method, a mixture of techniques, to estimate population by broad age groups. For example, school enrollment can be used to estimate or measure changes in the population under age 18, income tax returns for the population 18–64, and Medicare enrollment for the population over 65. The total population estimate is calculated by adding the estimates for the different age groups.[38]

Age-Specific Death Rate Method

A shortcut method for estimating population is the age-specific death rate method.[39,40] This simple method involves dividing the number of deaths in the postcensus year by the corresponding age-specific death rates for the census year. The result is an estimate of population in the postcensus year (P_2).

$$P_2 = \sum_a^f \left(\frac{Deaths}{fa} \times 1,000 \right)$$

where fa = Age-specific death rate per 1,000

This method, of course, has several limitations. For example, it assumes that the death rates have remained stable between the census year and the postcensus year of estimate. In small areas, however, death rates tend to fluctuate considerably from year to year. Using an average of the death rates for a period of several years (see Chapter 4) may alleviate this problem. In any case, the populations by age group that are computed to obtain the total estimate should not be used as estimates of individual age groups. Although this method has been quite accurate, even for relatively small areas (i.e., county level),[41] it should be used with great caution for very small areas (e.g., less than 30,000 population).

Statistical Methods

Several statistical methods can also be used to estimate population. In the ratio-correlation methods, regression techniques are used to relate changes in indirect indicators, such as automobile registration and school enrollment, to population change itself. The census-ratio methods project the ratio of such indirect indicators to the total population;[42] this ratio is calculated from the findings of the last census. Another statistical technique consists of simply extrapolating past growth, for example, the growth between the last three or four censuses. Finally, sample surveys are sometimes used.

Many statistical techniques for estimating population can be complex and time-consuming for making population estimates for small areas. Community health analysts should try first to obtain population estimates from outside sources, such as federal, state, county, or municipal governments. When such estimates are not available, the component methods and the housing unit method can be used. The age-specific death rate method can also be used, with caution, to estimate county or metropolitan populations.

Guidelines for Estimating Populations

Some of the methods for estimating populations are compared in Table 6-4. Probably the method used most often to estimate population for subcounty areas is the housing unit method. It is the most appropriate for estimating populations for small areas.

O'Hare offered some sound rules on evaluating population estimates.[43]

- Large populations can be estimated more accurately than can small populations.
- Moderately growing populations can be estimated more accurately than can rapidly growing or declining populations.
- Averaging several estimates of an area's population is usually more accurate than relying on one estimate.
- Adjusting estimates to match an independently derived control total reduces error.
- It is easier to estimate change over a short period of time than over a long period of time.
- The population of smaller places is more likely to be overestimated than is the population of large places.

Table 6-4 Comparing Methods for Estimating Populations

Method	Formula for Estimating Current Population	Advantage	Disadvantage
Censal ratio	Current population = last known population × (current symptomatic variable/past symptomatic variable)	Simple calculation, based on generally available data	Accuracy declines over time
Housing unit method	Current population = (current occupied housing units × average household size) + group quarters population	Simple calculation not dependent on old data	Data requirements can be tricky, tends to overestimate population
Component method	Current population = last known noninstitutional population + births − deaths + net migration* + group	Accounts for individual components of population change	Basing migration rates for population under age 65 on school enrollment may not be valid & tax records are not easily obtainable
Ratio correlation	Current population = $bX + a$	Can be based on a variety of symptomatic variables	Requires knowledge of higher mathematics
Age-specific death rate	$P_2 = \sum\limits_a^f \left(\dfrac{Deaths}{fa} \times 1{,}000 \right)$	Simple calculation data are readily available	Assumes death rates remain stable for small areas less than 30,000 population

*Migration is based on school enrollment or tax records for the population under age 65 and Medicare enrollment for the population aged 65 and older.

Source: Adapted from *American Demographics,* Vol. 11, No. 1, pp. 46–49, with permission of American Demographics, Inc., © 1989.

- Places that lost population between 1980 and 1990 are much more likely to be overestimated than are those that grew rapidly during the same period.

These rules should be used to evaluate the potential error of any population estimate that a community health analyst must use. The amount of error encountered may be as much as 35 percent for areas with less than 100 people and as little as 5 percent for areas with more than 100,000 people.

The actual use of these methods during the next few years will be limited, as the 1990 census data will become available. The rules for evaluating population estimates are always pertinent, however.

POPULATION PROJECTIONS

While population estimates are used to determine the number of people currently in a target area, population projections are used in attempts to determine how many people will be in the area in the future. Furthermore, projections differ from forecasts.[44] Population projections are based on certain assumptions about future trends in the rates of fertility, mortality, and migration. Demographers usually make low, medium, and high projections of the same population based on different assumptions as to how these rates will change.[45] A forecast, on the other hand, is a guess as to which of these projections is the most likely. To put it another way, all forecasts are projections, but not all projections are forecasts.[46]

There are five broad categories of methods for projecting population: (1) mathematical extrapolation methods, (2) ratio methods, (3) component and cohort component methods, (4) economy-based methods, and (5) land use methods. These categories are far from mutually exclusive, and a mix of principles and techniques from each is often used.

Mathematical Extrapolation Methods

As with population estimates, population projections can be reached simply by extending past growth into the future. These mathematical extrapolations are not usually considered very accurate, although large-scale applications of this method can become quite complex mathematically.[47] In general, however, mathematical extrapolation methods should be used only for rough approximations and only over a relatively short projected time period.

Ratio Method

In the ratio methods, an existing projection for a larger (parent) area and the ratio of the current population of a subarea to the current population of the parent area are used. The historical trend of the ratios is determined, projected into the future, and multiplied by the projection for the parent population.[48]

The projection of the future ratio is simply an extension of historical trends. Table 6-5 illustrates the calculation of the ratio projection for a hypothetical County A. As can be seen, the ratio of county population to state population has been increasing, but at a slowing rate. This trend has simply been extended to project that, after 1995, the county will simply maintain its share of the state population. Government agencies often use the ratio method, and health planners should find it easy to apply when population projections for larger (parent) areas are available.

Table 6-5 Ratio Method of Population Projection for County A

County A's Historical Population Ratio with the State

	State Population	County A Population	County A as a Ratio of State
1960	696,092	27,690	.0398
1965	722,245	29,863	.0413
1970	755,103	31,643	.0419
1975	780,994	33,130	.0424
1980	817,220	34,902	.0427
1985	873,089	37,542	.0430
1990	917,457	39,634	.0432

Ratio Projection of County A's Population

	State Projection	County A Projection	County A as a Ratio of State
1995	956,085	41,398	.0433
2000	986,195	42,702	.0433
2005	1,008,547	43,670	.0433

Source: Adapted from *How Communities Can Use Statistics* by Statistics Canada, June 1981, 54.

Component and Cohort Component Methods

The component method is essentially the same as the cohort component method, except that the former is based on total population and the latter is based on age groups (cohorts). In both methods, the components of population change (i.e., births, deaths, migration) are projected separately. In the cohort component method (also called the cohort survival method), the population is carried forward by cohort, with the survival rate and the migration rate calculated for that age-specific group. The population of each age group is projected individually. For example, the population aged 10–14 in 1980 is projected forward five years to 1985 by adjusting for deaths and migration. In 1985, this cohort will be 15–19. The process is repeated for every age group and for each future date desired.

Table 6-6 illustrates the calculation of a cohort component projection for a hypothetical county. Only calculations for females are shown. Projections for the male population would be done the same way, with the exclusion of the fertility rate columns. Total population projections would be obtained by summing the two. The calculations in the table are based on the assumption that the fertility rates, survival rates, and net migration between 1971 and 1975 will all remain unchanged in the succeeding time periods. If there were some reason to anticipate changes, the rates could be altered accordingly.

Table 6-6 Calculation of a Cohort Component Population Projection

Cohorts Females	Col. 1 1971 Actual Population	Col. 2 1971–75 Survival Rates per 1,000	Col. 3 1971–75 Fertility Rates per 1,000	Col. 4 1971–75 Births	Col. 5 1971–75 (Estimated 1976 Population)	Col. 6 1976 Actual Population	Col. 7 1971–75 Estimated Net Migration	Col. 8 1976–80 Births	Col. 9 1981 Survivors	Col. 10 1981 Projection Estimate	Col. 11 1981–85 Births	Col. 12 1986 Survivors	Col. 13 1986 Projection Estimate
0–4	1,290	982.2		.044	1,025	1,115	+ 90	1,326	1,302	1,392	1,542	1,514	1,604
5–9	1,750	998.5			1,288	1,355	+ 67		1,113	1,180		1,390	1,457
10–14	1,870	998.5			1,747	1,730	– 17		1,353	1,336		1,178	1,161
15–19	1,610	997.5	204.5	329	1,865	1,750	–115	357	1,726	1,611	352	1,337	1,222
20–24	1,135	997.5	599.0	680	1,606	1,390	–216	833	1,746	1,530	916	1,607	1,391
25–29	955	997.0	661.0	631	1,132	1,480	+348	978	1,386	1,734	1,146	1,525	1,873
30–34	980	996.0	340.0	333	951	1,160	+209	394	1,474	1,683	572	1,727	1,936
35–39	1,130	994.0	125.5	142	974	1,070	+ 96	134	1,153	1,249	157	1,673	1,769
40–44	1,220	990.1	28.0	34	1,119	1,190	+ 71	33	1,059	1,130	32	1,237	1,308
45–49	1,145	984.2	1.5	2	1,201	1,155	– 46	2	1,171	1,125	2	1,112	1,066
50–54	850	975.9			1,117	1,125	+ 8		1,127	1,135		1,098	1,106
55–59	605	962.4			818	760	– 58		1,083	1,025		1,092	1,034
60–64	420	943.0			571	565	– 6		716	710		967	961
65–69	350	912.4			383	425	+ 42		516	558		648	690
70–74	270	862.6			302	340	+ 38		367	405		481	519
75–79	225	780.2			211	280	+ 69		265	334		316	385
80–84	140	648.1			146	190	+ 44		181	225		216	260
85+	95	435.3			102	150	+ 48		148	196		183	231
	16,040			2,151 (× .4855)	17,063	17,230	+672	2,731 (× .4855)	17,886	18,558	3,177 (× .4855)	19,301	19,971

Notes:

Column 2: Calculated using death rates. This is done by taking the average annual death rate for the five-year period compounded at a declining rate, the result of which is multiplied by 1,000. In mathematical terms:

$$SR = 1,000 \times \frac{1}{(1+i)^n}$$

where SR = Survival rate

i = Annual average death rate

n = Number of years

In essence, this rate states the probability that a person who is in a certain age bracket will live from the beginning to the end of the particular time period. Published life tables are often used to calculate survival rates.

Column 4: Column 3 times Column 1. The entry opposite 0–4 indicates the total of all births factored by the number who will be female (48.55 percent). An alternative approach for this calculation would have been to apply the same fertility rates to the average midyear population:

$$\frac{\text{Population 1971} + \text{Population 1976}}{2}$$

Column 5: Column 2 times Column 1 with its cohorts dropped one age bracket, that is, the survival rate for the next succeeding age bracket is applied to the number in the cohort. For example, the 955 women ages 25 to 29 in 1971 are multiplied by the survival rate for the age bracket 30–34 to obtain the 1976 estimate (migration held aside for the moment). The births calculated in Column 4 are factored by the 0–4 survival rate.

Column 7: Column 6 minus Column 5. The result is assumed to be net migration, since Column 5 includes births and deaths of persons in 1971. This calculation also includes any error in census counts, fertility rate, and survival rate calculations of Columns 2 and 3. These errors are ignored, largely because they are impossible to measure. The calculation also includes births and deaths of migrants. With more work, the net migration could be recalibrated to extract these components, but [it was] decided to disregard this aspect.

Column 8: Column 3 times Column 6. The entry opposite 0–4 indicates the total of all births factored by the number who will be female (48.55 percent). Alternative calculation is possible, as noted for Column 4.

Column 9: Column 2 times Column 6 as for Column 5.

Column 10: The projection estimate calculated by taking Column 9 and adding Column 7. No survival rate or fertility rate calculations are made with the migration estimates, since these are assumed to be part of the residually derived estimates. If the estimates had been derived using another method, then it might have been necessary to apply separate fertility rate and survival rate calculations (usually at half the rate).

Column 11: Column 3 times Column 10. The entry opposite 0–4 indicates the total of all births factored by the number who will be female (48.55 percent). Alternative calculation is possible, as noted for Column 4.

Column 12: Column 2 times Column 10 as for Column 5.

Column 13: Column 12 plus Column 7 with same assumptions as in Column 10.

Source: Reprinted from *How Communities Can Use Statistics* by Statistics Canada, June 1981, 57.

The main advantage of the cohort component method is that it allows a detailed, age-specific analysis of future population trends. Births, deaths, and migration are all calculated and can be examined readily for each age group. As an alternative, the overall growth rates for each cohort between two censuses may be calculated and those rates applied to the new cohorts. The procedure is essentially the same, except that births, deaths, and net migration are combined into a single measure, the growth rate.

Economy-Based and Land Use Methods

Economy-based methods of population projection use projected economic data for the projection of migration. Births and deaths are projected by means of using other methods, while immigration and emigration are projected in relation to the future economy of an area (i.e., creation or loss of jobs). The land use methods are similar to the housing unit methods of population estimates. By calculating how many housing units can be built and determining the average household size, the likely additions to the population can be estimated—given a presumed rate of building to reach the saturation point.[49]

Evaluating Population Projections

The ratio and the cohort component methods are probably the easiest population projection measures for health planners to use. As in the case of population estimates, rules to evaluate population projections have been suggested.[50]

- The shorter the projection period, the more reliable (accurate).
- The larger the geographical area, the more reliable (accurate).
- The lower the current birth rate and the higher the current life expectancy, the lower the margin of error.

It always is advisable to use more than one method and to project the population under several different assumptions of birth, death, and migration rates. In every case, the reliability of the projections must be determined with some degree of certainty.

U.S. CENSUS

Most of the data required for demographic analysis of the population comes from vital and health statistics and from the census. Census publications contain an enormous wealth of information that health analysts too often ignore. All this information is compiled and readily available for every area of the United States. (Equivalent data are available in Canada from Statistics Canada.) In addition, private firms supply demographic data from the census.[51] These "demographic supermarkets" not only can compile all kinds of information for any given area, but also can provide computer graphics and population forecasts. They serve extremely useful functions, especially during the intercensal years.

POPULATION TRENDS

World Population

In mid-1989, the world population was approximately 5.2 billion and growing at 1.8 percent a year. If the growth rate remains constant, the world population will double in 39 years. This is quite amazing in view of the fact that it took 2 to 5 million years for the world to reach its first billion. It will take only until 1998 for the total population to reach 6 billion (Table 6-7).

Most of the current growth is taking place in the less developed regions of the world. Table 6-8 lists the ten largest cities in the world in 1950, 1980, and (projected) 2000. As can be seen, there will be a clear shift in their ranking. Differences in population growth rates in various regions, which are due primarily to differences in fertility behavior, are also evident in the age pyramids of populations in the developed and the developing regions of the world (Fig. 6-5). The age profile of the developing nations is clearly expansive, while that of the developed regions is nearly stationary.

Among the world's continents, Asia is by far the most populous—although its current rate of natural increase is third to those of Africa and Latin America

---

Table 6-7 Estimated Timing of Each Billion of World Population

	Time Taken To Reach	Year Attained
First billion	2–5 million years	About 1800 A.D.
Second billion	Approx. 130 years	1930
Third billion	30 years	1960
Fourth billion	15 years	1975
Fifth billion	12 years	1987
Projections:		
Sixth billion	11 years	1998

Source: Reprinted from *World Population: Toward the Next Century,* p. 3, with permission of Population Reference Bureau, © 1981.

Table 6-8 Ten Largest Cities in the World in 1950, 1980, and (Projected) 2000

1950	Population (in millions)	1980	Population (in millions)	2000	Population (in millions)
1. New York-N.E. New Jersey	12.3	1. New York-N.E. New Jersey	20.2	1. Mexico City	31.0
2. London	10.4	2. Tokyo-Yokohama	20.0	2. Sao Paulo	25.8
3. Rhine-Ruhr	6.9	3. Mexico City	15.0	3. Shanghai	23.7
4. Tokyo-Yokohama	6.7	4. Shanghai	14.3	4. Tokyo-Yokohama	23.7
5. Shanghai	5.8	5. Sao Paulo	13.5	5. New York-N.E. New Jersey	22.4
6. Paris	5.5	6. Los Angeles-Long Beach	11.6	6. Peking	20.9
7. Greater Buenos Aires	5.3	7. Peking	11.4	7. Rio de Janeiro	19.0
8. Chicago-N.W. Indiana	4.9	8. Rio de Janeiro	10.7	8. Greater Bombay	16.8
9. Moscow	4.8	9. Greater Buenos Aires	10.1	9. Calcutta	16.4
10. Calcutta	4.6	10. London	10.0	10. Jakarta	15.7

Source: Reprinted from World Population: Toward the Next Century, p. 2, with permission of Population Reference Bureau, © 1981.

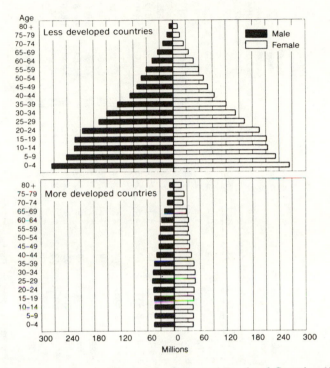

Figure 6-5 Population by Age and Sex for Developing and Developed Countries: 1989. *Source:* Reprinted from *Population Today,* Vol. 18, No. 1, p. 2, with permission of Population Reference Bureau, © 1990. Data from *World Population Profile: 1989, WP-89.*

(Table 6-9). Europe and North America have low rates of natural increase, and the percentage of their population over age 64 is correspondingly high. They also have the highest life expectancy at birth and the highest percentage of urban population. Per capita gross national product is highest in North America, Europe, and Oceania, while the crude death rate is lowest in Latin America followed by Oceania, North America, Europe, and the U.S.S.R.

The United States and Canada

In both the United States and Canada, the most striking recent demographic trend is the aging of the population. In 1980, the median age of the U.S. population was 30.2 years; that of the Canadian population was slightly below 29.9 years. The median ages were the same in 1950 before the postwar baby boom. As of 1980, the baby boom cohort was aged 20–34, and it is those age groups

Table 6-9 1989 World Population Data

Region or Country	Population Estimate Mid-1989 (millions)	Crude Birth Rate	Crude Death Rate	Natural Increase (Annual, %)	Population "Doubling Time" in Years (at Current Time)	Population Projected to 2000 (millions)	Population Projected to 2020 (millions)	Infant Mortality Rate	Total Fertility Rate	Percent Population under Age 15/65+	Life Expectancy at Birth (years)	Urban Pop. (%)	Percent Married Women Using Contraception (Total/Modern)	Per Capita GNP, 1987 (US$)
World	5,234	28	10	1.8	39	6,323	8,330	75	3.6	33/6	63	41	53/46	$ 3,330
More Developed	1,206	15	9	0.6	122	1,268	1,339	15	1.9	22/12	73	73	70/54	12,070
Less Developed	4,028	31	10	2.1	32	5,055	6,991	84	4.1	37/4	60	32	49/44	670
Less Developed (Excl. China)	2,924	35	11	2.4	29	3,763	5,468	93	4.7	40/4	58	36	38/30	820
Africa	646	45	15	2.9	24	898	1,523	113	6.3	45/3	51	30	—/—	610
Asia	3,061	28	9	1.9	36	3,743	4,883	78	3.6	34/5	62	29	53/48	1,170
Asia (Excl. China)	1,957	32	10	2.2	32	2,452	3,360	90	4.3	38/4	60	33	40/33	1,730
North America	275	16	9	0.7	97	297	325	10	1.9	21/12	75	74	68/64	18,110
Canada	26.3	15	7	0.8	92	28.4	30.2	7.9	1.7	21/11	76	77	73/69	15,080
United States	248.8	16	9	0.7	98	268.3	294.4	9.9	1.9	21/12	75	74	68/63	18,430
Latin America	438	29	7	2.1	33	535	705	55	3.6	38/5	66	68	54/46	1,820
Europe	499	13	10	0.3	269	507	502	12	1.7	20/13	74	74	73/47	9,700
USSR	289	20	10	1.0	70	312	355	25	2.5	25/9	69	66	—/—	8,375
Oceania	26	20	8	1.2	56	30	38	26	2.7	28/9	72	70	56/48	8,440

Source: Adapted from *World Population Data Sheet,* with permission of Population Reference Bureau, © 1989.

that showed the largest relative increases between 1970 and 1980. The number of young adults aged 20–24 increased by 30.1 percent during this period; the 25–29 and 30–34 groups increased by 44.7 percent and 53.5 percent, respectively. The number of people in the over-55 bloc also rose rapidly, with a greater relative gain for females than for males.[52]

In contrast, as of 1980, the number of children under 15 declined by 4.5 percent, with 4.8 percent fewer under 5, 16.4 percent fewer aged 5–9, and 12.3 percent fewer aged 10–14. The Depression cohort (babies born in the Depression years of low birth rates) were aged 40–49, so this group also decreased between 1970 and 1980.

In 1980, Canada's population was slightly younger, with 9.5 percent over 64 (up from 7.6 percent in 1961), 61.7 percent 17–64 (up from 53.5 percent in 1961), and 28.8 percent under 17 (down from 38.9 percent in 1961).

The changing age structure in both the United States and Canada is a result of changing fertility behavior. Both the crude birth rate and the general fertility rate decreased dramatically between 1950 and 1975, but increased slightly thereafter (Table 6-10). These changes in fertility can be observed at every age (Fig. 6-6).

The total fertility rate in the United States in the early 1980s was approximately 1.8 births per woman, in contrast to nearly 3.7 in the late 1950s. The average family size declined correspondingly, from a high of 3.67 in 1960 to 3.28 in 1980. Although fertility rates in the United States are low, teenage pregnancy rates are high in comparison to those in other industrialized countries (Table 6-11). Only East Germany had a higher rate than did the United States in 1976. Although teenage fertility rates in the United States decreased dramatically after

---

Table 6-10 Crude Birth Rates and General Fertility Rates, United States, 1950–1987

Year	Crude Birth Rate per 1,000 Population	General Fertility Rate per 1,000 Women 15–44
1950	24.1	106.2
1955	25.0	118.3
1960	23.7	118.0
1965	19.4	96.3
1970	18.4	87.9
1975	14.6	66.0
1980	15.9	68.4
1985	15.8	66.2
1986	15.6	65.4
1987	15.7	65.7

Source: Reprinted from Monthly Vital Statistics Report, Vol. 38, No. 3, p. 15, U.S. DHHS, 1987.

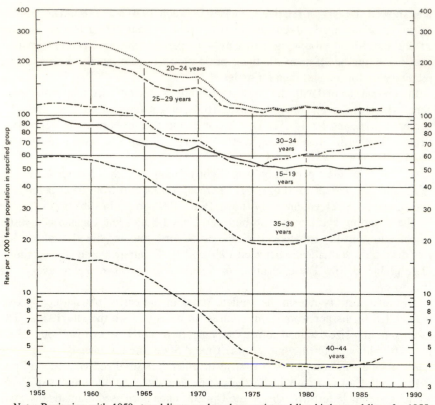

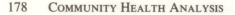

Note: Beginning with 1959, trend lines are based on registered live birth; trend lines for 1955–1959 are based on live births adjusted for underregistration.

Figure 6-6 Age-Specific Fertility Rates, United States, 1950–1987. *Source:* Reprinted from *Monthly Vital Statistics Report,* Vol. 38, No. 3, p. 3, U.S. DHHS, 1989.

1970 (Table 6-12) and even though the decline was more rapid for blacks than for whites, the fertility rates in 1986 remained considerably higher for black teenagers than for white teenagers.

The marriage rate in the United States decreased from 90.2 marriages per year per 1,000 unmarried women aged 15 and older in 1950 to 64.6 in 1981.[53] The divorce rate appeared to be leveling off at approximately 22.8 divorces per year per 1,000 married women aged 15 and over, after having more than doubled since 1967 and almost tripled since 1940.[54] The proportion of nonfamily households (i.e., individuals living alone or sharing living quarters with unrelated persons) increased from 18.8 percent in 1970 to 26.6 percent in 1980.

Table 6-11 Fertility Rates and Percentage of All Births for Women under 20 Years of Age

Selected Countries, Selected Years 1972–1976

Country and Year	Births per 1,000 Women under 20 Years	Percent of All Births
Canada (1975)	33.8	11.0
United States (1976)	54.7	18.0
Sweden (1976)	25.0	6.6
England and Wales (1976)	32.4	9.9
Netherlands (1976)	11.3	3.7
German Democratic Republic (1975)	61.6	21.8
German Federal Republic (1976)	19.9	7.5
France (1972)	28.8	6.7
Switzerland (1976)	12.4	3.9
Italy (1974)	50.7	11.3
Israel (1975)	43.7	7.2
Japan (1976)	3.7	0.8
Australia (1975)	40.9	10.4

Source: Reprinted from *Health, United States, 1980,* p. 19, U.S. DHHS, 1980.

Table 6-12 Race-Specific Teenage Fertility Rates, United States, 1970–1986

Years	Total			White			Black		
	10–14	*15–17*	*18–19*	*10–14*	*15–17*	*18–19*	*10–14*	*15–17*	*18–19*
1970	1.2	38.8	114.7	0.5	29.2	101.5	5.2	101.4	204.9
1975	1.3	36.6	85.7	0.6	28.3	74.4	5.1	86.6	156.0
1980	1.1	32.5	82.1	0.6	25.2	72.1	4.3	73.6	138.8
1981	1.1	32.1	81.7	0.5	25.1	71.9	4.1	70.6	135.9
1982	1.1	32.4	80.7	0.6	25.2	70.8	4.1	71.2	133.3
1983	1.1	32.0	78.1	0.6	24.8	68.3	4.1	70.1	130.4
1984	1.2	31.1	78.3	0.6	23.9	68.1	4.3	69.7	132.0
1985	1.2	31.1	80.8	0.6	24.0	70.1	4.5	69.0	137.1
1986	1.3	30.6	81.0	0.6	23.4	69.8	4.6	70.0	141.0

Source: Reprinted from *Health, United States, 1988,* p. 42, U.S. DHHS, 1989.

EFFECT OF DEMOGRAPHIC TRENDS ON UTILIZATION

Three important demographic pressures have had a significant impact on the health care system: (1) the post–World War II baby boom, (2) the aging of the population, and (3) the changing status of women.

Baby Boom

Between 1946 and 1964, 76.4 million babies were born in the United States, one-third of the present population. This postwar increase in the fertility rate occurred in many developed countries as well, including Canada, New Zealand, Australia, and the U.S.S.R. The baby boom created unusually large cohorts compared to those of the 1930s, the early 1940s, and the baby bust years of the 1960s and 1970s.[55] As Jones put it, the boom generated can be thought of "as a moving bulge in the population that, like a pig swallowed by a python, causes stretch marks and discomfort along the way"[56] (Fig. 6-7).

The great upsurge in fertility between 1945 and 1960 is affecting all aspects of the baby boomers' daily lives. In contrast to those in the Depression or the "good times" cohort, which, "by virtue of this smaller number, upon encountering each life cycle event, have experienced relative abundance,"[57] the baby boom cohort has been experiencing and can expect problems and frustrations as it passes through the life cycle.[58] Problems of overcrowded classrooms and shortages of teachers through the 1960s and 1970s, school closings and unemployment problems in the 1980s, and social changes in the 1990s are all related directly to the baby boom.

The recent increases in the number of births and in the crude birth rate are late effects of the baby boom of the 1950s. These so-called echo effects of the baby boom result simply from the fact that the women of that cohort are now in the prime childbearing ages of 20–29. Thus, annual birth totals were expected to rise during the late 1980s and early 1990s, even if the fertility rate remained at approximately 1.8 births per woman.[59] The number of births will remain high during the early 1990s, but, if fertility rates remain constant, the number of births should decrease when the women of the baby bust cohort reach their prime childbearing ages between 1995 to 2005. From then on, the number of births should remain constant at the early 1990s level, as the age-sex pyramid will assume a stationary, rectangular profile.

As the baby boom generation ages and fertility remains low, the median age of the population will rise. If the age-specific mortality and morbidity rates remain constant (see Chapter 5), it can be projected that the number of motor vehicle accidents, homicides, suicides, depressions, and heart diseases will increase through the 1990s, because the baby boom cohort will then be between 30 and 50. Similarly, if morbidity rates remain constant, the prevalence of cancer, heart disease, stroke, and respiratory conditions may increase during the early 2000s. The crude death rate will be artificially elevated.[60] When the baby boom cohort becomes elderly, starting in 2020, crude death rates will increase even more; some 15 percent of the population will then be 65 or over, compared to 11 percent in 1980.

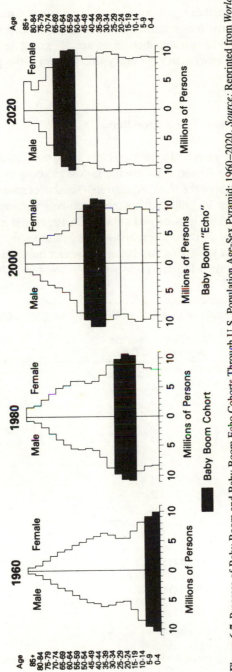
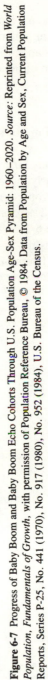

Figure 6-7 Progress of Baby Boom and Baby Boom Echo Cohorts Through U.S. Population Age-Sex Pyramid: 1960–2020. *Source:* Reprinted from *World Population, Fundamentals of Growth*, with permission of Population Reference Bureau, © 1984. Data from Population by Age and Sex, Current Population Reports, Series P-25, No. 441 (1970), No. 917 (1980), No. 952 (1984), U.S. Bureau of the Census.

Such trends as lengthening life expectancy, early retirement, increasing chronic medical patterns (environmental and lifestyle), rising rates of divorce, and women's labor force participation rates are all going to affect the needs and future care of the elderly in the twenty-first century—the present day baby boomers.

Aging of the Population: The Senior Boom

With declining birth rates and a progressively aging population, people 65 and over (particularly those 85 and over) are the fastest growing group in the United States.[61] The proportion of the U.S. population 65 and over rose from 4.1 percent in 1900 to 11.2 percent in 1980 and is expected to be approximately 12 percent in 1990 (Table 6-13). This growth will slow in the 1990s and in the first decade of the 2000s as the small Depression cohort reaches old age. Thereafter, however, the baby boom of the 1950s will become a senior boom and the proportion of the population over 65 will grow rapidly to 15 percent in 2020 and 18 percent

Table 6-13 Percent of Population 65 and Over, United States, 1900–2040

Year	% of Total Population Aged 65 and Over	Median Age of Total Population
	Estimates	
1900	4.1	22.9
1910	4.3	24.1
1920	4.7	25.3
1930	5.5	26.5
1940	6.9	29.0
1950	8.2	30.2
1960	9.3	29.5
1970	9.9	28.1
1980	11.2	30.2
	Projections	
1990	12.1 (11.7–12.6)*	32.8 (31.4–33.7)*
2000	12.2 (11.3–12.9)	35.5 (32.5–37.3)
2010	12.7 (11.1–13.9)	36.6 (31.1–40.2)
2020	15.5 (12.7–17.8)	37.0 (31.4–41.7)
2030	18.3 (14.0–22.1)	38.0 (31.2–43.2)
2040	17.8 (12.5–22.8)	37.8 (30.7–43.9)

*High and low rates of population projection.

Source: Reprinted from *Population Today,* Vol. 35, No. 4, p. 9, with permission of Population Reference Bureau, © 1980.

in 2030. After 2030, the number of people in the group will probably fall sharply again as the baby bust cohorts of the 1960s and 1970s become 65 and over.[62]

In the United States, life expectancy at age 65 for adults is 14.8 years for men and 18.7 years for women; for black males it is 13.4, and for black females it is 17.0.[63] Table 6-14 shows trends in life expectancy from 1900 to 1985 for those aged 65 and 85. Since 1979 life expectancy has increased almost minimally. Age-specific death rates for males 65 years and over declined by almost 30 percent between 1950 and 1986; for females, approximately 40 percent.[64]

The leading causes of death in the elderly were the same in 1986 as in 1950, with heart disease, cancer, and stroke accounting for 75 percent.[65] Mortality trends from heart disease parallel the decline for all causes combined. Death rates from stroke have been falling even more rapidly than those from heart disease. Death rates from cancer have been rising, however, with rapid increases in recent years resulting primarily from lung cancer.

Arthritis and rheumatism, followed closely by hypertension, are the most common causes of activity limitation at age 65 and over.[66] One study showed that 39 percent of more than 4,200 individuals aged 65 and older had some form of

Table 6-14 Trend in Expectation of Life and Chances of Surviving—Persons Aged 65 and 85—United States, 1900–02 to 1985

| | Expectation of Life (in Years) | | | | | | Chances per 1,000 of Surviving | | |
| | Age 65 | | | Age 85 | | | From Ages 65 to 85 | | |
Year	Both Sexes	Men	Women	Both Sexes	Men	Women	Both Sexes	Men	Women
1900–02	11.9	11.5	12.2	4.0	3.8	4.1	148	134	163
1909–11	11.6	11.2	12.0	4.0	3.9	4.1	139	126	152
1919–21*	NA	12.2	12.7	NA	4.1	4.2	NA	161	182
1929–31*	NA	11.8	12.8	NA	4.0	4.2	NA	143	181
1939–41	12.8	12.1	13.6	4.3	4.1	4.5	183	156	213
1949–51	13.8	12.7	15.0	4.7	4.4	4.9	234	191	279
1959–61	14.4	13.0	15.8	4.6	4.4	4.7	261	200	322
1969–71	15.0	13.0	16.8	5.3	4.7	5.6	291	205	371
1979–81	16.5	14.2	18.4	6.0	5.1	6.4	363	255	452
1982	16.8	14.5	18.8	6.3	5.3	6.8	378	271	467
1983	16.7	14.5	18.6	6.1	5.2	6.6	371	264	460
1984	16.8	14.6	18.6	6.1	5.2	6.5	374	268	461
1985†	16.8	14.5	18.6	6.0	5.0	6.5	375	272	460

*White population only.
†Estimated by Metropolitan Life Insurance Co.

Data from: Various reports by the Bureau of the Census and the National Center for Health Services. Statistical Bulletin, Trends in Longevity after Age 65, Jan-Mar 1987, p. 11.

hypertension and the condition was either untreated or poorly controlled in 25 percent of these cases.[67] Hearing disease affects 21 percent of the elderly population. The ten most common chronic conditions in the elderly are shown in Figure 6-8. Acute respiratory, digestive, and orthopedic impairments are common. Approximately half of elderly individuals have no teeth or dentures, wear dentures that fit poorly, or do not wear them at all, predisposing them to malnutrition and increasing their already high susceptibility to disease and disability.[68]

These patterns have undergone very little change in recent years, as reported in a 1988 study.[69] Neither do the patterns of impairment vary greatly by sex or race. These impairments are important, as they often lead to withdrawal, isolation, depression, further disability, and dependence.[70]

Not surprisingly, the utilization of health services is higher among the elderly population, especially after age 75, than among the general population. In 1980 in the United States, persons aged 65 and over averaged 6.4 physician visits during the year, compared to 5.1 for those 45–64 and 4.4 for those under 45. Rates of hospital utilization also are much higher for the elderly, who occupy more than 30 percent of acute care beds while comprising only 16 percent of the total population.[71] Although females in the general population have much higher rates of hospital utilization than do males, elderly females have much lower rates.[72]

It is not easy to determine which health changes result from age and which ones represent the development of disease.[73] Death, disease, and disability in the older population stem mostly from chronic conditions, which tend to originate early in life and develop gradually. This does not mean, however, that the elderly

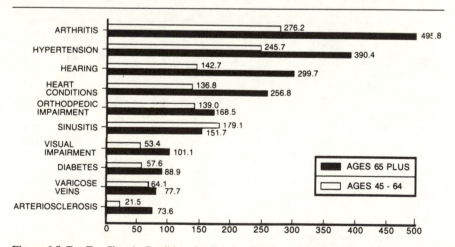

Figure 6-8 Top Ten Chronic Conditions for Elderly—Rates per 1,000 Persons: 1982. *Source:* Reprinted from *Aging America: Trends and Projections. 1985–1986,* p. 88, U.S. Senate Special Committee on Aging, 1986.

population in the years to come will be a sicker one. Some chronic illnesses can be postponed by changes in lifestyle. For example, the elimination of cigarette smoking greatly delays the date of onset of emphysema and reduces the risk of lung cancer. The recent decline in mortality rates, which is caused principally by a decrease in the incidence of arteriosclerosis and cerebrovascular disease, is the first demonstration of a national reduction in mortality rates from a major chronic disease. Most observers attribute it to changes in lifestyle (primary prevention) and to better treatment of hypertension (secondary prevention).[74] Fries suggested that, through further lifestyle changes, chronic illnesses may be postponed and morbidity may be compressed until near the end of the life span (which he calculated as, ideally, 85 years).[75]

Several issues regarding the care of the elderly have yet to be resolved. The elderly traditionally were cared for by family members, but, with most women in the labor force, the responsibility for care is being transferred to institutions. One estimate of the need for nursing home beds by the year 2000 suggested that one nursing home of 100 beds must be built every day until the year 2000 to satisfy the long-term care needs of the elderly. This is not the solution, however. It is essential to find alternatives to institutionalization, such as elderly foster homes, adult day care centers, custodial care, young elderly caring for the elder elderly, and government-sponsored centers run along the social model, rather than the medical model of care. Approximately 60 percent of the white aged and 50 percent of the black aged have no limitation. A certain portion of men and women, both black and white, do require help with everyday living events, such as dressing, eating, shopping, and washing. Our attitude toward support of these daily functions for the elderly is extremely varied.

A Japanese study that compared relationships among young and old family members in Japan, Thailand, Italy, Denmark, and the United States showed that Japan and Thailand had the highest percentage of three-generation families—58 percent and 66 percent, respectively—whereas the United States had the lowest percentage at 2.7 percent. When asked who the preferred care-giver should be, the U.S. respondents ranked family first, private agency second, and neighbor or friend third, with respective percentages of 69, 41, and 18.[76] In contrast, Japanese respondents ranked family and public agency first and second, representing 95 and 15 percent, respectively.[77] Certainly, the U.S. responses reflect the great mobility in our society and the entry of women into the labor force. As a result, according to a 1988 study, 30 percent of all elderly people in the United States live alone.[78]

The impact that the aging of the population will have on the future health care system, thus, is dependent on present health policy. An effective health care policy for the elderly should stress health maintenance and promotion; disease prevention; comprehensive and integrated health and social services; and personal autonomy, coping skills, and social interaction.[79-81]

Status of Women

The first two demographic pressures—the baby boom and the senior boom—are age phenomenon trends. The status of women is obviously gender-specific.

Women's Health Status

The only major area in which the female gender works a definite advantage is in health status. Women's life expectancy is longer by approximately seven years at birth, and lesser gains occur at other age groups (Fig. 6-9). The mortality rates for the five leading causes of death (1960–1986) by sex show major advantages for heart disease, cancer, accidents, and chronic obstructive pulmonary disease; however, there is only a slight advantage for cerebrovascular diseases (Fig. 6-10).

The analysis of morbidity reveals a different pattern. Although women live longer and are less susceptible to most of the top five causes of death, they generally have more short-term illnesses. In their daily lives, women report significantly more health problems than do men.[82] Furthermore, over a longer period women are more likely to have chronic conditions. Verbrugge noted that women

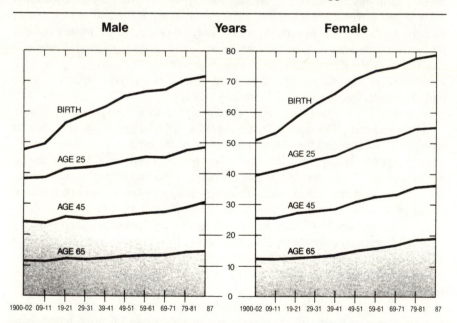

Figure 6-9 Expectation of Life at Selected Ages, United States, 1900–02 to 1987. *Source:* Reprinted from *Statistical Bulletin,* Vol. 69, No. 3, p. 13, with permission of Metropolitan Life Insurance Company, © 1988. Data from National Center for Health Statistics, 1900–1902 to 1979–1981; Metropolitan Life Insurance Company, 1987.

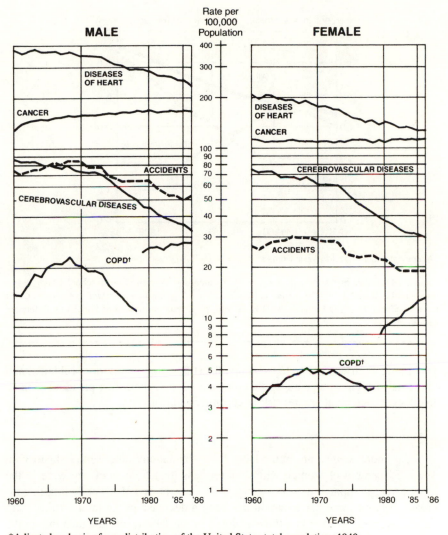

*Adjusted on basis of age distribution of the United States total population, 1940.
†Chronic Obstructive Pulmonary Diseases: The ninth revision in cause-of-death coding significantly affected comparability of data prior to 1979, hence the break in the trend line.

Figure 6-10 Age-Adjusted* Mortality Rate for the 5 Leading Causes of Death, by Sex, United States, 1960–1986. *Source:* Reprinted from *Statistical Bulletin*, Vol. 20, No. 2, p. 35, with permission of Metropolitan Life Insurance Company, © 1989. Data from various reports from the National Center for Health Statistics.

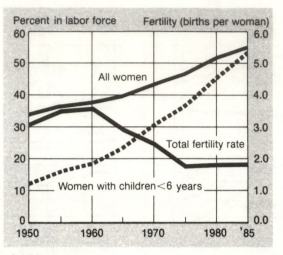

*Average number of children per woman.

Figure 6-11 Labor Force Participation for All Women and Women with Preschool Children and Total Fertility Rate,* 1950–1985. *Source:* Reprinted from *Juggling Jobs and Babies: America's Child Care Challenge* by M. O'Connell and D.E. Bloom, p. 3, with permission of Population Reference Bureau, © 1987.

---

experience injuries, stomach problems, heart trouble, respiratory problems, and anorexia in higher percentages than do men. Thus, there is a paradox: women live longer, but are at greater risk of chronic conditions.

Employment

Today more women are in the labor force than at any other time in history. In 1985, 55 percent of women with children less than 6 years of age were in the labor force, compared to approximately 11 percent in 1950. Paralleling this increase in labor force participation has been a decrease in the total fertility rate. On the average, women had three children in the 1950s, but less than two in the 1980s (Fig. 6-11). The labor force participation by age of the woman shows even greater changes. Labor force participation of women in the prime childbearing ages declined during the 1950s, 1960s, and 1970s, but not in the 1980s (Fig. 6-12). The increasing availability of child care has fostered this trend. Child care is not affordable to all women, however, as it can vary from $35.00 to $340.00 per week.[83]

An important fact related to this increase in the number of women in the labor force is the disparity in wages (Fig. 6-13). The greatest wage gap disparity was in 1973. Since 1982, women have outpaced men, but they still lag significantly.

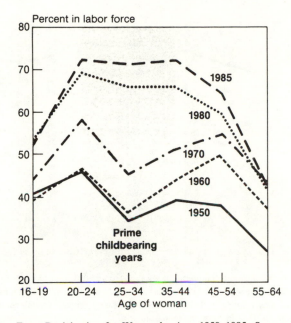

Figure 6-12 Labor Force Participation for Women by Age: 1950–1985. *Source:* Reprinted from *Juggling Jobs and Babies: America's Child Care Challenge* by M. O'Connell and D.E. Bloom, p. 5, with permission of Population Reference Bureau, © 1987.

Political Gaps

The struggle for women's suffrage has been an international one. The time elapsed between men's and women's right to vote has ranged from 1 year to 137 years, with an average delay of 47 years worldwide (Fig. 6-14).

In the United States, representation of women in the legislative and executive branches of government has been quite dismal, although it is improving. The country with the highest female participation in government in 1984 was the U.S.S.R.; those with the lowest participation were Uganda and South Africa.

The enrollment of women in U.S. institutions of higher education has increased since 1960. At that time, there were 59 women enrolled in such institutions for every 100 men enrolled; as recently as 1985, this ratio was 104:100.[84]

On the whole, the advances made by women worldwide have been modest, and those made in the United States have been less than desired. Women live longer, suffer more from chronic ailments, are not represented evenly in government, earn less for their positions, and must balance career and family. In sum, there is no major category, possibly with the exception of education, in which women have attained equality with men. Women are major resources who have been neglected too long. To quote Arnold, "If ever the world sees a time when

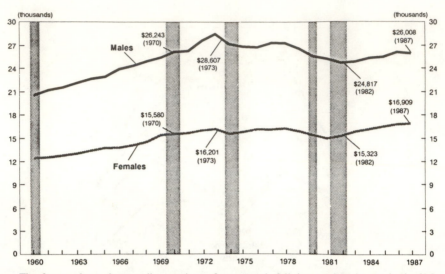

The figures above show median earnings of year-round, full-time workers by sex in the U.S., given in 1987 dollars; the shaded areas are recessions. Interestingly, in modern times the male-female income disparity was greatest in 1973 (57 cents for every dollar), and since 1982 females have outpaced males in terms of increase in real earnings.

Figure 6-13 The Male-Female Wage Gap. *Source:* Reprinted from *Population Today,* Vol. 17, No. 2, p. 2, with permission of Population Reference Bureau, © 1989. Data from U.S. Census Bureau, "Money Income and Poverty Status in the United States: 1987," *Current Population Reports,* P-60, No. 161.

women shall come together purely and strongly for the benefit of mankind, it will be a power such as the world has never known."[85]

CONCLUSION

Demography supplies the tools for the analysis of population composition and distribution, of changes in its components, and for the estimation and projection of its future. All these tools are essential for an epidemiological approach to community analysis since health, disease, and utilization all are related to population characteristics. Furthermore, any trend in population demographics has health care management and policy implications.

NOTES

1. E.M. Murphy, *World Population: Toward the Next Century* (Washington, D.C.: Population Reference Bureau, Inc., November 1981), 7.

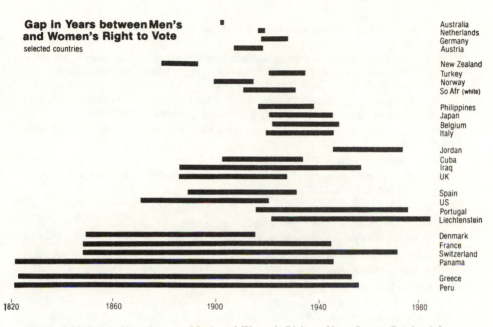

Figure 6-14 Gap in Years between Men's and Women's Right to Vote. *Source:* Reprinted from *Women: A World Survey* by R.L. Sivard, p. 29, with permission of World Priorities, © 1985.

2. U.S. Bureau of the Census, *The Methods and Materials of Demography,* 4th ed., prepared by Henry S. Shyrock, Jacob S. Siegel, and Associates (Washington, D.C.: U.S. Government Printing Office, June 1980), 91.

3. B. Robry, "Two Hundred Years and Counting: The 1990 Census," *Population Bulletin* 44, no. 1 (April 1989): 7.

4. A. Haupt and T.T. Kane, *Population Handbook,* int'l ed. (Washington, D.C.: Population Reference Bureau, Inc., 1980), 76.

5. Organization for Economic Co-operation and Development. (OECD), *Aging Populations—The Solving Policy Implications.* (Paris: OECD, 1980), 10–28.

6. Population Crises Committee, "Population Growth and Economic Development," *Population* 14 (February 1985): 1–8.

7. Haupt and Kane, *Population Handbook,* 14.

8. D. Ewbank and J.D. Wray, "Population and Public Health," in *Maxcy-Rosenau Public Health and Preventive Medicine,* 11th edition, ed. J.M. Last (New York: Appleton-Century-Crofts, Inc., 1980), 1512.

9. J. Coale, "How a Population Ages or Grows Younger," in *Population: The Vital Revolution,* ed. R. Freedman (New York: Anchor Press, 1964), 47–58.

10. U.S. Bureau of the Census, *Methods and Materials,* 299.

11. Ibid., 300.

12. World Population Data Sheet (Washington, D.C.: Population Reference Bureau, Inc., 1989).

13. Interchange, Where is Metropolitan U.S.? Vol. 16, No. 4 (December 1987) Population Reference Bureau.

14. U.S. Department of Health and Human Services, Public Health Service, *Geographic Patterns in the Risk of Dying and Associated Factors,* Vital and Health Statistics Analytical Studies, Series 3, no. 18 (Washington, D.C.: Public Health Service, 1980), 48.

15. G.C. Myers and K.G. Mantar, "The Structure of Urban Mortality: A Methodological Study of Hannover, Germany," *International Journal of Epidemiology* 6 (September 1977): 203–213.

16. A.S. Boote, "How To Get More from Demographic Analysis," *American Demographics* 3 (June 1981): 30–33.

17. U.S. Bureau of the Census, *Methods and Materials,* 462.

18. John Saunders, *Basic Demographic Measures—A Practical Guide for Users* (New York: University Press of America, 1988), 25–26.

19. Ibid., 27–28.

20. Ibid., 29.

21. U.S. Bureau of the Census, *Methods and Materials,* 472.

22. Saunders, *Basic Demographic Measures,* 30–32.

23. U.S. Bureau of the Census, *Methods and Materials,* 473.

24. Haupt and Kane, *Population Handbook,* 29.

25. Ibid.

26. Ewbank and Wray, "Population and Public Health," 1508.

27. U.S. Bureau of the Census, *Methods and Materials,* 579.

28. Ibid.

29. Haupt and Kane, *Population Handbook,* 48.

30. Saunders, *Basic Demographic Measures,* 21–24.

31. Haupt and Kane, *Population Handbook,* 50.

32. S.K. Smith, "How To Tally Temporary Population," *American Demographics,* July 1987, 44–45.

33. Haupt and Kane, *Population Handbook,* 54.

34. Ibid., 55.

35. World Population Data Sheet.

36. M.J. Batutis, "Estimating Population: I," *American Demographics* 4 (April 1982): 3–5.

37. M.J. Batutis, "Estimating Population: II," *American Demographics* 4 (May 1982): 38–40.

38. Batutis, "Estimating Population I," 3–5.

39. R.C. Atchley, "A Short-Cut Method for Estimating the Population of Metropolitan Areas," *Journal of the American Institute of Planners* 34 (1968): 259–262.

40. L.F. Bouvier, "Estimating Post-Censal Populations of Counties," *Journal of the American Institute of Planners* 37 (1971), 45–46.

41. Ibid.

42. U.S. Bureau of the Census, *Methods and Materials,* 752.

43. W.P. O'Hare, "How to Evaluate Population Estimates," *American Demographics* 10 (January 1988): 50–52.

44. J.V. Grauman, "Population Estimates and Projections," in *The Study of Population,* ed. P.M. Hauser and O.D. Duncan (Chicago: University of Chicago Press, 1959), 544–574.

45. Haupt and Kane, *Population Handbook,* 11.

46. U.S. Bureau of the Census, *Methods and Materials,* 771.

47. D.A. Kruekeberg and A.L. Silvers, *Urban Planning Analysis, Methods and Models* (New York: John Wiley & Sons, Inc., 1974), 259–273.

48. R. Irwin, "Methods on Data Sources for Population Projections of Small Areas," in *Population Forecasting for Small Areas,* proceedings of a conference of Oak Ridge (Tenn.) Associated Universities, October 1977, 15–26.

49. Statistics Canada, *How Communities Can Use Statistics* (Ottawa: Minister of Supply and Services, June 1981), 53.

50. C. Haub, "Understanding Population Projections," *Population Bulletin* 42, no. 4 (December 1987): 25.

51. F. Jill Charboneau, "The Best 100 Sources for Marketing Information: Who's Who from *American Demographics,*" *American Demographics* 11 (1989): 52.

52. Metropolitan Life Insurance Company, "Changes in the Age Profile of the Population," *Statistical Bulletin* 62, no. 3 (July/September 1981): 12.

53. Alvin P. Sanoff, "As Americans Cope with a Changing Population," *U.S. News & World Report,* 9 August 1982, 27.

54. J.A. Weed, "Divorce: Americans' Style," *American Demographics,* March 1982, 12–17.

55. Haupt and Kane, *Population Handbook,* 26.

56. L.Y. Jones, *Great Expectations: America and the Baby Boom Generation* (New York: Ballantine Books, 1982), 512.

57. C.L. Harter, "The 'Good Times' Cohort of the 1930s," *Population Reference Bureau Report* 3, no. 3 (April 1977): 4.

58. L.F. Bouvier, "America's Baby Boom Generation: The Fateful Bulge," *Population Bulletin* 35, no. 1 (April 1980): 17.

59. Ibid., 15.

60. M. Greenwald, "Bad News for the Baby Boom," *American Demographics* 11, no. 2 (February 1989): 34–37.

61. Beth J. Soldo, "America's Elderly in the 1980s," *Population Bulletin* 35, no. 4 (November 1980): 3.

62. Ibid., 7.

63. U.S. Public Health Service, *Health, United States, 1988* (Hyattsville, Md.: U.S. Department of Health and Human Services, National Center for Health Statistics, 1989), 61.

64. Ibid.

65. Ibid.

66. Metropolitan Life Insurance Company, "Health of the Elderly," *Statistical Bulletin* 63, no. 1 (January/March 1982): 3.

67. W.E. Hale et al., "Screening for Hypertension in an Elderly Population: Report from the Dunedin Program," *Journal of the American Geriatrics Society* 29 (1981): 123–125.

68. J.G. Ouslander and J.C. Beck, "Defining the Health Problems of the Elderly," *Annual Review of Public Health* 3 (1982): 55–83.

69. Metropolitan Life Insurance Company, "Older America's Health," *Statistical Bulletin* 69, no. 2 (April/June 1988): 10–16.

70. Ouslander and Beck, "Defining Health Problems," 65.

71. Soldo, "America's Elderly," 18.

72. L.O. Stone and S. Fletcher, *A Profile of Canada's Older Population* (Montreal: The Institute for Research on Public Policy, 1980), 39.

73. Ouslander and Beck, "Defining Health Problems," 60.

74. M.P. Stern, "The Recent Decline in Ischemic Heart Disease Mortality," *Annals of Internal Medicine* 91 (1979): 630–640.

75. J.F. Fries, "Aging, Natural Death, and the Compression of Morbidity," *The New England Journal of Medicine* 303, no. 3 (July 1980): 130–135.

76. L.G. Martin, "The Graying of Japan," *Population Bulletin* 44, no. 2 (July 1989): 43.

77. Ibid., 16.

78. J.D. Kasper, *Aging Alone—Profiles and Projections* (Baltimore: Report of the Commonwealth Fund, 1988), 26.

79. A.R. Somers, "Demographics Can Help Guide Health Policy," *Hospitals* 54 (May 1980): 67–72.

80. Soldo, "America's Elderly," 19–21.

81. Fries, "Aging, Natural Death," 130–135.

82. L.M. Verbrugge, "A Life and Death Paradox," *American Demographics* 10, no. 7 (July 1988): 34–37.

83. M. O'Connell and D.E. Bloom, "Juggling Jobs and Babies: America's Child Care Challenge," *Population Trends and Public Policy* 12 (February 1987): 9.

84. R.L. Sivard. *Women: A World Survey* (Washington, D.C.: World Pictures, 1985): 44.

85. Ibid., 39.

Chapter 7

Health Status Indicators and Indexes

The development of health status goals and objectives is essential to the construction of meaningful community health status indicators and indexes. The development of healthy public policy, as discussed in Chapter 2, is a prerequisite to the formulation of health status goals and objectives. The epidemiological model, together with a healthy public policy, outlines policy direction and analysis for the organization. The most beneficial aspect of these approaches is that they may be applied on a disease-by-disease or on a communitywide basis to provide information for program management and policy analysis.

HEALTH STATUS GOALS AND OBJECTIVES

It is impossible to develop responsible and realistic objectives without analyzing the community's population groups and the health services presently available to them. The major purpose of a community needs assessment by a health organization, therefore, is to determine (1) the characteristics and health status of the area's population, (2) the characteristics of existing health systems, (3) the areas that have the greatest potential for positive change, and (4) the health services that should receive priority in the health plan.[1] This needs assessment and the policy analysis of the social/epidemiological data are necessary in order to permit the construction of explicit statements of goals and objectives. Such an approach, embodying a healthy public policy that includes the concepts of holism and wellness, must guide the selection of health status indicators and indexes. (See Figures 2-1 and 2-2.)

In an approach of this type, the association of health status statistics with lifestyle, environment, education, socioeconomic factors, and biology will be useful in assessing the effect of the health services (health system goals) on the health and well-being (health status goals) of the population. Although it is not always easy to make such an association, an integrated statistical system is required.

The terms *goal* and *objective* have different meanings, cause indecisive debates, and involve time-consuming procedures. Program plans have been delayed six months or more because of an inability to reach a consensus on the definitions of these terms. Clarification of the terms is essential to the process of establishing meaningful health status measures.

> *Goals* are expressions of desired conditions of health status and health systems expressed as quantifiable, timeless aspirations. Goals should be both technically and financially achievable and responsive to community ideals.[2]

> *Objectives* should be prepared for goals which have been identified as high priority. Objectives generated from the goals contained in the health plan should express particular levels of expected achievements in health status or health system by a specific year.[3]

National Goals for the Year 2000

The U.S. Department of Health and Human Services (DHHS) has proposed five broad national goals for the year 2000 "to serve as overall measures of the Nation's health. Improvements in these measures will reflect the summed success of health promotion and disease prevention efforts."[4]

1. Reduce infant mortality to no more than 7 deaths per 1,000 live births.
2. Increase life expectancy to at least 78 years.
3. Reduce disability caused by chronic conditions to a prevalence of no more than 6 percent of all people.
4. Increase years of healthy life to at least 65 years.
5. Decrease disparity in life expectancy between white and minority populations to no more than 4 years.[5]

Furthermore, the DHHS noted that,

> although some continuity with the goals of the previous decade has been maintained, the goals for the year 2000 also reflect an increased emphasis on reducing preventable morbidity and disability, reducing health disparities between population groups, and improving the quality not just the quantity of life.[6]

The process of determining the goals and objectives for the year 2000 was a function of several national efforts completed over the past few years. As a result of these efforts, 21 priority areas were identified to serve as the basis for the year 2000 objectives (Table 7-1). The areas are grouped into four broad categories that define the principal type of preventive intervention: health promotion, health protection, preventive services, and system improvement. Within each of these groups and areas, there are five types of specific objectives.

1. *Health Status*—targets to reduce death, disease, and disability.
2. *Risk Reduction*—targets to reduce the prevalence or incidence of risks to health or to increase behaviors known to reduce such risks.
3. *Public Awareness*—targets to increase public awareness about health risks and/or appropriate preventive interventions.
4. *Professional Education and Awareness*—targets to increase the numbers of professionals aware of, trained to provide, and in some cases providing appropriate interventions.
5. *Services and Protection*—targets to increase comprehensiveness, accessibility, and/or quality of preventive services and protective interventions.[7]

Examples selected from the maternal and infant health priorities are presented in Exhibit 7-1.

The actual process of establishing health status goals and objectives involves several facets, depending on the current level of operations. In developing the draft year 2000 objectives, work groups were guided by the following eight criteria:[8]

1. *credibility.* Objectives should be realistic and should address the issues of greatest priority.
2. *public comprehension.* Objectives should be understandable and relevant to a broad audience, including those who plan, manage, deliver, use, and pay for health services.
3. *balance.* Objectives should be a mixture of outcome and process measures, recommending methods for achieving changes and setting standards for evaluating progress.
4. *measurability.* Objectives should be quantified.
5. *continuity.* Year 2000 objectives should be linked to the 1990 objectives where possible, but reflect the lessons learned in implementing them.
6. *compatibility.* Objectives should be compatible where possible with goals already adopted by Federal agencies and health organizations.
7. *freedom from data constraints.* The availability or form of data should not be the principal determinant of the nature of the objectives. Alternate and proxy data should be used when necessary.

Table 7-1 Year 2000 National Health Objectives, Priority Areas, and Public Health Service Lead Agencies

Priority Areas	Lead Agencies
Health Promotion	
1. Nutrition	Food and Drug Administration National Institutes of Health
2. Physical activity and fitness	President's Council on Physical Fitness and Sports
3. Tobacco	Centers for Disease Control
4. Alcohol and other drugs	Alcohol, Drug Abuse, and Mental Health Administration
5. Sexual behavior	Office of Population Affairs
6. Violent and abusive behavior	Centers for Disease Control
7. Vitality and functional independence of older people	National Institutes of Health
Health Protection	
8. Environmental health	National Institutes of Health Centers for Disease Control
9. Occupational safety and health	Centers for Disease Control
10. Unintentional injuries	Centers for Disease Control
Preventive Services	
11. Maternal and infant health	Health Resources and Services Administration
12. Immunization and infectious diseases	Centers for Disease Control
13. Human immunodeficiency virus infection	National AIDS Program Office
14. Sexually transmitted diseases	Centers for Disease Control
15. High blood cholesterol and high blood pressure	National Institutes of Health
16. Cancer	National Institutes of Health
17. Other chronic disorders	National Institutes of Health Centers for Disease Control
18. Oral health	National Institutes of Health Centers for Disease Control
19. Mental and behavioral disorders	Alcohol, Drug Abuse, and Mental Health Administration
System Improvement	
20. Health education and preventive services	Health Resources and Services Administration Centers for Disease Control
21. Surveillance and data systems	Centers for Disease Control

Source: Reprinted from *MMWR*. Vol. 38, No. 37, p. 631, U.S. DHHS, 1989.

Exhibit 7-1 Summary of Selected Objectives To Improve Maternal and Infant Health by the Year 2000

Health Status

1. Reduce the infant mortality rate (deaths of infants under 1 year) to no more than 7 per 1,000 live births. (Baseline: 10.4 per 1,000 live births in 1986)
   (a) Among blacks: 11/1,000 live births. (18/1,000 in 1986)
   (b) Among American Indians/Alaska Natives: 9/1,000 live births. (An estimated 13.8/1,000 in 1986)
2. Reduce the neonatal mortality rate (deaths of infants under 28 days) to no more than 4.5 per 1,000 live births. (Baseline: 6.7 per 1,000 live births in 1986)
   Special Population Target
   (a) Among blacks: (7/1,000 in 1986)
3. Reduce the postneonatal mortality rate (deaths of infants ages 28 days up to 1 year) to no more than 2.5 per 1,000 live births. (Baseline: 3.6 per 1,000 live births in 1986)
   Special Population Targets
   (a) Among blacks: 4/1,000 live births. (6.3/1,000 in 1986)
   (b) Among American Indians/Alaska Natives: 4/1,000 live births. (5.3/1000 in 1986)
4. Reduce the fetal death rate (20 or more weeks of gestation) to no more than 5 per 1,000 live births plus fetal deaths. (Baseline: 7.7 per 1,000 live births plus fetal deaths in 1986)
   Special Population Target
   (a) Among blacks: 7.5/1,000 live births plus fetal deaths. (12.5/1,000 in 1986)
5. Reduce to no more than 1 per 1,000 the prevalence of HIV infection among women giving birth to live-born infants. (Baseline: Approximately 1.4 per 1,000 in 1989)
   Special Population Target
   (a) Among blacks: 5/1,000 live births to black women. (18.8/1,000 in 1986)
6. Reduce to no more than 1 per 1,000 the prevalence of HIV infection among women giving birth to live-born infants. (Baseline: Approximately 1.4 per 1,000 in 1989)

Risk Reduction

7. Reduce low birth weight (less than 2,500 grams) to an incidence of no more than 5 percent of live births. (Baseline: 6.8 percent in 1986)
   Special Population Target
   (a) Among blacks: 9 percent of live births. (12.5 percent in 1986)
8. Reduce very low birth weight (less than 1,500 grams) to an incidence of no more than 1 percent of live births. (Baseline: 1.21 percent in 1986)
   Special Population Target
   (a) Among blacks: 2 percent of live births (2.66 percent in 1986)
9. Reduce severe complications of pregnancy to no more than 15 percent of live births, as measured by antenatal hospitalizations due to pregnancy-related complications. (Baseline: 24 percent of live births in 1986)

Source: Reprinted from *Promoting Health, Preventing Disease: Year 2000 Objectives for the Nation,* p. 11.3, U.S. DHHS, 1989.

8. *responsibility.* The objectives should reflect the concerns and engage the participation of professionals, advocates, and consumers,
as well as State and local health departments.

Presumably, the final document of goals and objectives will be stated as compre-
hensively as the draft document of goals and objectives.

Blum suggested that the analytical steps in qualitative goal analysis should
depend on whether the planning body has decided (1) to set a qualitative goal for
all (broadened to reflect the holistic model, that is, wellness) or (2) to study the
present delivery system in terms of the community problem that warrants priority.[9] These two approaches should be dovetailed. The use of the holistic model
entails the definition of quantitative goals related to the qualitative goals of good
care and wellness. With such an approach, each problem can be analyzed to
develop prevention and intervention measures to attack the causes and consequences of a disease. Not only do the objectives for the year 2000 appear to meet
Blum's concerns, but also the criteria developed by the task force are excellent
guides in the determination of appropriate and reasonable objectives.

Quantitative Goals and Objectives

A realistic level of attainment of goals and objectives may be determined on
the basis of committee or professional opinion as to what the level of attainment
should be, or it may be determined quantitatively by applying general, promulgated standards, such as national averages. The use of generally promulgated
standards to establish goal and objective levels has several advantages.[10]

1. Such standards serve as a quick reference to what is regarded as adequate.
2. By comparing standards to local conditions, local areas that fall significantly short of desired levels can demonstrate health gaps.
3. By comparing multiple health gaps (revealed by standards), a community
can identify gaps that are proportionately worse and, thus, may deserve
priority.
4. National standards are capable of demonstrating meaningful comparisons
of what "is" versus what "could be" or "should be."
5. Community comparisons of national standards can provide impetus to the
measurement of health status.

It is imperative that trends or standards be determined for specified health status
measures. Professional and committee opinion, a review of past trends, and
promulgated standards may all reveal appropriate targets or standards for the attainment of objectives.

When setting objectives, analysts must keep in mind that a rate may change within probability limits based on the standard deviation of the variables over time. For example, the use of an absolute value of 3 percent for a specific variable is misleading if a ± 1.00 standard deviation for the data set of observations is 1.5 percent. In this case, a more valid objective is a range of 1.5 to 4.5 percent. Many of the national objectives listed for the year 2000 include an effort to account for such potential variation. For instance, the observed data include the baseline, a trend is provided, a projection is made, and, finally, a target for the year 2000 is recommended (Fig. 7-1). Readjustment of objectives in the light of unforeseen issues that surface and affect the program is always feasible.

Kinds of Goals and Objectives

The selection of goals and objectives for inclusion in a health plan requires careful considerations. First, such goals and objectives are direct consequences of the adopted health policy (wellness and holistic). If the health policy is comprehensive (i.e., a healthy public policy)—including elements of the environment, human biology, lifestyle, education, socioeconomic factors, environment, and system of medical care organization—the goals and objectives should reflect

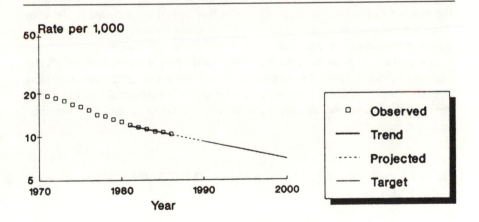

Infant mortality (logarithmic scale)

Note: **By the year 2000, reduce mortality to no more than 7 deaths per 1,000 live births.** (Baseone: In 1986, the infant mortality rate was 10.4 per 1,000 live births.)

Figure 7–1 Example of a Year 2000 Objective. *Source:* Reprinted from *Promoting Health, Preventing Disease: Year 2000 Objectives for the Nation,* p. 7, U.S. DHHS 1989.

such a policy. In the near future, however, the health agency must concentrate on more nontraditional goals and objectives. Those goals and objectives that have a decisive impact on changing disease patterns should have high priority. Second, national priorities should dictate to a health agency the types of goals and objectives to be included in the health plan. Third, a community needs assessment is necessary to identify disease and social patterns (i.e., problems that affect public health policy) for each health service or geographical area. Thus, the kinds of goals and objectives included in the plan are a function of the health agency's policy, national priorities, and a needs assessment—all of which form a very dynamic process.

Numbers of Goals and Objectives

There is no magic formula to determine how many goals and objectives should be listed in a health plan. One rational approach is based on the extent to which disease morbidity and mortality and social problems are crippling and killing the selected population. Proportional mortality ratios or specific death rates associated with such features as cause, age, sex, or race are health status indicators that may make it possible to set priorities and thereby limit the number of health goals and objectives within the plan. Other considerations, however, also affect the number of health goals and objectives that should be included in the plan. After determining proportional mortality ratios and specific death rates, for example, it is necessary to take into account a community's resources.

Not all national goals and priorities will become part of each community's plan because, obviously, not all problems are distributed evenly in the country. Thus, a needs assessment at the community level is critical to the process of identifying the number of goals and objectives that are appropriate to the problems identified in the community.

DEVELOPMENT OF HEALTH STATUS INDICATORS AND INDEXES

To measure the extent to which stated health status goals and objectives have been achieved, it is necessary to develop indicators and, if possible, an index relating to health status. The difference between a health status indicator and a health status index can be seen in the following definitions:

- A health status indicator is a single measure that is obtained from a single component (variable) and purports to reflect the health status of an individual or defined group—for example, infant mortality rate, proportional mortality ratio.

- A health status index is a composite measure that summarizes data from two or more components (variables) and, like an indicator, purports to reflect the health status of an individual or defined group[11]—for example, a Z-score model or Gender Gap Index.

Criteria for Selection

Several criteria for a health status indicator or index must be considered before a specific type is chosen.[12] Although some of the data may be inappropriate and the measures of health status imperfect, the health agency must use the data, indicators, or indexes that are currently available. Consequently, the agency should use basic health status indicators or simplified applications of a health status index. Whichever approach is followed, it is important to comply with basic criteria for selecting appropriate indicators or an index to reflect the health status of the population being investigated. Failure to follow a standardized procedure for selecting a health status indicator or index will result in invalid comparisons or differences in results and, potentially, erroneous conclusions.

Data Availability. The mere existence of data does not ensure that they are ready for incorporation into a health plan. The manipulation required may be as simple as collapsing categories or as complex as abstracting subset categories. Generally, the data should not require additional detailed, complex investigations.

Level of Analysis. The unit of investigation or level of analysis must be specific enough to determine geographical variations of the phenomenon being studied (Table 7-2). Thus, if the universe to be investigated is a particular health service area, the level of analysis for investigation should be the township, enumeration district, other subcounty geographical area, or city.

Level of Measurement. In using a health status indicator or in providing summary statements (which are usually of more practical value than the complete distribution), the level of measurement is important. Four levels of measurement may characterize a set of data.[13]

1. *nominal.* In nominal data, one data element is distinguished from another, but no direction is implied. Examples include male and female; health service areas A, B, and C; and religion categories, such as Baptist, Lutheran, and Mormon. Nominal data may be displayed in bar charts and pie charts. Appropriate statistics are the mode and frequency counts.

Table 7-2 Levels of Analysis in Rank Order for Identifying Health Needs and Resources

Universe	Levels of Analysis for Investigation
World	Continents
Continent	Countries
Country	States
State	Counties
	Health Service Areas
County	Townships
Health Service Area	Enumeration Districts
	Cities
City	Neighborhoods
Neighborhood	Census Tracts
Census Tract	Blocks
Block	Households
Household	Families
Family	Individuals

2. *ordinal.* In ordinal data, the data items are ranked. The level shows that one value is more or less than another value, but does not indicate by how much. For example, health service areas may be ranked according to high, medium, or low socioeconomic status. Appropriate statistics include the median, percentile, Spearman r_s, and Kendall$_\tau$.
3. *interval.* In interval data, the data items are characterized by identical distance between adjacent points on a scale. Interval scales reflect not only the number of points between two values, but also direction. Appropriate statistics are the mean, standard deviation, Pearson product-moment correlation, multiple correlation, and t and F tests.
4. *ratio.* Because the ratio is represented by a true zero, a value of 20 can be conceived as being twice the value of 10. Ratio measurement is the highest level of measurement, and any statistical test is usable. Appropriate statistics that require knowledge of true zero are the geometric mean and the coefficient of variation.

Data Quality. Every effort should be made to ensure that the data represent comparable time periods and geographical areas. The planner should carefully examine the data for gaps that may be detrimental to their usefulness.

Comprehensiveness. The health status index may cover a broad range of diseases and conditions that have a decided impact on the health levels of a population (e.g., a Q index), or it may focus on a specific disease and all risk factors associated with that disease (e.g., a regression model). It should be clear, however, that such an index indicates only a general level of well-being, and its application to program evaluation, resource allocation, and the setting of goals and objectives is limited.

Specificity. The health status index should be as disease-specific as possible. It is recommended that an index relate to a specific population subgroup, such as an infant health status index.[14] The more specific the index, the more useful it will be in program analysis and resource allocation.

Indicator or Index Calculation. The indicator or index should be calculated by the simplest method feasible. It should not be expensive in terms of resources required.

Usefulness. If an indicator or index is to have maximum utility, it should be widely accepted and easily reproduced. Above all, it must have practical applicability.

Data Requirements for Health Status Measurement

The adoption of the wellness or holistic approach to planning for health will make it necessary to consider the use of nontraditional, as well as traditional, data for health status measurement. Therefore, health data must be available to reflect broad categories, such as community health status, the health system, lifestyle, human biology, the environment, social indicators, and overall quality of life.[15,16] Within these categories there is a need for specific data sets.

- Community health status data. These data provide a community health diagnosis. Although these traditional health status indicators reflect deeply entrenched belief systems, they are important for developing indicators for acceptable goals and objectives. Appropriate measures include
  1. mortality rates
  2. disability rates (workday loss)
  3. incidence and prevalence of specific diseases
  4. morbidity rates
- Health system data. Changes in lifestyle, biology, and the environment will affect health status and, in turn, the health system. The health system will also have a limited impact on health status. Selected specific categories of health system data are
  1. health service utilization data
     (a) hospital admissions
     (b) discharges
     (c) visits for ambulatory care
     (d) patient origin data

(e) residential data

(f) accessibility in terms of geographical, economic, and cultural factors, or distance to facilities in terms of time, mileage, social aspects, and cost

2. facility and management data (availability)

(a) institutional resources, such as hospital beds, nursing homes, health access stations (primary care), and county health departments

(b) human resources, such as physicians, nurses, dentists, and other essential personnel

3. cost data

(a) diagnosis and care costs

(b) indirect costs of lost wages and lost productivity

(c) indirect costs attributed to investment in individuals, that is, premature illness or death

(d) government subsidies, such as Medicare and Medicaid

● Lifestyle data. Generally, but not always, lifestyle or health behavior data must be collected by a survey instrument.

1. reasons for seeking health care

2. barriers to health care

3. spatial restrictions

4. lifestyle components, such as drugs, nutrition, carelessness (alcohol, driving behavior), and risk taking (smoking, obesity, level of exercise)

5. marriage

6. divorce

● Human biology data. These data are necessary to identify target groups at risk of a disease or to provide health information via health marketing, promotion, and awareness programs.

1. demographic characteristics, such as age, sex, race, and ethnic group

2. genetic risks

3. intelligence

● Environmental data

1. air, water, and soil conditions (toxic wastes)

2. general climatic conditions

3. prevalence of rats and other pests that present disease risks

4. general environmental quality

5. housing data to reflect the quality and type of housing

(a) crowding

(b) plumbing facilities

(c) social restrictions due to inadequate planning

(d) psychological needs and satisfactions

(e) neighborhood quality

6. occupational health

● Socioeconomic indicators data
1. income, distribution of wealth, employment status, poverty levels, and income supplements
2. living environment, including housing, the neighborhood, and the physical environment
3. physical and mental health
4. education in terms of achievement, duration, quality (literacy), and dropout rates
5. social order (or disorganization) indicated by personal pathologies, family breakdown, crime and delinquency, and public order and safety
6. social belonging (alienation and participation) reflected in democratic participation, criminal justice, and segregation/desegregation
7. recreation and leisure in terms of facilities, culture and the arts, and leisure available[17-19]

The health agency should use this list of data requirements as a guide to present and future data needs. Data in some of the categories will not be available for some time; until they are, the agency should concentrate on the more traditional categories.

Types of Health Status Indicators

Many indicators have been developed to measure the health status of a population. Some are simple and easily applied, while others are quite advanced and require considerable sophistication. By applying the definition of a health status indicator cited earlier to a review of the types of indicators available, a health agency can choose an indicator that is consistent with its skills and abilities.

Age-Specific Death Rates

Differences in the magnitude of age-specific death rates in time and place suggest "poor" and "good" areas of health status. This type of rate approximates the risk of death from a specific condition and is perhaps the most important epidemiological indicator available. It may be expanded to include rates specific to other factors (e.g., sex, race, occupation, cause), as well as adjusted or standardized rates. The crude rate and the adjusted rate can be compared to the state rates for a particular disease category. If the crude rate of a county or a community has been stable for several years, a community diagnosis can be determined by comparing it with the adjusted rate (Table 7-3).

To obtain an age-adjusted rate, for example, the age-specific rate is multiplied by a factor that is the proportion of population of each group in a standard million. The standard chosen should closely resemble the population being investi-

Table 7-3 Community Health Diagnosis Using Crude and Adjusted Rates

Relative Crude Rate	Status of Adjusted Rate	Community Diagnosis
Low	Low	Low mortality is not due to age, race, and sex factors; other mortality conditions are favorable.
Low	High	Low mortality is due to favorable age, race, and sex factors; other mortality conditions are unfavorable.
High	Low	High mortality is due to unfavorable age, race, and sex factors; other mortality conditions are favorable.
High	High	High mortality is not due to age, race, and sex factors; other mortality conditions are unfavorable.

Source: Reprinted from *North Carolina Vital Statistics*, Vol. 2, p. 8, 1977.

Table 7-4 Age-Adjusted Death Rate for Cancer, Utah, 1972–1976

Age Group	Average Deaths	Age Group Population	Age-Specific Rate*	Proportion of Population in a Standard Million	Expected Deaths*
	(1)	(2)	(3)	(4)	(5)
≤4	6.2	132,459	4.6807	.08536	.3995
5–9	7.2	115,683	6.2239	.09931	.6181
10–14	5.0	121,299	4.1220	.10346	.4265
15–19	8.8	128,005	6.8747	.09350	.6428
20–24	8.8	120,715	7.2899	.07600	.5540
25–29	12.8	101,072	12.6642	.06569	.8320
30–34	11.4	74,362	15.3304	.05593	.8575
35–39	14.2	59,477	23.8748	.05436	1.2980
40–44	24.6	54,896	44.8120	.05922	2.6542
45–49	49.0	55,091	88.9437	.06011	5.3464
50–54	79.2	52,986	149.4734	.05517	8.2474
55–59	105.8	48,295	219.0703	.04961	10.8694
60–64	132.6	40,204	329.8179	.04288	14.1432
65–69	168.4	32,824	513.0392	.03479	17.8511
70–74	158.4	24,021	659.4230	.02709	17.8643
75–79	144.2	17,336	831.7951	.01907	15.8694
80–84	118.0	10,322	1,142.1893	.01136	12.9975
85+	83.6	6,196	1,349.2576	.00700	9.4485
		State Age-Adjusted Death Rate		(6)*	120.9198

*(3) = (1)/(2) · 100,000 = Age-Specific Rate; (5) = (4) · (3) = Expected Deaths; (6) = sum of all values of (5) = Age-Adjusted Death Rate.

gated. Multiplying the factor by the age-specific rate gives the number of expected deaths, and the sum of all expected deaths provides the age-adjusted death rate. This is the direct method of computation (Table 7-4). The resulting state rates are those that can be expected. Differences found in the adjusted rates must be due to differences in age-specific rates. Table 7-5 shows the advantages and disadvantages of crude, specific, and adjusted rates as health status indicators.

Proportional Mortality Ratio

Because it refers to total deaths, not to the population at risk, the proportional mortality ratio is not a rate. The ratio indicates what proportion of deaths is attributable to a specific disease. It is useful because it permits an estimation of the number of lives that may be saved by reducing a given cause of death. The proportional mortality ratio may be calculated by (1) dividing the number of deaths from a given cause in a specified period by the total number of deaths in the same time period and (2) multiplying the result by 100.

Table 7-5 Advantages and Disadvantages of Using Crude, Specific, and Adjusted Rates for Health Status Indicators

Health Status Indicators	Advantages	Disadvantages
Crude rates	Easy to calculate. Summary rates. Widely used for international comparisons (despite limitations).	Because population groups vary in age, sex, race, etc., the differences in crude rates are not directly interpretable.
Specific rates	Applied to homogeneous subgroups. The detailed rates are useful for epidemiological and public health purposes.	Comparisons can be cumbersome, if many subgroups are calculated for two or more populations.
Adjusted rates	Represents a summary rate. Differences in composition of groups reviewed, allowing unbiased comparison.	Not true rates (fictional). Magnitude of rates is dependent upon the standard million population chosen. Trends in subgroups can be masked.

Source: Adapted from *Epidemiology: An Introductory Text* by J. S. Mausner and A. K. Bahn, p. 138, with permission of W. B. Saunders Company, © 1974.

Indicator of Unnecessary Deaths

Using mortality data, it is possible to calculate an indicator of unnecessary deaths.[20,21] This indicator is useful in demonstrating variations between death rates in two populations. The indicator is simply the difference between an expected death rate and the actual death rate of the population under study:

$$UD = DR_A - DR_E$$

where UD = Unnecessary deaths

DR_A = Actual death rate

DR_E = Expected death rate

In the case of an infant mortality rate in a county where the state is selected as a standard, for example

$$UD_{County} = DR_A \text{ (county)} - DR_E \text{ (state)}$$

To make statistically valid comparisons, the death rates should be specific, although crude rates may be used if it is reasonably certain that the age and sex structures of the population under investigation are similar. The expected death rate may be the rate for the national, regional, or state population, or it could be another calculated rate.

The unnecessary death indicator may be quite useful to a health agency in setting objectives to reduce the number of such deaths and in determining the success of its programs. Because of the relatively clear expression of the frequency of deaths, the indicator may also serve as a tool to educate the community and to support resource allocation decisions. Finally, the indicator may also be used as a community-rating scale when various counties are compared to determine overall health statuses.

Years of Life Lost

Health planners can use the number of deaths at different ages from a specific cause, such as acute myocardial infarction, to calculate estimated total years of life lost[22,23] (Table 7-6). The years of potential life lost (YPLL) can be calculated by using age 65 as the end point (Table 7-7) or by using the total life expectancy remaining at the time of death as the end point (Table 7-8). (A comparison of these two methods to the crude mortality rate is presented in Table 7-9.)

The Centers for Disease Control suggested at least the following uses for YPLL:[24]

● Geographical variations can be a useful tool for health planning at the state or local level.

Table 7-6 Estimated Years of Life Lost from Acute Myocardial Infarction

Age Group	Deaths		Average Years of Life Lost*	Estimated Total Years of Life Lost
35–49	81	×	30	2,430
40–44	201	×	25	5,025
45–49	433	×	20	8,660
50–54	692	×	15	10,380
55–59	1,101	×	10	11,010
60–64	1,426	×	5	7,130
Total	3,934			44,635

*Based on a life expectancy of 69 years.

Table 7-7 Estimated Years of Potential Life Lost (YPLL) before Age 65 and Mortality, by Cause of Death, United States, 1984

Cause of Mortality (Ninth Revision ICD)	YPLL (in thousands) for Persons Dying in 1984	Cause-specific Mortality (Rate/100,000)
All causes Total	11,761	866.7
Unintentional injuries (E800-E949)	2,308	40.1
Malignant neoplasms (140-208)	1,803	191.6
Diseases of the heart (390-398, 402, 404-429)	1,563	324.4
Suicide and homicide (E950-E978)	1,247	20.6
Congenital anomalies (740-759)	684	5.6
Prematurity (765, 769)	470	3.0
Sudden infant death syndrome (798)	314	2.0
Cerebrovascular diseases (430-438)	266	65.6
Chronic liver diseases and cirrhosis (571)	233	11.3
Pneumonia and influenza (480-487)	163	25.0
Chronic obstructive pulmonary diseases (490-496)	123	29.8
Diabetes mellitus (250)	119	15.6

Source: Reprinted from *MMWR*, Vol. 35, No. 25, p. 25, U.S. DHHS, 1986.

Table 7-8 Estimated Years of Potential Life Lost (YPLL)* and Mortality, by Cause of Death in United States, 1984

Cause of Mortality (Ninth Revision ICD)	YPLL (in thousands) for Persons Dying in 1984	Cause-specific Mortality (Rate/100,000)
All causes (Total)	33,581	866.7
Diseases of the heart (390-398, 402, 404-429)	9,400	324.4
Malignant neoplasms (140-208)	7,171	191.6
Unintentional injuries (E800-E949)	3,381	40.1
Suicide and homicide (E950-E978)	1,833	20.6
Cerebrovascular diseases (430-438)	1,735	65.6
Chronic obstructive pulmonary diseases (490-496)	903	29.8
Congenital anomalies (740-759)	820	5.6
Pneumonia and influenza (480-487)	691	25.4
Chronic liver diseases and cirrhosis (571)	585	11.3
Prematurity (765, 769)	548	3.0
Diabetes mellitus (250)	525	15.6
Sudden infant death syndrome (798)	361	2.0

*Calculated by the remaining-life-expectancy method.

Source: Reprinted from MMWR, Vol. 35, No. 25, p. 35, U.S. DHHS, 1986.

- A delineation of the pattern of YPLL rates among varied populations can provide an accurate description of the causes of premature mortality for the persons at highest risk of premature death.
- State/local-specific rates of YPLL can be used for planning and evaluating local public health interventions.
- Efforts can be made to target and monitor those populations at highest risk.
- Information can be helpful in the establishment of research and resource priorities.

Table 7-9 Rankings of the 10 Leading Causes of Mortality and Years of Potential Life Lost (YPLL), by Method of Calculation, United States, 1984

Ranking	Crude Mortality Rate	YPLL—0–65 Years	YPLL—Life Expectancy
1	Heart disease	Unintentional injuries	Heart disease
2	Malignant neoplasms	Malignant neoplasms	Malignant neoplasms
3	Cerebrovascular disease	Heart disease	Unintentional injuries
4	Unintentional injuries	Suicide and homicide	Suicide and homicide
5	COPD*	Congenital anomalies	Cerebrovascular disease
6	Pneumonia/influenza	Prematurity	COPD
7	Suicide and homicide	Sudden infant death syndrome	Congenital anomalies
8	Diabetes	Cerebrovascular disease	Pneumonia/influenza
9	Cirrhosis	Cirrhosis	Cirrhosis
10	Congenital anomalies	Pneumonia/influenza	Diabetes

Source: Reprinted from *MMWR*, Vol. 35, No. 25, p. 45, U.S. DHHS, 1986.

- Temporal trends in premature mortality can be monitored.
- This simple approach makes it possible to target health education efforts to the sections of the general population most in need of public health interventions.

Additionally, this indicator may be applied to disability statistics to determine productive workday loss.

Health agencies may also use this type of analysis to set priorities in terms of specific ages and particular diseases. Goals and objectives may be established in terms of clear quantitative statements. Because the requisite data are usually readily available to an agency, this indicator should be easy to use.

Other Health Status Indicators

Several other measures are traditionally used as health status indicators. The general format for these indicators is a numerator over a denominator multiplied by a constant:

$$(x/y)(k)$$

where x, y, and k are defined as in Table 7-10.

Table 7-10 Health Status Indicators Most Frequently Used for Describing Natality, Morbidity, and Mortality

No.	Description of Indicator	Numerator (x)	Denominator (y)	Expressed per Number at Risk (k)
Natality				
1	Birth Rate Crude; specific for age of mother, sex of child, socioeconomic status, etc.	Number of live births reported during a given time interval	Estimated mid-interval population	1,000
2	Fertility Rate Crude; specific for age of mother, race, socioeconomic status, etc.	Number of live births reported during a given time interval	Estimated number of women in age group 15–44 years at mid-interval	1,000
3	Low Birth Weight Ratio Crude; specific for age of mother, race, socioeconomic area, etc.	Number of live births under 2,500 grams (or 5½ lbs.) during a given time interval	Number of live births reported during the same time interval	100 (%)
Morbidity				
1	Incidence Rate Crude by cause; specific for age, race, sex, socioeconomic area, state of disease, etc.	Number of new cases of a specified disease reported during a given time period	Estimated mid-interval population	Variable: 10^x where $x = 2, 3, 4, 5, 6$
2	Attack Rate Crude by cause; specific for age, race, socioeconomic area, etc.	Number of new cases of a specified disease reported during a specific time interval	Total population at risk during the same time interval	Variable: 10^x where $x = 2, 3, 4, 5, 6$
3	Point Prevalence Rate (Ratio) Crude by cause; specific for age, race, sex, socioeconomic area, stage of disease, etc.	Number of current cases, new and old, of a specified disease existing at a given point in time	Estimated population at the same point in time	Variable: 10^x where $x = 2, 3, 4, 5, 6$

Table 7-10 continued

No.	Description of Indicator	Numerator (x)	Denominator (y)	Expressed per Number at Risk (k)
4	Period (Case Load) Prevalence Rate (Ratio) Crude by cause; specific for age, race, sex, socioeconomic area, stage of disease, etc.	Number of current cases, new and old, of a specified disease occurring during a given time interval	Estimated mid-interval population	Variable: 10^x where $x = 2$, 3, 4, 5, 6

Mortality

No.	Description of Indicator	Numerator (x)	Denominator (y)	Expressed per Number at Risk (k)
1	Crude Death Rate Crude; specific for age, race, sex, socioeconomic area, etc.	Total number of deaths reported during a given time interval	Estimated mid-interval population	1,000
2	Cause-Specific Death Rate Crude by cause; specific for age, race, sex, socioeconomic area, etc.	Number of deaths assigned to a specific cause during a given time interval	Estimated mid-interval population	100,000
3	Proportional Mortality Ratio Crude by cause; specific for age, race, sex, socioeconomic area, etc.	Number of deaths assigned to a specific cause during a given time interval	Total number of deaths from all causes reported during the same interval	100 (%)
4	Case Fatality Rate (Ratio) Crude; specific for age, race, sex, socioeconomic area, etc.	Number of deaths assigned to a specific disease during a given time interval	Number of new cases of that disease reported during the same time interval	100 (%)
5	(a) Fetal Death Rate I Crude; specific for age of mother, race, socioeconomic area, etc.	Number of fetal deaths of 28 weeks or more gestation reported during a given time interval	Number of fetal deaths of 28 weeks or more gestation reported during the same time interval plus the number of live births occurring during the same time interval	1,000

continues

Table 7-10 continued

No.	Description of Indicator	Numerator (x)	Denominator (y)	Expressed per Number at Risk (k)
	(b) Fetal Death Rate II Crude; specific for age of mother, race, socioeconomic area, etc.	Number of fetal deaths of 20 weeks or more gestation reported during a given time interval	Number of fetal deaths of 20 weeks or more gestation reported during the same time interval plus the number of live births occurring during the same time interval	1,000
6	(a) Fetal Death Ratio I Crude; specific for age of mother, race, socioeconomic area, etc.	Number of fetal deaths of 28 weeks or more gestation reported during a given time interval	Number of live births reported during the same time interval	1,000
	(b) Fetal Death Ratio II Crude, specific for age of mother, race, socioeconomic area, etc.	Number of fetal deaths of 20 weeks or more gestation reported during a given time interval	Number of live births reported during the same time interval	1,000
7	(a) Perinatal Mortality Rate I Crude; specific for age of mother, race, etc.	Number of fetal deaths of 28 weeks or more gestation reported during a given time interval plus the reported number of infant deaths under 7 days of life during the same time interval	Number of fetal deaths of 28 weeks or more gestation reported during the same time interval plus the number of live births occurring during the same time interval	1,000
	(b) Perinatal Mortality Rate II Crude; specific for age of mother, sex, socioeconomic area, etc.	Number of fetal deaths of 20 weeks or more gestation reported during a given time interval plus the reported number of infant	Number of fetal deaths of 20 weeks or more gestation reported during the same time interval plus the number of live births occurring	1,000

Table 7-10 continued

No.	Description of Indicator	Numerator (x)	Denominator (y)	Expressed per Number at Risk (k)
		deaths under 28 days of life during the same time interval	during the same time interval	
8	Infant Mortality Rate Crude; specific for race, sex, socioeconomic area, birth weight, cause of death, etc.	Number of deaths under one year of age reported during a given time interval	Number of live births reported during the same time interval	1,000
9	Neonatal Mortality Rate Crude; specific for race, sex, socioeconomic area, birth weight, cause of death, etc.	Number of deaths under 28 days of age reported during a given time interval	Number of live births reported during the same time interval	1,000
10	Postneonatal Mortality Rate Crude; specific for race, sex, socioeconomic area, cause of death, etc.	Number of deaths from 28 days of age up to, but not including, one year of age, reported during a given time interval	Number of live births reported during the same time interval	1,000
11	Maternal Mortality Rate Crude; specific for age of mother, race, socioeconomic area, etc.	Number of deaths assigned to causes related to pregnancy during a given time interval	Number of live births reported during the same time interval	10,000

Source: Reprinted from *Descriptive Statistics, Rates, Ratios, Proportions, and Indices*, pp. 3–8, U.S. DHHS, CDC.

Types of Health Status Indexes

Where possible, health agencies should develop health indexes to provide a composite description of health status. Such indexes have several uses for community and individual diagnosis (Table 7-11). They may be used to demonstrate community health status on a community rating scale (e.g., the index derived from regression analysis). A health index may also be used as a baseline or

Table 7-11 Uses of Health Status Indexes

Use	Community	Individual
Comparison	Social indicators	Clinical status
Evaluation	Program trials	Clinical trials, peer review
Allocation	Program planning	Patient management
Baseline measurement	Program planning	Patient management

Source: Adapted from *Health Services Research*, Vol. 8, No. 2, p. 154, with permission of the Hospital Research and Educational Trust, © 1973.

benchmark measure if the methodology is standardized so that future comparisons will be valid.

To be useful, an index must satisfy certain practical requirements. It must be simple in construction, use, and application. It should be acceptable to both respondents and users. It should be economical and make use of available data or data that are readily gathered. Clearly, under these requirements and under the definition of health index given earlier, many forms of indexes can be constructed. For any index, however, four points should be considered.

1. What is the purpose of the index?
2. What are the exact components of the index?
3. What is the form of interpretation?
4. What are the limitations of the index?

There has been a great deal of concern about health-status index development.[25] The general impression of the state of the art in the development of health status indexes is one of ferment. Some work is methodologically sophisticated; some is naive. Certain approaches offer immediate programmatic uses; others appear too complex or conceptually confused to be used readily in policy analysis and planning. One lesson is clear: solid results require competent methodological input.

Berger pointed out that the measurement of health status has changed through the years.[26] In the early 1960s, mortality was the key indicator; in the late 1960s, morbidity became the important indicator of health status measurement. The 1970s produced aggregated indexes that made use of population level data and indexes that focused on dysfunction and disability. The future role of community analysts in health status measurements is likely to involve the aggregation of other health indicators into a single index; the utilization of weights and specific preferences for health states; and the wider use of health status measures for resource allocation, evaluation, program delivery, and certainly health care planning.

Wellness Appraisal Index

The data from a wellness index developed for individuals may be aggregated to reflect populations at a small-area analysis level. The wellness index centers on the four main components of self-responsibility, nutrition, stress control, and physical awareness.[27] From several detailed questionnaires on these four components, the answers to 16 wellness index questions can be summarized (Table 7-12). The responses of "rarely," "sometimes," or "very often" may also be portrayed graphically. Figure 7-2 shows a blank pie chart, divided into quarters that represent the four dimensions of wellness. The inner broken circle corresponds to "rarely," the middle broken circle to "sometimes," and the outer broken circle to "very often." When a person fills in the appropriate areas according to the answers to each question, the resulting shape on the figure provides an evaluation of that person's level of wellness.

This approach may be modified by inserting percentages to broaden the categories beyond "rarely," "sometimes," and "very often." The result is a numerical index that, through a minor statistical analysis, reflects levels of wellness for population groups. For example, a health agency can apply this wellness evaluation to the employees in a section or unit to determine the overall level of wellness in the organization. If the results reveal any problems, the director can provide the employees with appropriate solutions. Simple telephone or newspaper surveys utilizing this approach can provide results or measures on a community basis. This health status index on wellness is obviously consistent with the epidemiological model and the development of a healthy public policy.

Health Risk Appraisal Index

Also based on wellness and holistic principles is the health risk appraisal index. The basic aim of a health risk appraisal is to obtain information from individuals concerning their personal lifestyles. In each case, an attainable age is calculated based on responses to the questions. To help individuals reach their attainable ages, recommendations may include more exercise, cessation of smoking, and the loss of weight, with benefits measured in years. If known, certain medical facts, such as blood pressure, cholesterol level, and triglyceride levels, are also weighted in the final recommendations.

In a community survey, the health risk appraisal may be administered to a random sample in a health service area that encompasses several counties. Questions may address the average risk reduction by county, the average benefit in years from an exercise program, and the average patient risk by county for comparable age and sex groups. Essentially, this procedure is an application of an individual clinical questionnaire to a community population. The results from each county can be tabulated and an index constructed.

Table 7-12 Wellness Appraisal Index: Questions and Evaluation Criteria

Area	Question No.	Wellness Evaluation Questions	Categories	Evaluation Criteria	Survey Instrument	Response
Nutrition	1	I am conscious of the food ingredients I eat and their effect on me.	R, S, VO	Conscious about nutrition	Eating Habits Survey (64 questions)	VO
	2	I avoid overeating and abusing alcohol, caffeine, nicotine, and other drugs.	R, S, VO	Awareness of overuse of substances	Eating Habits Survey	VO
	3	I minimize my intake of refined carbohydrates and fats.	R, S, VO	Reduced carbohydrate and fat intake	Computerized Nutrition Survey	VO
	4	My diet contains adequate amounts of vitamins, minerals, and fiber.	R, S, VO	Adequacy of vitamins, minerals, fiber	Computerized Nutrition Survey	S
Physical awareness	5	I am free from physical symptoms.	R = >10 S = 5-10 VO = <5	Absence of physical symptoms	Symptom Checklist	VO
	6	I get aerobic cardiovascular exercise.	R, S VO = 12-20 min. 5 times/ wk.	Aerobic exercise level (running, swimming, bicycling)	Wellness Inventory	VO
	7	I practice yoga or some other form of limbering/stretching exercise	R, S, VO	Body flexibility and training	Wellness Inventory	S
	8	I nurture myself. (Nurturing means pleasuring and taking care of oneself; e.g., massages, long walks, buying presents for oneself, sleeping late without feeling guilty.)	R, S, VO	Awareness of self-nurturing	Wellness Resource Book (Part 3) Survey Questions	R

Stress control	9	I pay attention to changes occurring in my life and am aware of them as stress factors. (A score of 300 from the Life Change Index is considered very stressful.)	R, S, VO	In control of life changes	Life Change Index	S
	10	I practice relaxation regularly. (20 minutes a day, "centering" or "letting go" of thoughts, worries, etc.)	R, S, VO	Regular relaxation needs		R
	11	I am without excess muscle tension.	R, S, VO	Levels of muscle tension, stress	Body Stress Assessment	S
	12	My hands are warm and dry.	R, S, VO	Tense, uptight	Body Stress Assessment	VO
Self-responsibility	13	I am both productive and happy.	R, S, VO	Productivity and aliveness	Wellness Resource Book (Part I)	VO
	14	I constructively express my emotions and creativity.	R, S, VO	Enlightenment and happiness	Wellness Resource Book (Part 6)	VO
	15	I feel a sense of purpose in life, and my life has meaning and direction.	R, S, VO	Purpose in life directed and clear	Purpose in Life Test	VO
	16	I believe I am fully responsible for my wellness or illness.	R, S, VO	Locus of control internal versus external	Wellness Work Book (Part 4) Summary Questions	VO

R = Rarely, S = Sometimes, VO = Very Often.

Source: Adapted from *Wellness for Helping Professionals* by John W. Travis, with permission of the Wellness Associates, © 1977, 1981, 1990.

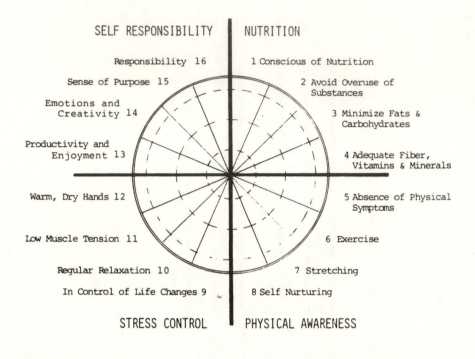

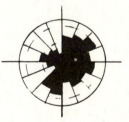

Completed Wellness
Appraisal Index Graph

Figure 7-2 Wellness Appraisal Index Graphs. *Source:* Reprinted from *Wellness for Helping Professionals* by John W. Travis, with permission of the Wellness Associates, © 1977, 1981, 1990.

The health risk appraisal index provides (1) a community diagnosis, (2) baseline measurements, (3) an excellent educational and awareness program, and (4) an evaluation of health status. The only potential drawback to this approach is the funding needed. In most cases, however, analysis can be completed for a few dollars. The health risk appraisal index is indeed nontraditional and can address very effectively the holistic and wellness epidemiological policies of life-style, environment, human biology, and medical care system.

Standard Scores (Z-Score Additive Model)

In statistical analysis, a Z-score or standard score is defined as

$$Z_j = X_j - \bar{X} / S$$

where Z_j = Standard score for county j

X_j = Original value for county j. This could be an infant mortality rate, a hyper-tension death rate, or another specific mortality, morbidity, natality, fertility, or disability rate.

$\bar{X}$ = Average or mean of the death rate(s) for the nation, state, or health agency

S = Standard deviation of the death rate(s) for the nation, state, or health agency

To translate a set of *n* measures into standard scores, each value is expressed as a deviation from the mean of the distribution; then each county deviation is divided by the standard deviation of the distribution. Some of the Z-scores are negative in sign, because some of the scores are smaller than the mean. These standardized values reflect a distribution with a mean of 0 and a standard deviation of 1. The Z-score for infant mortality for a county in a health service area thus becomes

$$Z_{county/HSA} = X_{county/HSA\ infant\ mortality} - (\bar{X})_{infant\ mortality} / S_{infant\ mortality}$$

where HSA = Health Service Area

This process is continued in each county of the health service area for as many mortality rates as are to be included in the health status index.

At this point, the health planner can either weight the mortality rates equally or weight the individual mortality rates in terms of importance by using known standards. The sets of weighted or unweighted standard scores obtained by this method are then summed in the Z-score additive model as follows:

$$D_j = \sum_{i=1}^{K} Z_{ij}$$

where D_j = Sum of all weighted or unweighted standard scores for each disease for that county (j), giving a health status index value for that county (j)

Z_{ij} = Weighted or unweighted standard score for each disease (i) for that county or health service area (j)

K = Number of diseases used in determining the health status index

The results obtained from this model are expressed as Z-scores.

The Z-score additive model is relatively simple and easily applied. It is meaningful in the interpretation and comparison of geographical areas concerning disease, personnel, or facility distribution. It is important to remember, however, that changing a set of scores to standard or Z-scores does nothing to alter the shape of the original distribution; the only change is to shift the mean to 0 and the standard deviation to 1.

Q Index

Developed by the Indian Health Service, the Q index has been used by management to decide program priorities.[28] The index combines measures of mortality and morbidity. It is statistically defined as follows:

$$Q = [(Mi/Ma)\,(DP)] + (274A + 91.3B) / N$$

where

Mi = Age- and sex-adjusted mortality rates for the target population (e.g., census tract, county)

Ma = Age- and sex-adjusted mortality rates for the reference population (e.g., state, nation)

D = Crude mortality rate (per 100,000 population) for the target population

P = Years of life lost using life expectancy to age 65 for the target population

A = Hospital days for the target population

N = Number of individuals in the target population

274 and 91.3 = Constants to convert A and B to years per 100,000 population (i.e., three outpatient visits are equated in time to one hospital day)

The Q index is greatly affected by the crude mortality and the years of life lost measures. Donabedian has shown that the rankings of mortality by these measures are quite similar to the ranking of mortality in the Q index.[29] Thus, the dominant measurement in the Q index is mortality, with the hospital activity having little influence on the rankings. Because of this and because of the difficulty that agencies often have in obtaining data on hospital days and outpatient visits, it is recommended that an alternative form of the Q index be used:

$$Q = (Mi / Ma)\,(DP)$$

When Q is computed by either method for each of several diseases, the rank order of the most prevalent disease may be determined. This information is obviously helpful to planners, although final program priorities must weight political and community attitudes.

Life Expectancy and Weighted Life Expectancy

Variation in life expectancy is a result of variation in the relative impact of disease and death. Therefore, variation in life expectancy may be used as a measure to demonstrate variation in health status[30,31] (Fig. 7-3). Life expectancy data may also be used as a variable in a regression model to analyze the determinants of health status or to identify areas of need for programs such as urban or rural health initiatives.

A weighted life expectancy is based on a prorated age-specific disability value that may be determined from survey findings (Table 7-13). For this reason, it may be difficult for a health agency to apply this index in local-area analysis. The major advantage of a weight value for life expectancy is that it can represent either individuals or populations.

Regression Analysis

Disease variables and their respective values may be subjected to a multiple regression analysis to determine the interrelationship of the diseases as a measure

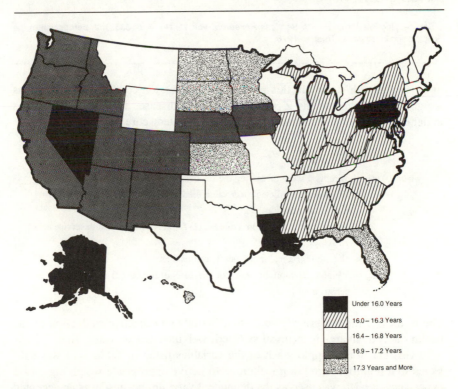

Figure 7-3 Expectation of Life at Age 65, by State, United States, 1979–1981. *Source:* Reprinted from *Statistical Bulletin,* Vol. 68, No. 1, p. 12, with permission of Metropolitan Life Insurance Company, © 1987.

Table 7-13 Weighted Life Expectancy Table

Ages	Hypothetical Average Value of Life	Weighted Life Years
0–4	0.91	3.64
5–14	0.94	9.40
15–24	0.93	9.30
25–44	0.90	18.00
45–64	0.88	17.60
65–74	0.85	8.50
75+	0.80	
		66.44

Note: The total of 66.44 weighted life-years represents the value of life expectancy for an individual with a 75-year life expectancy at birth. It is equivalent to saying that the value of 74 years of life with the average amount of infirmity and disability is roughly equal to 66.44 years of a fully healthy life. Similarly, a life expectancy of, say, 24 years under these circumstances would be equal to $(.91 \times 4)$ + $(.94 \times 10)$ + $(.93 \times 10)$, or 22.34 years of healthy life. This type of weighted life expectancy is based on current experience. That is, life and disability tables are created from the current disease and disability rates in given age ranges.

Source: Reprinted from *Health Services Research*, Vol. 11, No. 4, p. 335, with permission of the Hospital and Educational Trust, © 1976.

---

of existing health status. In this process, the regression coefficients are used as weights and applied to the Z-score value of all diseases for each of the areas under consideration. The method provides a weighted score for each area:

$$H_j = W_1 Z_{1j} + W_2 Z_{2j} + \ldots + W_i Z_{ij}$$

where
H_j = Weighted score measuring the relative health status of area j

W_1 = Regression coefficient or b value used as a weight for the first mortality rate in the equation

Z_{1j} = Mortality rate for the first disease (1) for the county or health service area j

j = Notation for a real unit (county, census tract)

$W_2 Z_{2j}$ = Weight and mortality rate for the second disease (2) in the county or census tract j

The result is a ranked priority score that permits an objective evaluation of the health status of an area in terms of selected, weighted disease categories.

In Georgia, for example, each of the variables listed in Table 7-14 was subjected to a multiple regression technique to derive appropriate weightings. Life expectancy at birth was used as the dependent variable, because it is an accepted indicator of health status. The six independent variables, classified as morbidity/

Table 7-14 Health Status Indicators Used in Developing Priority Ranking for a Health Status Index

Health Index	Independent Variables	Health Status Indicators
Morbidity/ Mortality	Z_1	Infant mortality
	Z_2	Age-adjusted death rates from motor vehicle accidents
	Z_3	Age-adjusted death rates from acute myocardial infarction
	Z_4	Live birth rates
	Z_5	Immature birth rates
	Z_6	Median household buying power

Source: C.M. Plunkett and G.E.A. Dever, Division of Physical Health, Georgia Department of Human Resources, Health Services Research and Statistics, Atlanta, Georgia. Adapted from "Rural Health Initiative," 1977, p. 3.

mortality indicators and median household buying power, proved to be significantly related to the dependent variable. To arrive at a weighted measure, the morbidity/mortality measures were transformed into standardized Z-scores, multiplied by their respective weights, and summed. The values were rank-ordered from 1 to 159 (the number of Georgia counties). Thus, for each county, the following morbidity/mortality measure was developed:

$$W_1 Z_{1j} + W_2 Z_{2j} + W_3 Z_{3j} + W_4 Z_{4j} + W_5 Z_{5j} + W_6 Z_{6j}$$

where W_1 = Regression weight for mortality rate (1)

Z_{1j} = Standardized Z-score for mortality rate (1), county j

After each county's ranking for morbidity/mortality was derived, the county ranks were divided into five approximately equal groups of 32 each (31 in group 5). Group 1 represented counties with the highest priorities. Thus, the priority scores became quantitative inputs into the decision-making process for the need and location of primary health care centers. In conjunction with other more subjective criteria, they can help to establish priorities related to health status.

Factor Analysis

Health analysts may use factor analysis to deduce relationships among diseases in such a way that highly interrelated diseases are combined to form a new factor.[32,33] The basic purposes of factor analysis are

1. to delineate a distinct cluster of interrelated health status data
2. to group interdependent disease variables into descriptive health status categories
3. to provide weightings by dividing health status characteristics into independent sources of variations so that each factor becomes a method for applying weights to the original values of each variable

The result is a composite index for each observation (health service area, county) on each of the factors.

To map the pattern of variations uncovered by factor analysis, the weights provided by the factor score coefficient matrix are multiplied by the Z-scores of the original values on each variable. This yields a weighted score for each observation. The model is as follows:

$$H_j = W_1Z_{1j} + W_2Z_{2j} + \ldots + W_iZ_{ij}$$

where H_j = Magnitude of the health status indicator in county j for the factor in question
W_1 = Factor score coefficient (weight) for the first disease (1) of the factor in question
Z_{1j} = Standard score for the first disease (1) in county j

The computation of an index using factor analysis is a rather complicated task, but statistical computer packages that employ standard software are available to simplify the actual calculations.[34] Critical aspects of this approach are in satisfying the assumptions of the statistical test and in understanding the significance of the results.

Mortality Index

In 1951, Yerushalmy introduced the mortality index as an alternative to techniques that can be unduly influenced by population composition and that summarize absolute rather than relative differences in specific rates.[35,36] For a comparison of schedules of age-specific rates, Yerushalmy proposed a simple unweighted average of ratios that assigns equal weight to the ratio at each year of life and summarizes the relative difference in weights (Table 7-15). The mortality index can be expressed by the following formula:

$$MI = \Sigma[n_i(c_i/c_{si})] / \Sigma n_i$$

where n_i = Number of years in the ith age interval
c_i/c_{si} = Ratio of specific rates

In order to compare Groups A and B, it is necessary to calculate the mortality index for each group and take the ratio as the index of comparison. If an external

Table 7-15 Mortality Index Using an Unweighted Average of Ratios

Age Group	Weights	Specific Ratios Male/Total Population	Product
<10	10	0.81/0.81 = 1.00	10.00
10–24	15	0.59/0.85 = 0.69	10.35
25–34	15	4.54/4.50 = 1.01	15.15
35–44	15	14.81/16.48 = 0.90	13.50
45–54	15	47.11/43.32 = 1.09	16.35
55–64	15	161.11/149.19 = 1.08	16.20
65–74	15	482.49/434.48 = 1.11	16.65
75+	15	1548.37/1417.44 = 1.09	16.35
Sum	115		114.55

Note: MI = 114.55/115 = 0.99: no sex differential in mortality.

Source: Adapted from *American Journal of Public Health*, Vol. 41, pp. 901–908, with permission of American Public Health Association, © 1951.

---

standard population is used, it is not difficult to show that the ratio of age-adjusted death rates obtained by using the direct method for the two groups has the same form as the ratio of the mortality indexes obtained by using the number of deaths in the standard population as weights. Full acceptance of the mortality index, however, is unlikely, because it assumes an equal importance to each year of life.

Socioeconomic Status Index

By using rank-order correlation,[37] the socioeconomic status index can be applied to mortality rates. Data from the 1980 and 1990 U.S. Census on median education, median income, and occupation for each geographical unit may be mathematically combined to determine the socioeconomic status index for each unit. These variables are operationally defined as follows:

1. *median education:* years of school completed by males and females who are 25 years old and over
2. *median income:* the median income of families and unrelated individuals
3. *occupation:* the ratio of employed professional, technical, and kindred workers, managers, and administrators to the total work force

The method used to obtain the index score follows the approach used by Nagi and Stockwell,[38] as well as by Donabedian and colleagues.[39] Because education, income, and occupation have different ranges, it is necessary to standardize the three variables (or any others selected) so that all scores are treated with equal weight. Otherwise, income, which is measured in thousands, would carry more weight than education, which is measured in a range of scores from 0 to 16+ school years, and occupation, which is measured as a percentage. Scores may be standardized by the following formula:

$$\text{Standardized score} = (M_v - L_v) / (H_v - L_v) \times 100$$

where M_v = Individual county score for median education, median income, or occupation
　　　L_v = Lowest score for the variable being standardized
　　　H_v = Highest score for the variable being standardized

An example of standardized scores of three variables for a selected county in Georgia is presented in Table 7-16.

The three standardized scores are added together and divided by 3 to obtain the combined score for a socioeconomic status index for the county:

$$S_c = (E + I + O) / 3$$

where S_c = Socioeconomic status index
　　　E = Standardized score for education
　　　I = Standardized score for income
　　　O = Standardized score for occupation

Table 7-16 Standardizing Scores for a Selected County, Georgia

Variables	Median Scores (M_v)	Highest Scores (H_v)	Lowest Scores (L_v)
Education	9.5 years	12.6 years	7.8 years
Income	$5,284	$12,137	$3,384
Occupation	15.24	34.75	8.45

Variables		Calculations		Standardized Scores
Education (E)	=	$\dfrac{9.5 - 7.8}{12.6 - 7.8} \times 100$	=	35.42
Income (I)	=	$\dfrac{\$5,284 - \$3,384}{\$12,137 - \$3,384} \times 100$	=	21.70
Occupation (O)	=	$\dfrac{15.24 - 8.45}{34.74 - 8.45} \times 100$	=	25.83

Source: Reprinted from *Socioeconomic Analysis of the Disease Patterns of the 70s*, pp. 3–4, Division of Physical Health, Georgia Department of Human Resources, 1977.

Therefore, from Table 7-16, the combined score for the socioeconomic status index is

$$(35.42 + 21.70 + 25.83) / 3 = 27.65$$

This method may be followed for all county units, with 100 the maximum score and 0 the minimum score.

Rank-Order Correlation Analysis

Spearman's rank-order correlation can be used to test the hypothesis that, as an area's socioeconomic status index increases, its mortality rates also increase, that is, they show a direct corresponding relationship with socioeconomic status. Spearman's rank-order correlation focuses on the differences (D_i) between paired rankings of two variables $(X_i$ and $Y_i)$. Thus, the equation $D_i = X_i - Y_i$ measures the extent to which the paired rankings of mortality rates and socioeconomic statuses depart from a perfect direct or inverse correlation. The formula for determining Spearman's rank-order correlation is as follows:

$$r_s = 1 - 6\Sigma D_i^2 / n(n^2 - 1)$$

where $r_s = r$ values of Spearman's rank-order correlation

Σ = Sum of

D_i^2 = Difference between the socioeconomic status rankings (X_i) and the mortality rate rankings (Y_i) for the areas, squared $(D_i$ is squared because some of the differences will be negative.)

n = Number of observations or areas

With the use of Spearman's rank-order correlations, a perfect direct relationship between a mortality rate and socioeconomic status will yield an r_s value of $+1$, while a perfect inverse relationship will yield an r_s value of -1. The procedure for testing r_s for significance depends on the sample size. The statistic $Z = r_s\sqrt{n - 1}$ is computed and compared with appropriate values of the standard normal distribution.

It may be necessary to normalize socioeconomic scores by transforming the scores to the log 10 to ensure that all scores, even those on the extreme ends of the distribution, fall into a more normal curve. The score results may be divided into five socioeconomic groups (Fig. 7-4).

Each socioeconomic group can be characterized in terms of education, income, and occupation. For example, Group 3 in Table 7-17 has 9.4 median school years completed, a median income of $6,395, and 15.7 percent of its occupations classified as professional.

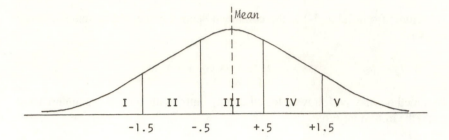

Where:

    Group I   = less than -1.5 standard deviation from the mean
    Group II   = -1.5 to -.5 standard deviation from the mean
    Group III = -.51 to +.5 standard deviation from the mean
    Group IV   = +.51 to +1.5 standard deviation from the mean
    Group V   = greater than +1.5 standard deviation from the mean

Figure 7-4 Breakdown of Socioeconomic Groups. *Source:* Health Services Research and Statistics, *Socioeconomic Analysis of the Disease Patterns of the 70s,* Series 2, Vol. 4 (Aug. 1977), p. 51.

Table 7-17 Socioeconomic Status Index Levels by Variables

Variable	Mean	Socioeconomic Groups				
		1	2	3	4	5
Median education	9.5	7.9	8.5	9.4	10.3	11.9
Median income	$6,526	$3,766	$4,038	$6,395	$8,089	$10,035
Occupation (professional)	15.7	11.4	13.0	15.7	18.9	25.6
SES Score	32.7	14.8	21.1	31.7	45.3	70.1

Source: Reprinted from *Socioeconomic Analysis of the Disease Patterns of the 70s,* p. 9, Division of Physical Health, Georgia Department of Human Resources, 1977.

Not all the 11 mortality variables correlated directly with the socioeconomic status of these Georgia groups when analyzed by Spearman's rank-order correlation coefficient (Table 7-18). Of the 11 mortality categories, 9 correlated at the 0.5 level of significance or better; 2 of the 9 were direct correlations, as hypothesized: ischemic heart disease and cancer of the trachea, bronchus, and lung. The two causes of mortality that showed no significant relationship to socioeconomic status when analyzed by Spearman's rank-order correlation coefficient were acute myocardial infarction (except for occupation) and other forms of heart disease.

Table 7-18 Spearman's Rank-Order Correlation and Coefficients of Mean Mortality Rates, Combined Socioeconomic Index, Median Education, Median Income, and Occupation, Georgia

Mortality Categories	Combined Socioeconomic Status		Median Education		Median Income		Occupation	
	"r" Value	Significance	"r" Value	Significance	"r" Value	Significance	"r" Value	Significance
Total mortality	−.6203	.001	−.5001	.001	−.7233	.001	−.2561	.001
Other accidents	−.3630	.001	−.3271	.001	−.4515	.001	−.1590	.05
Motor vehicle accidents	−.3250	.001	−.3542	.001	−.2936	.001	−.2326	.01
Infant mortality	−.2762	.001	−.1772	.05	−.3357	.001	−.1611	.05
Ischemic heart disease	.2116	.01	.2424	.01	.1376	NS	.1866	.05
Influenza and pneumonia	−.1885	.05	−.1917	.05	−.2193	.01	−.0498	NS
Cancer of the trachea, bronchus, and lung	.1812	.05	.1657	.05	.0936	NS	.2189	.01
Cerebrovascular disease	−.1754	.05	−.1116	NS	−.2472	.01	−.0400	NS
Homicide	−.1581	.05	−.0961	NS	−.2350	.01	−.0292	NS
Acute myocardial infarction	−.1461	NS	−.1000	NS	−.1482	NS	−.1615	.05
Other forms of heart disease	.0186	NS	.0066	NS	.0070	NS	.0457	NS

Note: NS = Not significant.

Source: Reprinted from *Socioeconomic Analysis of the Disease Patterns of the 70s,* p. 10, Division of Physical Health, Georgia Department of Human Resources, 1977.

Index of Demographic Pressure

The dramatic changes occurring now and expected to continue into the year 2000 in population structures (e.g., age, sex) and migration patterns are likely to create demographic pressures that can be detrimental to health. In a recent study of 120 countries, five indicators were used to form an index of demographic pressure:[40]

1. Population increment (a 20-, 30-, or 40-year growth measure that includes immigration and emigration expressed as a percentage of the base year) measures the potential buildup of pressure from overall population growth.
2. Age structure is measured as the percentage of total population less than 15 years of age. A disproportionate share of young people in a population can have negative or destabilizing impacts on economic and political systems.
3. Urbanization is measured by the rate of urbanization for 20-, 30-, or 40-year periods as a percentage of a base year. Rates of urbanization have dramatic potential for social and political destabilization.
4. Labor force growth is calculated as the labor force growth rate between two time periods.
5. Heterogeneity, the existence of major ethnic, religious or language divisions, has the potential to create an explosive climate when combined with demographic trends.

These five indicators were scaled from 1 to 20 to give each of the 120 countries five scores that were added together to create an overall index of demographic pressure. Countries that ranked high included Kenya, Saudi Arabia, Libya, and Uganda (Table 7-19). Low-ranking countries were Denmark, Sweden, Greece, Switzerland and Italy. The United States ranked low (98 of 120), meaning that the demographic index reflected a relatively stable situation. Although this index was applied on a world scale, it can be applied on a state or county basis to identify areas within the state or county at risk for instability or destabilization because of demographic pressure.

Index of Destabilization

Associated with the index of demographic pressure is the destabilization index, which is an attempt to evaluate the problems of governance. Five indicators were combined to produce this index:[41]

1. *change of government*. Countries were scored based on a 27-year history (1962–1989) of changeover in control. Scores were low when change was

Table 7-19 Highest and Lowest Rankings of World Countries by Index of Demographic Pressure

	Country	Increment of Pop. Growth 1960–1990[1] Scale: 1–20	Percent Pop. under 15 Mid-1988[2] Scale: 1–20	Rate of Urbanization 1960–1990[3] Scale: 1–20	Growth of Labor Force 1985–1990[4] Scale: 1–20	Heterogeneity of the Population: Ethnic, Religious, Language[5] Scale: 1–20	Index of Demographic Pressure 1–100
	Kenya	19	20	20	16	13	88
H	Cote d'Ivorie	18	18	15	12	19	82
I	Saudi Arabia	20	17	17	17	7	78
G	Tanzania	14	19	20	13	12	78
H	Botswana	15	19	20	14	7	75
	Libya	19	17	20	16	3	75
	Uganda	15	19	11	13	16	74
	Argentina	6	9	2	6	3	26
	Canada	5	4	2	5	10	26
	Czechoslovakia	2	6	2	3	13	26
	United States	4	4	1	5	12	26
	Spain	3	5	2	5	10	25
	Australia	6	5	2	8	3	24
	Romania	3	6	2	4	9	24
	Uruguay	3	7	1	4	8	23
	Belgium	1	3	1	2	14	21
	Netherlands	3	3	1	5	7	19

continues

Table 7-19 continued

Country	Increment of Pop. Growth 1960–1990[1] Scale: 1–20	Percent Pop. under 15 Mid-1988[2] Scale: 1–20	Rate of Urbanization 1960–1990[3] Scale: 1–20	Growth of Labor Force 1985–1990[4] Scale: 1–20	Heterogeneity of the Population: Ethnic, Religious, Language[5] Scale: 1–20	Index of Demographic Pressure 1–100
United Kingdom	1	3	1	2	12	19
Norway	2	3	4	4	5	18
Poland	3	7	2	3	3	18
Bulgaria	2	4	3	1	7	17
Japan	3	4	2	4	4	17
France	2	4	1	3	6	16
Hungary	1	4	2	2	7	16
Portugal	2	5	2	4	3	16
Germany, East	1	3	1	1	9	15
Germany, West	1	1	1	2	10	15
Italy	2	3	1	3	5	14
Switzerland	2	2	1	2	7	14
Greece	2	4	2	2	3	13
Sweden	2	2	1	2	5	12
Denmark	2	2	1	3	3	11

(L O W)

[1]United Nations, World Population Prospects. Estimates and Projections as Assessed in 1984.
[2]Population Reference Bureau, 1988 World Population Data Sheet.
[3]United Nations. The Prospects of World Urbanization, Revised as of 1984–85.

[4]International Labor Office, Economical Active Population–Estimates and Projections, 1950–2025.
[5]World Almanac Book of Facts, 1989.

Source: Reprinted from *Population Pressures: Threat to Democracy* by S. L. Camp, with permission of Population Crisis Committee, © 1989.

peaceful, and high when change was associated with turmoil. Most African countries scored high, while Western countries scored low.

2. *political freedoms*. Countries were rated as they relate to each other rather than to standards; 11 measures were used (e.g., fair election laws, multiple political parties).
3. *civil liberties*. There were 25 measures considered in rating civil liberties. They included political censorship, imprisonment, freedom of speech, and freedom from gross socioeconomic inequality.
4. *communal violence*. Based on 1975–1988 U.S. State Department data, indicators such as violent conflicts between ethnic and/or religious groups were used.
5. *dissatisfied youth/frustrated expectations*. The percentage change in youth educational attainment and per capita growth in the gross national product, expressed as a ratio, produced measures of expectations. Low scores reflected a modest increase in the percentage of young people in secondary school, while the gross national product increased 10 to 20 times. High scores resulted from large increases in young people attending secondary school, while the gross national product grew only by a factor of 5 or less. Japan, Korea, and Taiwan reported low scores; Zaire, Ethiopia, and Zimbabwe reported high scores.

Scores of each of the indicators were ranked, and their combined scores resulted in an index of destabilization (Table 7-20).

The relationship between the index of destabilization and the index of demographic pressure is quite clear. The correlation showed that demographic pressures and patterns generally reflect past political performance and potential instability. In fact, of the 120 countries studied by the population crisis committee, there was a positive relationship between demographic pressure and destabilization in 101. Table 7-21 shows the results of the two indexes for selected countries. The application of these health status indexes in the United States by country and/or county would be most appropriate. Furthermore, by using projected and estimated populations, it may be possible to predict areas where demographic pressure could lead to future instability or destabilization. If so, the identification of potential priority areas would be of tremendous benefit not only to health planners, but also to social planners.

Index on the Status of Women

Perhaps the most important index is the index on the status of women. First, the status of women in the world and in the United States has been ignored for too long. Second, the combination of several important indicators into five indexes truly epitomizes a healthy public policy approach.

Table 7-20 Highest and Lowest Ranking of World Countries by Index of Destabilization

		Selected Indicators					
	Country	*Change of Government 1962–1989[1] Scale: 1–20*	*Political Rights 1973–1987[2] Scale: 1–10*	*Civil Rights 1973–1987[3] Scale: 1–10*	*Communal Violence 1975–1988[4] Scale: 1–20*	*Dissatisfied Youth 1965 and 1985[5] Scale: 1–40*	*Index of Destabilization Scale: 1–100*
	Mauritainia	20	9	9	20	37	95
H	Ethiopia	20	10	10	20	27	87
I	Zaire	20	10	9	10	34	83
G	Burundi	20	10	9	20	22	61
H	Sudan	20	8	9	20	25	61
	Netherlands	1	1	1	10	16	29
	Jamaica	1	2	3	1	21	28
	Costa Rica	1	1	1	1	21	25
	Venezuela	1	1	2	1	19	24
	Germany, West	1	1	2	1	18	23
L	Belgium	1	1	1	1	18	22
O	Sweden	1	1	1	1	18	22
W	Australia	1	1	1	1	17	21
	Denmark	1	1	1	1	17	21
	Italy	1	1	2	1	16	21
	Switzerland	1	1	1	1	16	20
	Norway	1	1	1	1	14	18
	Japan	1	1	1	1	9	13

[1]United States Department of State. Background Notes.
[2]Raymond D. Gastil, Freedom in the World—Political Rights and Civil Liberties, 1987–1988, New York, 1988.
[3]Ibid.
[4]United States Department of State, Country Reports on Human Rights Practices, 1987.
[5]Principal source of GNP—Population Reference Bureau, World Population Data Sheet, 1968 and 1987, Principal sources for Education—World Bank, World Development Report, 1988, and UNESCO Statistical Yearbooks.

Source: Reprinted from *Population Pressures: Threat to Democracy* by S. L. Camp with permission of Population Crisis Committee, © 1989.

Table 7-21 Scores for the Index of Demographic Pressure and the Index of Destabilization for Selected Countries

Country	Index of Demographic Pressure	Index of Destabilization
Afghanistan	70	73
Albania	42	52
Algeria	61	53
Angola	59	77
Argentina	26	48
Australia	24	21
Bangladesh	57	73
Belgium	21	22
Benin	71	68
Bolivia	56	53
Botswana	75	30
Brazil	46	52
Bulgaria	17	37
Burkina Faso	57	61
Burma	42	79
Burundi	59	81
Cameroon	65	44
Canada	26	30
Cen. African Rep.	55	66
Chad	70	78
Chile	36	62
China	36	57
Colombia	45	46
Sweden	12	22
Switzerland	14	20
Syria	67	74
Taiwan	38	34
Tanzania	78	53
Thailand	43	53
Togo	67	59
Tunisia	47	64
Turkey	45	50
Uganda	74	78
United Kingdom	19	41
United States	26	31
Uruguay	23	43
USSR	32	56
Venezuela	55	24
Vietnam	50	72
Yemen, North	69	72
Yemen, South	53	67
Yugoslavia	34	45
Zaire	61	83
Zambia	72	48
Zimbabwe	70	63

Source: Reprinted from *Population Pressures: Threat to Democracy* by S. L. Camp with permission of Population Crisis Committee, © 1989.

Table 7-22 Factors and Indicators Used To Determine the Gender Gap Index and Index on the Status of Women

Factor	Indicator/Definition
Health	**Female infant and child mortality,** technically infant and child mortality, is the percent of girls born who die before their fifth birthday.
	Female mortality—childbearing years is the percent of all women aged 15 who will die before they reach the age of 45, based on current age-specific death rates for women.
	Female life expectancy at birth is the average number of years a woman may expect to live at the time she is born.
	Gender gap: female/male differential life expectancy is the difference in years between female and male life expectancy at birth. A small differential or higher male life expectancy may indicate a gender gap in health status.
Marriage and children	**Adolescent marriage** refers to the percent of women aged 15 to 19 who have been married.
	Total fertility rate refers to the average number of children a woman will have in her lifetime, based on current age-specific fertility rates.
	Contraceptive prevalence is the percentage of women married or living in union who are using contraception, including traditional methods.
	Gender gap: widowed, divorced or separated refers to the ratio of widowed, divorced or separated women to widowers and divorced or separated men. In every country, those households in which women are the sole source of support for themselves and their families tend to be at the bottom of the socioeconomic ladder.
Education	**Primary and secondary school enrollment** indicates the number of girls in primary and secondary school as a percentage of all girls of primary and secondary school age.
	Women secondary school teachers indicates the percentage of all secondary school teachers who are women. In countries scoring well on overall women's status, about half of all secondary school teachers are women.
	University enrollment indicates the number of all women enrolled in a university as a percent of all women aged 20 to 24.
	Gender gap: differential literacy for men and women measures the gap between literacy rates for men and women aged 15 to 44 years, a gap which has largely closed in high and upper middle income countries.
Employment	**Employed women** measures the number of women who are working for pay as a percentage of all adult women aged 15 years and over. In the industrialized countries, where virtually all households are part of the money economy, it is a good measure of women's economic participation, although not of their real earning power.
	Self-employed women measures the percent of women aged 15 or older who appear as self-employed in official statistics, whether they work in agriculture, commerce, manufacturing or a profession and whether or not they hire employees. For some developing countries the measure may largely reflect the diligence with which governments have attempted to quantify women's work.

Table 7-22 continued

Factor	Indicator/Definition
	Professional women measures the number of women in professional, technical, managerial and administrative occupations as a percent of all women aged 15 years and over.
	Gender gap: women's share of paid employment measures the percent of the official paid work force that is female.
Social equality	**Political and legal equality** measures the degree to which women can expect legal protection against all types of discrimination based on sex and the degree to which they have and exercise political rights, including their representation in political office.
	Economic equality measures the degree to which women can expect equal treatment with male co-workers in their place of work and whether they are in other ways free to participate equally in economic life, including the right to own, manage, and inherit real property.
	Equality in marriage and the family covers the right to enter freely into marriage, equal rights in divorce, and other issues involving family law.
	Gender gap: societal equality: The absence of discrimination against in society, 1986–1988, representing total of social equality variables.

Source: Reprinted from *Country Rankings of the Status of Women: Poor, Powerless, and Pregnant*, Population Briefing Paper No. 20, p. 10, with permission of Population Crisis Committee, © 1988.

Five factors, each represented by several indicators, are summed to produce a gender gap index and an index on the status of women (Table 7-22).[42] Each factor has a variable that is considered a gender gap variable. Thus, the addition of scores for female/male life expectancy differential; the ratio of widowed, divorced, or separated women to widowers and divorced or separated men; female/male literacy rate differential; women's share of paid employment; and societal equality produce the gender gap index. The remaining variables for each factor represent the index on the status of women. Because each of the 20 measures has a maximum of 5 points (highest), the maximum score possible is 100—75 for women's status and 25 for the gender gap index. The combination of the two gives the final score for the index on the status of women.

The distribution of the world's countries from excellent to extremely poor in terms of women's status is shown in Figure 7-5. In more than 60 percent of countries, the status of women index is ranked poor, very poor, or extremely poor. No countries are ranked excellent. A comparison of the status of women in Sweden, one of the highest ranking countries, and Bangladesh, one of the lowest ranking countries, is presented in Table 7-23. The comparison is shocking. The United States ranks third on the status of women index.

The gender gap index for the 12 best and 12 worst countries is presented in Table 7-24. Again, Bangladesh is the worst; however, Sweden ranks second. The United States ranks fifth for this index. A major factor in the country rankings in

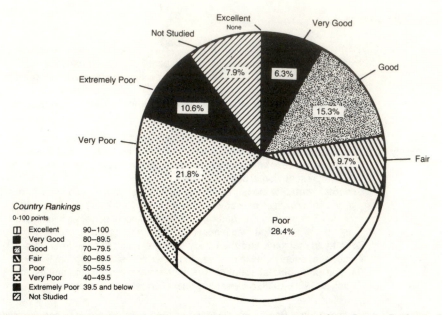

Figure 7-5 Status of Women by Country Rankings. *Source:* Reprinted from *Country Rankings of the Status of Women: Poor, Powerless, and Pregnant,* Population Briefing Paper No. 20, p. 2, with permission of Population Crisis Committee, © 1988.

Table 7-23 Women's Status in Highest and Lowest Ranked Countries

In Sweden . . . (Population: 8.4 million, Area: 173,730 square miles)	In Bangladesh . . . (Population: 109.5 million, Area: 55,598 square miles)
Female life expectancy is 81 years.	Female life expectancy is 49 years.
One in 167 girls dies before her fifth birthday.	One in five girls dies before her fifth birthday.
One in 53 15-year-olds will not survive her childbearing years. (One percent of these deaths relates to pregnancy and childbirth.)	One in six 15-year-olds will not survive her childbearing years. (About one-third of these deaths relate to pregnancy and childbirth.)
Fewer than one percent of 15–19 year old women have already been married.	Almost 70 percent of 15–19 year old women have already been married.
Women bear one to two children on average.	Women bear five to six children on average.
Over three-fourths of married women use contraception.	One-fourth of married women use contraception.
Virtually all school-aged girls are in school.	One in three school-aged girls is in school.
Female university enrollment is 37 percent of women aged 20–24.	Female university enrollment is less than 2 percent of women aged 20–24.
About half the secondary school teachers are women.	One in ten secondary school teachers is a woman.
Three out of five women are in the paid labor force.	One in 15 women is in the paid labor force.

Table 7-23 continued

In Sweden . . . (Population: 8.4 million, Area: 173,730 square miles)	In Bangladesh . . . (Population: 109.5 million, Area: 55,598 square miles)
Two out of five women are professionals.	Only 3 out of 1,000 women are professionals.
Women live an average of seven years longer than men.	Women live an average of two years less than men.
Women and men have similar literacy rates.	Some 24 percent more women are illiterate than men.
About half of the paid work force is female.	Only 14 percent of the paid work force is female.
In 1988, women held 113 seats in Sweden's 349-member parliament.	In 1988, women held 4 seats in Bangladesh's 302-member parliament, out of 30 reserved for them.

Source: Reprinted from *Country Rankings of the Status of Women: Poor, Powerless, and Pregnant,* Population Briefing Paper No. 20, p. 10, with permission of Population Crisis Committee, © 1988.

Table 7-24 Gender Gap Scores

12 Worst		12 Best	
Country	*Score*	*Country*	*Score*
Bangladesh	5.5	Finland	23.5
Saudi Arabia	6.5	Sweden	23.0
Egypt	7.5	USSR	23.0
Syria	8.5	Norway	22.0
Nigeria	8.5	USA	22.0
Libya	9.0	Australia	21.5
Pakistan	9.5	Bulgaria	21.5
Morocco	9.5	Canada	21.5
Yemen, North	10.0	Czechoslovakia	21.5
Sudan	10.0	Denmark	21.5
Mali	10.0	Germany, East	21.5
Kuwait	10.0	Hungary	21.5

Source: Reprinted from *Country Rankings of the Status of Women: Poor, Powerless, and Pregnant,* Population Briefing Paper No. 20, p. 8, with permission of Population Crisis Committee, © 1988.

terms of the overall status of women and the resulting index scores is the number of births. Clearly, the lower a country ranks in the index, the greater number of births per woman. In the lowest ranking countries, women have an average of about 5.9 children (infectious disease cycle), while women in the highest ranking countries average 1.9 children (transformation disease cycle) (Fig. 7-6).

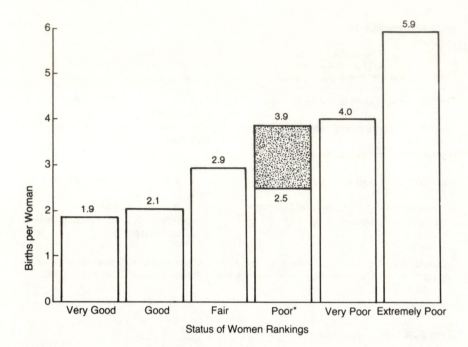

Births per Woman: Average number of children per woman (total fertility rate).

*The inclusion of China, the largest nation in the world, with over half a billion women and low fertility (2.1 births per women) brings down the total average in this category. The shaded area shows the increase in average births per woman when China is excluded from this group of countries.

Figure 7-6 Births per Woman Compared to Status of Women. *Source:* Reprinted from *Country Rankings of the Status of Women: Poor, Powerless, and Pregnant,* Population Briefing Paper No. 20, p. 9, with permission of Population Crisis Committee, © 1988.

This analysis serves as an excellent model to evaluate the status of women in the United States either by state or by county within the state. Furthermore, the essence of this approach can be expanded to address other groups that are faced with disparities in their everyday living as a result of ageism or racism, for example. Zero Population Growth, Inc. recently used a similar appraisal process to study urban stress in the United States.[43]

CONCLUSION

The holistic and wellness approach to health status analysis will guide a health agency to a conceptual framework (like the one presented in Chapter 2) and a clearer understanding of what should be included in an index. The basic difficulty in measuring health status stems from a lack of sensitive data, not from a lack of methodology by which to apply data. It is hoped that these examples provide the impetus for health and community analysts to begin to think of health not as the outcome, but rather consider health as a resource in the ongoing analysis and development of a healthy public policy.

NOTES

1. G.E. Alan Dever, *Considerations in the Measurement of Health Status,* DHEW Contract #HRA 232-78-0109 (Houston: Region VI Center for Urban Research, June 1978), 46.

2. U.S. Department of Health, Education and Welfare, Bureau of Health Planning and Resource Development, *Guidelines Concerning the Development of Health Systems Plans and Annual Implementation Plans* (Washington, D.C.: U.S. Government Printing Office, December 23, 1976), 22.

3. Ibid., 26.

4. U.S. Department of Health and Human Services, *Promoting Health/Preventing Disease: Year 2000 Objectives for the Nation: Draft for Public Review and Comment* (Washington, D.C.: U.S. Government Printing Office, September 1989), 23–24.

5. Ibid., 7.

6. Ibid.

7. Ibid., 3.

8. Ibid., 2.

9. H.L. Blum, *Planning for Health—Development and Application of Social Change Theory* (New York: Human Sciences Press, 1974), 223–224.

10. Ibid.

11. National Center for Health Statistics, Clearinghouse on Health Indexes, *Correlated Annotations, Oct. 1973–Dec. 1974,* DHEW Pub. No. (HRA) 76-1225 (Washington, D.C.: U.S. Government Printing Office, 1976). NCHS volumes are extremely helpful to anyone involved in the issues of health status measurement.

12. K.N. Lohr and G.A. Mock, *Advances in the Assessment of Health Status* (Washington, D.C.: Council of Health Care Technology, Institute of Medicine, National Academy of Science, 1989).

13. For an excellent discussion on the different levels of measurement, see S. Siegel, *Nonparametric Statistics for the Behavioral Sciences* (New York: McGraw-Hill Book Co., 1956), 21–34.

14. Georgia Department of Human Resources, Division of Physical Health, Health Services Research and Statistics, *Infant Health Status: A Quality of Life Analysis,* series 2, vol. 2 (Atlanta: Georgia Department of Human Resources, January 1976), 37.

15. G.E.A. Dever and M.R. Lavoie, "Data Base—Identification of Needs," in *A Companion to the Life Sciences,* ed. Stacey B. Day (New York: Van Nostrand Reinhold Co., 1979), 16–19.

16. G.B. Hill and J.M. Romeder, "Health Statistics in Canada" (Paper presented at the Society for Epidemiological Research, Toronto, Ontario, June 18, 1976), 11.

17. D.M. Smith, *The Geography of Social Well-Being in the U.S.: An Introduction to Territorial Social Indicators* (New York: McGraw-Hill Book Co., 1973), 144.

18. K.C. Land and S. Spilerman, *Social Indicators Models* (New York: Russell Sage Foundation, 1975), 411.

19. Environmental Protection Agency, Office of Research and Monitoring, Environmental Studies Division, *The Quality of Life Concept—A Potential New Tool for Decision Makers* (Washington, D.C.: Environmental Protection Agency, March 1973).

20. U.S. Department of Health, Education and Welfare, *A Data Acquisition and Analysis Handbook for Health Planners,* Health Planning Information series no. 4, vol. 1 (Washington, D.C.: U.S. Government Printing Office, October 1976), 142–143.

21. D.O. Rutstein et al., "Measuring the Quality of Medical Care," *New England Journal of Medicine* 229, no. 11 (1974): 603–610.

22. J.M. Romeder and J.R. McWhinnie, "Potential Years of Life Lost between Ages 1 and 70: An Indicator of Premature Mortality for Health Planning," *International Journal of Epidemiology* 6, no. 2 (1977): 143–151.

23. Janet D. Perloff et al., "Premature Death in the United States: Years of Life Lost and Health Problems," *Journal of Public Health Policy* (June 1984): 167–184.

24. Centers for Disease Control, "Premature Mortality in the U.S.: Public Health Issues in the Use of Years of Potential Life Lost," *Morbidity and Mortality Weekly Report,* supplement to vol. 35, no. 25 (December 19, 1986): 10S.

25. Papers of the 1976 Health Status Indexes Conference, *Health Services Research* (Winter 1976): 340.

26. M. Berger, "Measurement of Health Status," *Medical Care* 23, no. 5 (May 1985): 696–704.

27. J.W. Travis, *Wellness for Helping Professionals* (Mill Valley, Calif.: Wellness Associates, 1977, 1981, 1990).

28. J.E. Miller, "An Indicator To Aid Management in Assessing Program Priorities," *Public Health Reports* 85, no. 8 (April 1970): 725–731.

29. Avedis Donabedian, *Aspects of Medical Care Administration: Specifying Requirements for Health Care* (Cambridge, Mass.: Harvard University Press, 1973), 649.

30. Georgia Department of Human Resources, Division of Physical Health, Health Services Research and Statistics, *Life Expectancy, Current Trends and Potential Gains,* series 2, vol. 3 (Atlanta: Georgia Department of Human Resources, January 1976), 7.

31. R.L. Berg, "Weighted Life Expectancy as a Health Status Index," *Health Services Research* (Summer 1975): 153–156.

32. Georgia Department of Human Resources, Division of Physical Health, Health Services Research and Statistics, *Nonwhite Disease Patterns—Black Health Status in Georgia,* series 2, vol. 1 (February 1975), 99.

33. W.L. Hightower, "Development of an Index of Health Utilizing Factor Analysis," *Medical Care* 16, no. 3 (March 1978): 245–255.

34. The most commonly used statistical package is SPSS (Statistical Package for the Social Sciences); BMD (Biomedical) is also usually available. An excellent example of the application of factor analysis to derive an index is in J.C. Maloney, *Social Vulnerability in Indianapolis* (Indianapolis: Community Services Council of Metropolitan Indianapolis, July 1973), 53.

35. J. Yerushalmy, "A Mortality Index for Use in Place of the Age-Adjusted Death Rate," *American Journal of Public Health* 51 (August 1951): 901–908.

36. Some of the material presented in this section is modified from Course No. 401 of the Applied Statistical Training Institute, Washington, D.C.

37. Georgia Department of Human Resources, Division of Physical Health, Health Services Research and Statistics, *Socioeconomic Analysis of the Disease Patterns of the '70s,* series 2, vol. 4 (August 1977), 51.

38. M.H. Nagi and E.G. Stockwell, "Socioeconomic Differences in Mortality by Cause of Death," *Health Services Reports* 88, no. 5 (May 1973): 449–450.

39. Avedis Donabedian et al., "Infant Mortality and Socioeconomic Status in a Metropolitan Community," *Public Health Reports* 80, no. 12 (December 1965): 1083–1094.

40. S.L. Camp, *Population Pressures—Threat to Democracy* (Washington, D.C.: Population Crisis Committee, 1989).

41. Ibid.

42. Population Crisis Committee, "Country Rankings of the Status of Women: Poor, Powerless, and Pregnant." Population Briefing Paper no. 20 (Washington, D.C.: June 1988), 10.

43. Zero Population Growth, "Rating U.S.: Urban Stress," Washington, D.C., 1988, summary, *Population Today* 17, no. 1 (January 1989): 9.

Chapter 8

Marketing Community Health

The management of health services in public, private, and community health agencies should be population based; thus, demography, epidemiology, and marketing offer principles and methods to guide management decision making. The market analysis of programs and policies should determine the best strategies for the identification of clients and/or patients (i.e., targeting—a who, where, and when risk profile) and the most appropriate strategies for providing services. Such an approach requires a knowledge of demographic trends, psychographic and socioeconomic behavior, physician distribution, public health clinic services and distribution, incidence rates for diagnosis-related groups (DRGs), facility data, and agency client profile data.

The same basic principles lie behind both the marketing and epidemiological approaches to the management of health programs and services, and the combination of the two can lead to optimal population-based planning. Both aim at strengthening the fit between the health services offered and the needs of the population. Both thus provide a set of principles and tools that can be used to manage the delivery of health services in a more equitable, appropriate, effective, and efficient way.

WHAT IS MARKETING?

Marketing can be conceived of as a set of methods designed to reconcile the resources and production capacity of an organization with the needs and preferences of the consumers. Marketing theory is based on a systemic view of organizations in which their functioning is viewed in terms of exchanges.

In order to have an exchange relationship, an organization requires two things:[1] (1) a constituency, that is, some person, group, or organization with whom an exchange is to be accomplished; and (2) a value, that is, "something" to exchange. In other words, an exchange relationship involves the offering of something of value, such as a product or service, to someone who is willing to exchange it for something else of value, such as money or time.[2] Marketing offers a structure to analyze, predict, and manage exchanges for the benefit of all concerned. In this usage, marketing is defined simply as the conscious, systematic approach to the planning, implementation, and evaluation of the exchange relationships of an organization.[3]

Marketing is based on the fundamental assumptions that, if each constituency can be identified and analyzed, and if each exchange can be examined and controlled, the organization will attain its objectives (profit or other) more effectively. An important corollary of the model is that exchanges are maximized if—and only if—the product (or service) of the organization coincides with the needs, wants, and desires of the consumers. As Drucker wrote, "the aim of marketing is to make selling superfluous."[4] Similarly, Kotler stated that "marketing is the philosophical alternative to force."[5]

The negative connotation often attached to this subject—that marketing creates needs—results from a misconception of its modern orientation. Although it may well be possible to find situations in which production precedes marketing, organizations with a product orientation are likely to fail because they are trying to impose on a market a product (or service or idea) that is not matched to the consumer's needs or wants. For example, are family planning programs matched to needs? Are statewide high-risk mother programs matched to needs? Are women, infants, and children (W.I.C.) programs matched to needs? The answer is usually no. As a result, many community and public health programs and/or agencies, having a service system orientation rather than a community capacity building orientation, have failed in many respects. Modern theory holds that marketing's only effective form involves consumer orientation through a strategic or integrated approach in which the marketing function precedes and embodies production and in which the product is matched to needs. This is the challenge in community health.

Another inherent feature of modern or strategic marketing is the identification and selection of specific subgroups of the constituency, or target markets. Any attempt to serve every market will undoubtedly be in vain, yet this is the goal of health services in the United States (i.e., health for all by the year 2000). The resources are simply not available to accomplish this goal. Therefore, it is essential to develop a healthy public policy that makes it possible to determine the best distribution of resources to meet the needs of those most in need. The correct marketing process is one that focuses on the market segments that can *best* be served. Eventually, with the use of this strategy, health for all may become a reality; at least, the overall general health status of the U.S. population will improve.

MARKETING TERMINOLOGY

There are three particularly important marketing concepts: (1) the organization's publics, (2) its markets, and (3) its marketing mix.

The Public of an Organization

A public is any distinct group that has an actual or potential interest in or impact on an organization, in this instance, the community/public health agency.[6] The publics are all of the internal and external individuals or groups that influence or potentially could influence the organization.[7] The sum of all the publics constitutes the entity's immediate environment.

The Markets of an Organization

A market is a public that is involved (or may realistically be expected to become involved) in an exchange relationship with the organization. It is composed of a distinct set of people and/or entities that have or will have resources (values) that they want to exchange (or may be willing to exchange) for something they want and that the organization has (or will have). In the health care field, markets are often referred to as constituencies.[8] Both of these terms are used interchangeably here.

As Kotler wrote:

> If the organization wishes to attract certain resources from that public through offering a set of benefits in exchange, then the organization is taking a "marketing viewpoint" toward that public. Once the organization starts thinking in terms of trading values with that public, it is viewing the public as a market.[9]

Community health agencies trade services for improved health status; however, they must shift from their traditional service system, which tends to build dependencies and deficiencies in the market, to a community orientation in which the community builds capacity and strength in the market.

A health care organization has four types of markets: (1) external markets, (2) internal markets, (3) client markets, and (4) competitor markets.[10] External markets include supporters, suppliers, regulators, and the community at large. Internal markets include the board of trustees, the employees, the physicians, and the volunteers. Client markets include patients and other consumers of services such as physical examinations, laboratory tests, and blood tests. Other publics that benefit indirectly from the agency's services, such as relatives of patients and members of the constituency whose health is affected by the agency's environmental, occupational, prevention, and health education programs, can also be considered client markets.

The competitors or colleagues markets, which include other health care providers or the producers of health-related services and products, pose a basic problem for a public health agency. Because such an agency has no real competitors, it has little incentive to utilize marketing approaches to do a better job, to reach the most vulnerable, and to be efficient in the allocation of resources. Even without competitors and consumer pricing, however, public health agencies must identify their markets by means of demographics, psychographics, socioeconomic lifestyles, and epidemiology. Government resources are becoming more scarce; therefore, resources must be allocated on the basis of marketing techniques, as well as demographic and epidemiological methods and principles.

A marketing program should be considered for each of these constituencies. The community/public health agency can engage in patient marketing, community marketing, and public health marketing, for example. A public health agency short of nurses can engage in nurse marketing. Although the focus here is on patient marketing, precisely the same process can be used to develop effective exchange relationships with any markets.

The Marketing Mix

The marketing process involves four distinct groups of elements, together referred to as the marketing mix. They represent forces or variables that the organization can control or influence to achieve its objectives in the target market.[11] The four groups of elements are known traditionally as the four Ps; product, place, price, and promotion. The organization can devise different combinations of these to optimize exchanges with a given target market. The marketing mix, of course, must be adapted to each target. The concept suggests that results will be effective only with careful consideration and adaptation of the product, the place of exchange, the price, and finally the promotion, to the target market.

Under the term *product* are included all the characteristics of that which the organization offers to exchange with the target market, such as quality, features, options, styles, brand names, packaging, sizes, warranties, and returns. Each of these should be carefully adapted to the needs, wants, and desires of the target. In community health marketing, or more precisely in patient program marketing, the products are the services to be delivered. These should be geared to the health needs of the constituency, of high quality, and adapted to the patients' social characteristics (e.g., culture, ethnicity, language), for example. Clearly, this approach requires a knowledge of descriptive epidemiology (person) and psychographic analysis.

Place refers to the location where the product or services are delivered (exchanged). Such variables as geographical and temporal accessibility and availability (see Chapter 5) are important in patient health services marketing. Again, descriptive epidemiology—place and time—plays a role in marketing.

Price includes all the direct and indirect costs that the patient must bear in the exchange of services.

Finally, promotion refers to the organization's causal, informative, or persuasive communication with the target market. The institution consciously develops its messages (e.g., through publicity or advertising) to have a calculated impact on the attitude and/or behavior of the target market.[12] Promotion generally has four objectives.[13]

1. to inform and educate consumers as to the existence of a product (or service) and its capabilities (what do community/public health agencies have to offer)
2. to remind present and former users of the product's continuing existence (quality and quantity [e.g., prenatal care services])
3. to persuade prospective purchasers that the product is worth buying (improved health status)
4. to inform consumers where and how to obtain and use the product (accessibility, location, and time)

MARKETING PROCESS

Strategic or integrated marketing (consumer-oriented as opposed to product-oriented) can be defined as a planning process of identifying, analyzing, choosing, and exploiting marketing opportunities to fulfill the organization's mission and objectives.[14] Although no two authors describe the marketing process in exactly the same way, all definitions include three fundamental components or steps.

1. a research and analysis component in which the environment, the competition, and the potential markets are identified and analyzed and in which target markets are selected
2. an implementation or operational component in which programs are elaborated and the marketing mix is developed
3. an evaluation and control component in which the exchange relationship is monitored and appropriate corrective actions are taken as needed

These three basic components are illustrated in Figure 8-1. As can be seen, the research and analysis component includes many different analyses: of the environment; of the market, including its structure, opportunities, and targeting; of the competition; and of the organization's resources. Furthermore, all of these serve as inputs into the analysis of the organization's portfolio. Programs are then set up and the marketing mix developed. The last stage of the marketing process consists of the monitoring, control, and evaluation of the exchanges (delivery of services). The research and analysis component of the strategic marketing process is of particular importance to community/public health programs.

Market Structure Analysis

The first step in a market structure analysis is the identification and analysis of the organization's markets. For a hospital, the actual markets can be determined with a patient origin study, while the potential markets can be ascertained on a geographical/political basis or on a service capacity basis. For community/public health programs, the actual markets can be determined by analyzing program data to identify client profiles; potential markets are established by specific program standards that are set by state or federal agencies. For example, a program created to provide prenatal care to all women at 150% of the poverty level has these women as its potential market.

If possible, actual and potential markets should be broken down into distinct and homogenous subgroups. This process is called market segmentation. Its aim is to facilitate the analysis of actual and potential exchanges in an effort to improve their effectiveness. The criteria of segmentation should be the homogeneity within each segment and the heterogeneity among the different segments. A market segment is a grouping of individuals whose behavior may be expected to differ from that of another market segment in the exchange relationship.

Three classes of variables can be used for market segmentation.

1. Geographical segmentation refers to the grouping of people according to their locations of residence or work. This can be done either on a simple geographical basis or according to another variable, such as population density or climate.[15]
2. Demographic segmentation is the grouping of individuals on the basis of such variables as age, sex, income, occupation, education, religion, or race (see Chapter 6).
3. Psychographic segmentation is based on such criteria as personal values, attitudes, opinions, personality, behavior, and lifestyle.[16-18]

Psychographic segmentation is often the most useful, and several demographic vendors have recently made psychographic data readily available. Health man-

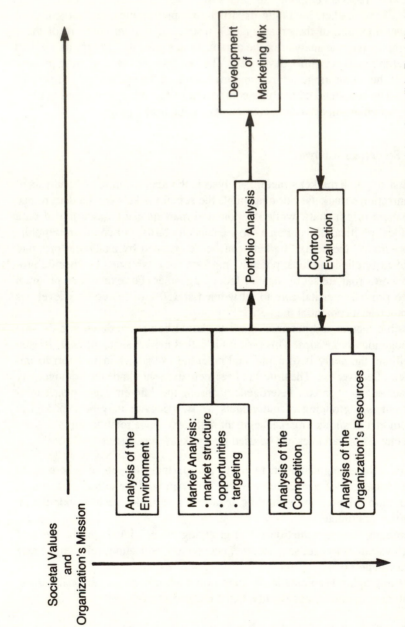
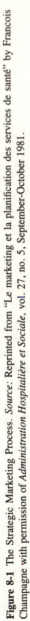

Figure 8-1 The Strategic Marketing Process. *Source:* Reprinted from "Le marketing et la planification des services de santé" by Francois Champagne with permission of *Administration Hospitalière et Sociale*, vol. 27, no. 5, September–October 1981.

agers may prefer to use a combination of geographical, demographic, and psychographic segmentation.

Marketing Analysis: Demographics

The understanding of marketing and demographics is most essential to the development and targeting of community/public health programs. Programs in community health are quite different from those in the business world. Basically, community health agencies hope to market products/services that are purchased because of their net return (i.e., improved health status). Generally, the programs are provided at no cost to the consumer or patient. Community health programs basically promote or sell such products as (1) smoking cessation, (2) low fat diets, (3) exercise programs, (4) prenatal care, (5) hypertension screening, (6) prevention of acquired immune deficiency syndrome (AIDS), (7) cancer prevention, (8) seat belt use, (9) family planning, and (10) infant mortality reduction. This list is by no means exhaustive.

The role of the community/public health agency is to analyze the demographics of the areas that are served or targeted by these programs in order to identify their clients. The information needed may be categorized as follows: (1) total population of the area that the program is intended to serve, (2) rate of change of population, (3) age/sex distribution, (4) racial/ethnic composition, (5) socioeconomic status, (6) housing information, and (7) fertility patterns. Each of these factors and their dynamics should be analyzed relative to the market of the particular program. Probably, the most important of these to community health programs are the age distribution of the population, the fertility rates, and the trends or changes over the next five to ten years. Thus, the analysis of births, deaths, migration and trends over time are critical factors to be considered in the marketing of community health programs.

The health agency must specifically track the more important demographic events. At least four such events are critical to community health programs: (1) the baby boom population, (2) the elderly population, (3) the women's market, and (4) the changing nature of the birth rate in an area. These events and how they change should be part of a marketing strategy for the development and expansion or contraction of a health program.

Public health programs are most sensitive demographically to women, infants, and the elderly. These three groups dominate the patient profile in most public and community health programs. Because the public health system is driven by the need to provide services to these groups, community health analysts should examine the public health market from these vantage points. Most health agencies provide services to small areas; therefore, it is appropriate to analyze public health markets by using small-area analysis or community health analysis techniques.

One of the most significant demographic events to be monitored is the baby boom population. They represent almost one-third of the U.S. population and include approximately 77 million individuals who were born between 1946 and 1964. A knowledge of their character, magnitude, and location is essential to public health markets. In 1986, the first baby boomer turned age 40, and, in 2029, the last baby boomer will become 65. The changing nature of the baby boom generation is shown in Figure 8-2. The increases and/or decreases in various age groups as the baby boomers progress through them affect program development and the just allocation of resources so that areas of future need can be considered. For example, the entry of baby boom females into the work force in large numbers has increased the need for child care services and programs in public health. The baby boomlet in the 1980s occurred because baby boomers postponed births to the mid-1980s. The future aging of the U.S. population is also directly related to the aging of baby boomers.

The wise yet cautious health organization will monitor and analyze these trends and pay particular attention to these population groups as they progress through the various life cycles. The marketing of community/public health programs requires demographic analysis. In order to improve infant mortality, increase the success of family planning, reach more children for nutrition services, or simply promote disease prevention and health education, it is essential to know the demographics of these groups: who they are, where they are, what they need, how much is required, and what changes in their composition are likely to take place over time.

Marketing Analysis: Psychographics

In the marketing of public health programs, psychographics permits community health analysts to go one step beyond demographic analysis. Psychographics is the addition of psychology to demographics to determine consumer wants and needs. This relationship between psychology and demographics produces values and lifestyles that may be useful in the marketing of health programs and the understanding of various lifestyles as they relate to disease and health.

A Values and Lifestyle (VALS) typology was introduced in 1978 and has been recently updated to produce VALS 2 (Fig. 8-3).[19] Alley, Dever, and Wade correlated the original VALS typology with changes in disease patterns in order to determine the relationship of various lifestyles to disease and to identify the demographic and lifestyle groups that succumb to different diseases.[20] The identification of the geographical concentration of these demographic and lifestyle groups could make it possible to predict pockets of disease and, thereby, to market health programs in areas where the most benefit or most improvement in health status would be obtained.

In the original VALS typology, there were four major groups: (1) those with

Tracking the Baby-Boom Generation

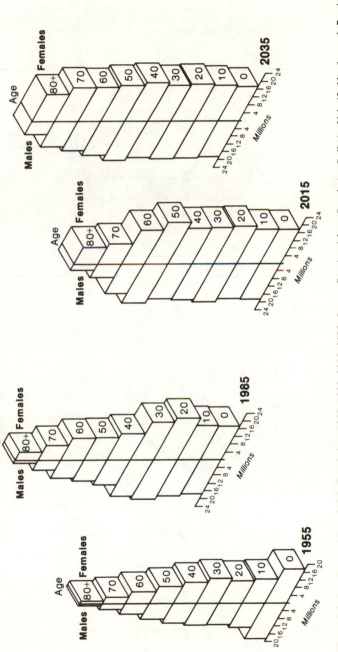

Figure 8-2 Age Composition of U.S. Population, 1955, 1985, 2015, 2035. *Source:* Reprinted from *Population Bulletin*, Vol. 43, No. 1, pp. 6–7, with permission of Population Reference Bureau, © 1988. Data from Bureau of the Census.

Old & New

The nine original VALS psychographic segments have been replaced by
eight new psychographic groups. In the new system, the groups are arranged
vertically by their resources and horizontally by their self-orientation.

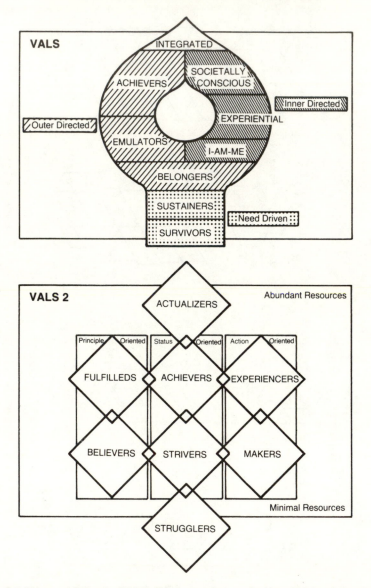

Figure 8-3 Value and Lifestyle (VALS) Typologies. *Source:* Courtesy SRI International, Menlo Park, CA.

need-driven lifestyles, who are dominant in the infectious disease model; (2) those with outer-directed lifestyles, who prevail in the chronic disease model; (3) those with inner-directed lifestyles, who will become the major force in the social transformation disease model; and (4) those with integrated lifestyles, who will not be a major factor until the distant future, although individuals who fit the integrated profile will gradually play a more important role in future societies (Fig. 8-4).

Need-Driven/Infectious Disease Model. The need-driven group comprises 11 percent of the U.S. population[21] and is concentrated in pockets of rural and urban poverty. Because this group lives in poverty, it is motivated by the basic needs for food, shelter, and security. Within this group are two subgroups, survivors and sustainers. Although both groups are in need, they are different in significant ways.[22]

Survivors are the poorest U.S. group, with a median household income of less than $10,000 per year. They are older than the general population (i.e., median age of 66); 37 percent have an eighth-grade education or less, and 79 percent have not gone to school beyond high school. Women make up 77 percent of the group, and nearly half of all survivors (47 percent) are retired. The group contains a high concentration of minorities (28 percent).[23] Survivors are resigned to their situation and are the most conservative group in the typology. They are outside the mainstream and know it, which leads to despair in many cases.

Sustainers, on the other hand, have hope. They are slightly more affluent than survivors, but they are still struggling financially, with a median household income under $15,000. Relatively young (half of them are under 33), most sustainers have not gone beyond high school (81 percent). There are more people looking for work in this group (15 percent) than in any other group in the typology. Sustainers also have the highest proportion of minorities (36 percent).[24] Even though sustainers are hopeful, they, too, feel left out of society. Consequently, they are resentful, distrustful, and likely to disregard rules if they feel it benefits them.

The need-driven group is at greater risk than any other for the health problems in the infectious disease model. For the most part, they have not entered into the industrial economy and are subject to pre-industrial and agrarian societal influences. This correlation between the need-driven group and the infectious disease model is much more apparent in underdeveloped countries and some intraurban areas that are still battling to control infectious disease problems. Recently, for example, the disease patterns in Manhattan have been shown to be as bad as those in Bangladesh.[25] Specifically, life expectancy for some groups was lower in Manhattan than in Bangladesh.

Outer-Directed/Chronic Disease Model. The outer-directed group is the largest segment of U.S. society, making up 67 percent (108 million) of the adult

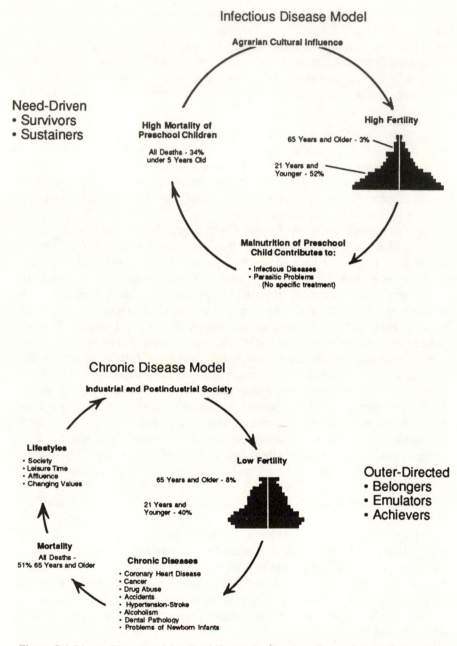

Figure 8-4 Disease Patterns and Levels of Human Development. *Source:* Reprinted from *Social Transformation Model: Human Development and Disease Patterns,* Datalog File No. 87-1153 by J.W. Alley, G.E.A. Dever, and T.E. Wade, p. 19, with permission of SRI International, © 1986.

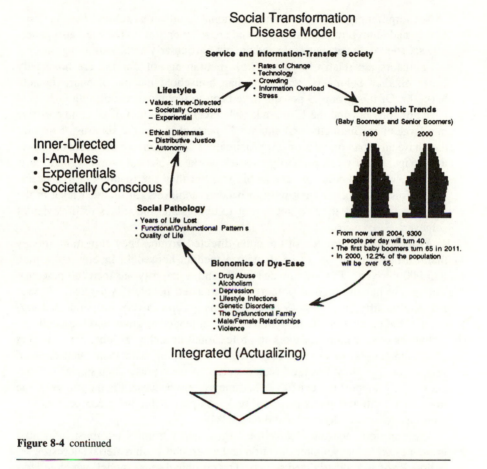

Social Transformation Disease Model

Service and Information-Transfer Society
- Rates of Change
- Technology
- Crowding
- Information Overload
- Stress

Lifestyles
- Values: Inner-Directed
  - Societally Conscious
  - Experiential

- Ethical Dilemmas
  - Distributive Justice
  - Autonomy

Inner-Directed
- I-Am-Mes
- Experientials
- Societally Conscious

Social Pathology
- Years of Life Lost
- Functional/Dysfunctional Patterns
- Quality of Life

Bionomics of Dys-Ease
- Drug Abuse
- Alcoholism
- Depression
- Lifestyle Infections
- Genetic Disorders
- The Dysfunctional Family
- Male/Female Relationships
- Violence

Demographic Trends
(Baby Boomers and Senior Boomers)

1990   2000

- From now until 2004, 9300 people per day will turn 40.
- The first baby boomers turn 65 in 2011.
- In 2000, 12.2% of the population will be over 65.

Integrated (Actualizing)

Figure 8-4 continued

population.[26] They react to perceived or real signals from others. The values of this group emphasize tradition, status, established institutions, and material possessions. They are the mainstream of U.S. culture. Within this group are three distinct levels with differing average incomes and educational backgrounds: the belongers, emulators, and achievers.[27]

Belongers are a little older than the general population, with a median age of 52. A majority are female (68 percent), with a moderate-to-low median household income of $15,000 a year. Among belongers, 74 percent have a high-school education or less, and only 7 percent have completed college or attended graduate school. Over half live in rural areas or small towns, the largest proportion of any level. A higher than average segment is retired (20 percent). Belongers who are working tend to be self-employed workers, clerical workers, machine operators, crafts workers, and homemakers.[28,29]

Not surprisingly, belongers share traditional, conformist values. They hold the family and church in highest regard and are very patriotic. They are also generally satisfied with the status quo and are not particularly ambitious as a group.[30]

Emulators are relatively young (i.e., median age of 27) and are financially better off than belongers, with a median household income of approximately $20,000. Of this group, 9 percent have been to technical school, although most have not gone beyond the 12th grade (63 percent). One-half of all emulators live in a large or medium city, and another 37 percent live in the suburbs; therefore, they have an urban orientation. Approximately 21 percent are members of minority groups. They work primarily as sales workers, clerical workers, and crafts workers.[31,32] Emulators are very ambitious, but they see roadblocks to success, which frustrates them. They wish to become achievers, at the next level in the typology; however, they do not appear to understand the values or lifestyles of achievers.[33]

Achievers are at the top of the outer-directed group. They earn more money than do those at any other level, with a median household income more than $35,000 per year. The average age is 43, and a majority are men (60 percent). This group has the highest proportion of married people (83 percent). Almost half live in suburban areas (49 percent). This group is a very well-educated segment of the population; 60 percent has either attended or graduated from college. Achievers most commonly work in professional or technical jobs, are managers or administrators, or are self-employed.[34] In keeping with their outer-directed orientation, people at this level seek material success, power, and status. Achievers strongly support the existing economic system because it is the source of the material wealth and status that they seek. As part of the most competitive segment, achievers are decisive and direct.[35,36]

The outer-directed are clearly the largest and currently the most influential group in U.S. society. Outer direction and an emphasis on material successes are hallmarks of an industrialized society. The chronic disease model, which reflects the influences of industrialization, illustrates the diseases and health problems of this group. Although outer-directed values are still dominant in the United States, the society is rapidly moving toward inner direction and a new disease cycle.

Inner-Directed/Social Transformation Disease Model. The past four decades have seen a trend toward inner direction, "one of the most significant sociological phenomena of the post–World War II Period."[37] The inner-directed group currently makes up 20 percent (32 million) of the U.S. population.[38] People in this group are driven by internal values and needs. This group has three levels: I-am-me, experiential, and societally conscious.

The I-am-me group is the youngest segment of any level (i.e., median age of 21) and has the highest concentration of students (44 percent). Many have either gone to college or graduated from college (58 percent). Nearly all are single (98 percent). The median income is low (less than $10,000), probably because I-am-mes are young and, in many cases, still in school.[39] I-am-mes are spontaneous and often flamboyant. They have not thought seriously about social issues, preferring to concentrate on their personal lives and self-awareness. They are quick to accept new ideas and situations. The I-am-me stage is nearly always a transition period that lasts only four or five years. Often I-am-mes grow into the next level, the experientials.

Experientials are older than I-am-mes (i.e., median age of 27), with a moderately high household median income of $26,000 a year. They are very well educated; 26 percent are college graduates, and an additional 12 percent have been to graduate school. Although 53 percent are married, 9 percent are not married but living with someone, the highest percentage of any level. In this group, 27 percent are in professional or technical jobs, 13 percent are self-employed, and 12 percent are homemakers.[40,41] Experientials participate personally in events. They are emotional and open to experience. They are the most inner-directed of the inner-directed group. They are less self-centered and more self-reliant than I-am-mes, however. This segment is more likely than any other to explore the mystical ideas or Eastern religions in search of personal insight.[42]

The societally conscious are concerned primarily with events and issues in the larger society. Their median age is 39, and their median household income is $32,000 a year. They are relatively mature and successful, and they are very well educated; 39 percent have attended graduate school. Societally conscious people typically hold professional or technical positions (59 percent).[43,44] They believe strongly in social responsibility and promote consumer interests, conservation, and environmental protection. This group's activism largely reflects its lack of confidence in the current outer-directed leadership, both in government and business. Societally conscious people believe that power is concentrated in too few hands.[45]

As the United States continues to move from an industrial society to a service and information transfer society, different psychological, social, genetic, and lifestyle preconditions will affect disease patterns. The infectious disease and chronic disease models will continue to be a reality, but the influences of industrialized society and the needs of a relatively younger population will no longer be dominant. Furthermore, financial rewards will cease to be as important to many people, who will look more for inner, intangible rewards. Consequently, the inner-directed group may become the majority by the year 2000, depending on societal and future factors. The social transformation disease model reflects the cultural patterns and health problems of a society strongly influenced by this inner-directed group.

Integrated Group. Because the integrated group makes up such a small portion of the adult population (2 percent) Mitchell was unable to develop a statistical profile of them. In theory, those in the integrated group blend inner-directed and outer-directed perspectives, using the best attributes of each. They bring balance and probably would score high as both achievers and societally conscious individuals.[46] Mitchell described them as people "who seem to have a kind of inner completeness, a kind of deep-core certainty, that commands respect, admiration, sometimes awe, and not infrequently love. These are people one truly trusts and seeks to be like. These are people who seem to have more wisdom than the rest of us."[47]

Although the integrated group probably numbers only 3 million in the United States, they are significant contributors to all sectors of the society. They probably will never become a large segment of the population. In all likelihood, however, they will play critical roles as leaders and facilitators.

VALS 2. Since the original analysis of disease patterns in relation to lifestyles, the VALS 2 segmentation was developed (see Figure 8-3). The VALS 2 features eight new psychographic groups arranged vertically by resources and horizontally by self-orientation: principle-oriented, status-oriented, or action-oriented. The earlier segments (VALS) were based on a population in their 20s and 30s in 1978; the new classification was created because of the "demographic and economic shifts, the aging of the baby boom, the increasing diversity of the population, the rise of the global economy, and the decline in consumers' expectations for the future."[48]

The VALS 2 apparently reveals unchanging psychological stances rather than shifting values and lifestyles as outlined in VALS. These data are quite appropriate for buying and media behavior; however, a blend of the original segmentation with the VALS 2 information seems appropriate for programs that target disease prevention and health education and promotion. In any event, the community health analyst should monitor and research the VALS and VALS 2 trends as they relate to the marketing of health programs.

Futures and Marketing Analysis

Of significance to the marketing of health programs, it is potentially possible to identify the dominant disease patterns and the changes in human development that will occur as a result of the projected future. There are four possible futures for the year 2000: hard times, bouncy prosperity, transition, and plain living. Table 8-1 shows the relationship of these futures to the original VALS typology and the dominant model of disease patterns for the 1980s, 1990s, and 2000s.

Hard Times

In the hard times future, the economic, social, and cultural climate will become increasingly unstable.[49] This instability will increase the proportion of

Table 8-1 Futures: Human Development and Disease Patterns—1980, 1990, 2000

Levels of Human Development	1980	1990 (Percent)	2000*	Dominant Model
Hard Times Future				
Need-driven	11	25	35	Infectious
Outer-directed	67	60	53	Chronic
Inner-directed	20	12	8	Social transformation
Integrated	2	3	4	Social transformation
Bouncy Prosperity Future				
Need-driven	11	7	3	Infectious
Outer-directed	67	77	87	Chronic
Inner-directed	20	14	8	Social transformation
Integrated	2	2	2	Social transformation
Transition Future				
Need-driven	11	10	9	Infectious
Outer-directed	67	60	53	Chronic
Inner-directed	20	26	32	Social transformation
Integrated	2	4	6	Social transformation
Plain Living Future				
Need-driven	11	10	9	Infectious
Outer-directed	67	52	37	Chronic
Inner-directed	20	33	46	Social transformation
Integrated	2	5	8	Social transformation

*Data from J.W. Alley, G.E.A. Dever, and T. Wade, "Social Transformation Model: Human Development and Disease Patterns," SRI International. Datalog File No. 87-1153, 1987, Menlo Park CA.

Source: Adapted from *The Nine American Lifestyles* by Arnold Mitchell, pp. 206–233, with permission of Warner Books, © 1984.

need-driven people from 11 percent to 35 percent of the U.S. population. The outer-directed group will show a corresponding downward shift from 67 percent to 53 percent. Thus, by the year 2000, 88 percent of the population will be in these two groups. In addition, the infectious and chronic disease models will be dominant. This scenario is the only one of the four in which the infectious disease model will increase in importance. Furthermore, if this future is realized, public health programs must be poised for a massive increase in the use of community/public health services.

Bouncy Prosperity

In the bouncy prosperity future, the economy will greatly expand, with the business community taking on most of the social responsibilities. The role of government will decline, and cultural activity will be at a low ebb. With increased prosperity, the society will become much more outer directed; this group will account for up to 87 percent of the population, with the need-driven and inner-directed groups decreasing accordingly. This shift will support the chronic disease model. Community/public health agencies will be doing business as usual, as represented by the health programs during most of the 1960s, 1970s, and early 1980s.

Transition

There will be movement toward a more inner-directed society in a transition future. In this scenario, the outer-directed group will still be the majority (53 percent in the year 2000). The inner-directed group will increase to 32 percent by the year 2000. These two shifts suggest that the chronic disease model will predominate; however, the social transformation disease model will emerge as a major factor toward the year 2000. Because of this shift, the following trends will appear:[50]

- decentralization of decision making
- personal involvement with work and national issues
- appreciation of other people, other ways, other ideas, and of the strengths and weaknesses of both inner direction and outer direction
- attention to spiritual and artistic needs

Economic, demographic, and social trends may bring a decade of the "real thing" (more direct living). The resulting values will range from the "new conservatism to a more personal involvement in artistic expression."[51] This future is the most difficult for health agencies, because the emerging transformation disease patterns are, in many instances, outside the purview of public health. This is one of the futures that will move society rapidly to a healthy public policy, however.

Plain Living

The major difference between the transition and the plain living futures is a shift of the outer- and inner-directed groups. The inner-directed group dominates in the plain living future, while the outer-directed group decreases in size and importance. Thus, this future most closely parallels the social transformation disease model. Although this disease model will dominate, others will continue to operate to a lesser degree. The plain living future will be an era of decentralization and "voluntary simplicity," a term coined by Mitchell.[52] The plain living future will foster inner-directed lifestyles, emphasizing the "ecologic ethic," "small is beautiful," "rights of the Earth," and the "right to personhood" (i.e., the right of each person to society's support in his or her search for self-realization).[53] Such a society will consciously move from the industrial era into the service and information transfer society; and a growing integrated group (the largest percentage of integrated people in any of the scenarios) will certainly promote this movement.

The social transformation disease model is particularly applicable to this future, in which rapid rates of change, demographic trends, the bionomics of disease, and lifestyles will bring a simpler, more direct, and more mature approach to living. It appears that the plain living future is becoming a reality as the year 2000 approaches. Concerns about the environment, education, technology, ecology, and society's overall value systems seem to set the stage for a more simple "back to basics" approach to problems. Community and public health agencies in this future need to become advocates for change and promoters of health to foster the move from public health policy to a healthy public policy.

Implications

Societal events and demographic shifts lay the groundwork for future health and quality of life. The responses of individuals and of society as a whole will determine the dominant disease models and lifestyles. Community health analysts can prepare for the future by closely monitoring changes in events, in the population, and in diseases. They will be able to predict much of what will happen. If they fail to monitor such changes, however, the health care system, especially the public health care system, will be in jeopardy and may even become obsolete.

The social transformation disease model demonstrates the need for a healthy public policy approach, one that recognizes education, environment, socioeconomic factors, poverty, and illiteracy as elements of a community/public health marketing approach.

Marketing Analysis Targeting and Forecasting

The most important aspect of marketing community and public health programs is the ability to target groups for health promotion in terms of their geography, demography, and psychography. Health agencies may use the interrelationships of these factors to target areas that match their health program risk profiles. This type of analysis is helpful not only in targeting those at risk, but also in (1) carrying out strategic planning, (2) developing health marketing media strategies, (3) examining the feasibility of direct mailing of health promotion materials, (4) selecting a site for a new community/public health clinic, (5) re-

Table 8-2 The Forty PRIZM® Lifestyle Clusters: Block Group Model

Group Codes	Descriptive Titles	Numbers	Nicknames	% of 1987 U.S. HH's*
S1	Educated, Affluent Executives and Professionals in Elite Metro Suburbs	28 8 5	Blue Blood Estates Money and Brains Furs and Station Wagons	1.13 0.94 3.19
S2	Pre- and Post-Child Families and Singles in Upscale, White-Collar Suburbs	7 25 20	Pools and Patios Two More Rungs Young Influentials	3.42 0.74 2.86
S3	Upper-Middle, Child-Raising Families in Outlying, Owner-Occupied Suburbs	24 30	Young Suburbia Blue-Chip Blues	5.40 6.04
U1	Educated, White-Collar Singles and Ethnics in Upscale, Urban Areas	21 37 31 23	Urban Gold Coast Bohemian Mix Black Enterprise New Beginnings	0.48 1.14 0.76 4.32
T1	Educated, Young, Mobile Families in Exurban Satellites and Boom Towns	1 17 12	God's Country New Homesteaders Towns and Gowns	2.71 4.16 1.15
S4	Middle-Class, Post-Child Families in Aging Suburbs and Retirement Areas	27 39 2	Levittown, U.S.A. Gray Power Rank and File	3.05 2.94 1.41
T2	Mid-Scale, Child-Raising Blue-Collar Families in Remote Suburbs and Towns	40 16 29	Blue-Collar Nursery Middle America Coalburg and Corntown	2.24 3.19 1.93
U2	Mid-Scale Families, Singles and Elders in Dense, Urban Row and High-Rise Areas	3 36 14 26	New Melting Pot Old Yankee Rows Emergent Minorities Single City Blues	0.90 1.59 1.72 3.35
R1	Rural Towns and Villages Amidst Farms and Ranches Across Agrarian Mid-America	19 34 35	Shotguns and Pickups Agri-Business Grain Belt	1.85 2.09 1.24
T3	Mixed Gentry and Blue-Collar Labor in Low-Mid Rustic, Mill, and Factory Towns	33 22 13 18	Golden Ponds Mines and Mills Norma Rae-Ville Smalltown Downtown	5.25 2.84 2.34 2.44

Table 8-2 continued

Group Codes	Descriptive Titles	Numbers	Nicknames	% of 1987 U.S. HH's*
R2	Landowners, Migrants and	10	Back-Country Folks	3.43
	Rustics in Poor Rural	38	Share Croppers	3.98
	Towns, Farms, and	15	Tobacco Roads	1.22
	Uplands	6	Hard Scrabble	1.50
U3	Mixed, Unskilled Service and	4	Heavy Industry	2.73
	Labor in Aging, Urban Row	11	Downtown Dixie-Style	3.37
	and Hi-Rise Areas	9	Hispanic Mix	1.88
		32	Public Assistance	3.10
			TOTAL U.S.	100.0

Note: Seen above are the 40 PRIZM® Lifestyle Clusters, organized into 12 broad Social Groups. The Groups are coded "S" for Suburban, "U" for Urban, "T" for Towns, and "R" for Rural, and are shown from top to bottom in descending socioeconomic rank, with the Group numbers (S1, S2, S3, etc.) indicating these ranks.

 * HH's = Households. Numbers = 1 through 40 for PRIZM® groups.

Source: Courtesy of Claritas Corporation, The Target Marketing Company, Alexandria, VA.

cruiting physicians (i.e., matching potential employee geography, demography, psychography characteristics with an area of similar characteristics), (6) determining a basic demographic/psychographic profile of the community/public health service area, and (7) determining the appropriate mix of health programs to offer based on demographics (e.g., concentration of elderly, children, infants, and women).

The information needed to perform these activities related to the marketing of health programs may be obtained from any one of several demographic vendors. Most vendors build on the VALS typology to separate consumers by differences and then cluster them with similar consumers. The vendors that sell the demographic/psychographic cluster systems are Claritas, Donnelley Marketing Information Services, CACI, and National Decision Systems. Each of these marketing vendors has a clustering system that groups individuals on the basis of like characteristics. For instance, Claritas has the PRIZM® system that identifies 12 social groups categorized into 40 lifestyle clusters (Table 8-2). Table 8-3 highlights three lifestyle clusters of consumers (i.e., blue blood estates, new melting pot, and Norma Rae-ville), including their likes and dislikes for several variables.

Donnelley Marketing Information Services has formulated the cluster PLUS system, which targets 47 unique consumer groups by lifestyle clusters (Table 8-4). Each cluster represents distinct lifestyle patterns that are ranked from

Table 8-3 Preferences of Consumers in Three Lifestyle Clusters

Variable	What They Like . . .	And Don't Like . . .
Blue Blood Estates		
Automobiles	Jaguar	Monte Carlo
Electronics	Home Computers	CB radios
Fast food	Friendly's	Pizza Hut
Investments	Treasury notes	Christmas Cl
Leisure/sports	Skiing	Pro wrestling
Magazines	*Barron's*	*Grit*
Package goods	Frozen pastry	TV dinners
TV programs	"Cheers"	"Gimme a Break"
Vacation/travel	Foreign travel	Camper/trail
VALS type	Achievers	Survivors
New Melting Pot		
Automobiles	Mitsubishi	Ford Escort
Electronics	Portable radios	Hair curlers
Fast food	Arthur Treacher	Popeye's
Investments	Certificates of deposit	Credit union
Leisure/sports	Horse racing	Hunting
Magazines	*Metro. Home*	*True Story*
Package goods	Yogurt	Pizza mixes
TV programs	"Hill St. Blues"	"20/20"
Vacation/travel	By railroad	Cruise ships
VALS type	Experientials	Sustainers
Norma Rae-Ville		
Automobiles	Bonneville	Saab
Electronics	Hair irons	Slide projectors
Fast food	Hardee's	Ponderosa
Investments	Personal loan	Brokerage A
Leisure/sports	Roller Derby	Live theatre
Magazines	*National Enquirer*	*Forbes*
Package goods	Canned hash	English muffin
TV programs	"A-Team"	"Family Ties"
Vacation/travel	By bus	Passports
VALS type	Survivors	Experiential

Note: VALS, Values and Lifestyle typology.

Source: Courtesy of Claritas Corporation, The Target Marketing Company, Alexandria, VA.

---

highest to lowest by socioeconomic status. CACI has developed A Classification of Residential Neighborhoods (ACORN), a clustering system and target marketing tool. Their premise is that people who have similar demographic, housing, and socioeconomic characteristics tend to live in homogenous neighborhoods

Table 8-4 Cluster PLUS Classifications

Cluster Code	Demographic Characteristics
01	Highest SESI, Highest Income, Prime Real Estate Areas, Highest Education Level, Professionally Employed, Low Mobility, Homeowners, Children in Private Schools
02	Very High Household Income, New Homes and Condominiums, Prime Real Estate Areas, Highly Mobile, High Education Level, Professionally Employed, Homeowners, Families with Children
03	High Income, High Home Values, New Homes, Highly Mobile, Younger, High Education Level, Professionally Employed, Homeowners, Married Couples, High Incidence of Children, Larger Families
04	High Income, High Home Values, High Education Level, Professionally Employed, Married Couples, Larger Families, Highest Incidence of Teenagers, Homeowners, Homes Built in 60s
05	High Income, High Home Values, High Education Level, Professionally Employed, Low Mobility, Homeowners, Homes Built in 50s and 60s
06	Highest Incidence of Children, Large Families, New Homes, Highly Mobile, Younger, Married Couples, Above Average Income and Education, Homeowners
07	Apartments and Condominiums, High Rent, Above Average Income, High Education Level, Professionally Employed, Mobile, Singles, Few Children, Urban Areas
08	Above Average Income, Above Average Education, Older, Fewer Children, White Collar Workers
09	Above Average Income, Average Education, Households with Two or More Workers, Homes Built in 60s and 70s
10	High Education Level, Average Income, Professionally Employed, Younger, Mobile, Apartment Dwellers, Above Average Rents
11	Above Average Income, Average Education, Families with Children, High Incidence of Teenagers, Homeowners, Homes Built in 60s, Small Towns
12	Highly Mobile, Young, Working Couples, Young Children, New Homes, Above Average Income and Education, White Collar Workers
13	Older, Fewer Children, Above Average Income, Average Education, White Collar Workers, Homeowners, Homes Built in 50s, Very Low Mobility, Small Towns

continues

Table 8-4 continued

Cluster Code	Demographic Characteristics
14	Retirees, Condominiums and Apartments, Few Children, Above Average Income and Education, Professionally Employed, High Home Values and Rents, Urban Areas
15	Older, Very Low Mobility, Fewer Children, Above Average Income and Education, White Collar Workers, Old Housing, Urban Areas
16	Working Couples, Very Low Mobility, Above Average Income, Average Education, Homeowners, Homes Built in 50s, Urban Areas
17	Very Young, Below Average Income, High Education Level, Professionally Employed, Highly Mobile, Singles, Few Children, Apartment Dwellers, High Rent Areas
18	High Incidence of Children, Larger Families, Above Average Income, Average Education, Working Couples, Homeowners
19	High Incidence of Children, Larger Families, Above Average Income, Average Education, Younger, Married Couples, Homeowners, Homes Built in 60s and 70s, Primarily Rural Areas
20	Areas with High Proportion of Group Quarters Population, College Dormitories, Homes for the Aged, Mental Hospitals and Prisons, Other Institutions
21	Average Income and Education, Blue Collar Workers, Families with Children, Homeowners, Lower Home Values, Rural Areas
22	Below Average Income and Education, Older, Fewer Children, Single Family Homes, Frequently Located in the South
23	Below Average Income, Average Education, Low Mobility, Married Couples, Old Homes, Farm Areas, Frequently Located in the North Central Region
24	Highly Mobile, Young, Few Children, Low Income, Average Education, Ethnic Mix, Singles, Apartments, Urban Areas
25	Younger, Mobile, Fewer Children, Below Average Income, Average Education, Apartment Dwellers
26	Older, Mobile, Fewer Children, Below Average Income, Average Education, Mobile Homes, Retirees, Primarily Rural Areas
27	Average Income and Education, Single Family Homes, Lower Home Values, Homes Built in 50s and 60s

Table 8-4 continued

Cluster Code	Demographic Characteristics
28	Below Average Income, Lower Education Level, Younger, Mobile, High Incidence of Children, Mobile Homes, Primarily Rural Area
29	Older, Low Mobility, Ethnic Mix, Average Income, Below Average Education, Old Home and Apartments, Urban Areas, Frequently Located in Northeast Region
30	Low Income, Lowest Education Level, Families with One Worker, Farms, Rural Areas
31	Older, Fewer Children, Low Income, Low Education Level, Low Mobility, Retirees, Old Single Family Homes
32	Old, Few Children, Low Income, Below Average Education, One-Person Households, Retirees
33	Below Average Income, Low Education Level, Blue Collar Workers, Manufacturing Plants, Homes Built in 50s and 60s, Very Low Mobility, Low Home Values
34	Older, Below Average Income, Average Education, Blue Collar Workers, Low Mobility, Rural Areas
35	Old Housing, Low Income, Average Education, Younger, Mobile, Fewer Children, Apartment Dwellers, Small Towns
36	Average Income, Low Education Level, Blue Collar Workers, Hispanics, Families with Children
37	Average Income, Below Average Education Level, Blue Collar Workers, Manufacturing Areas, High Unemployment, Frequently Located in the North Central Region
38	Old, Lowest Incidence of Children, Very Low Income, Low Education Level, Apartment Dwellers, One-Person Households, Retirees, Urban Areas
39	Older, Very Low Mobility, Very Old Housing, Below Average Income and Education, Blue Collar Workers, Manufacturing Areas
40	Older, Very Low Income, Low Education Level, One-Person Households, Retirees, Few Children, Old Homes and Apartments
41	Below Average Income, Low Education Level, Blue Collar Workers, Manufacturing Plants, High Unemployment, Rural Areas

continues

Table 8-4 continued

Cluster Code	Demographic Characteristics
42	Low Income, Lowest Education Level, Low Mobility, Blue Collar Workers, Manufacturing Plants, Rural Areas
43	Low Income Blacks, Families with Children, Single Family Homes, Low Mobility, Low Education Level, Unskilled Workers, High Unemployment
44	Urban Blacks, Very Low Income, Low Education Level, High Unemployment, Singles, Mobile, Apartment Dwellers, Large Metro Areas
45	Urban Blacks, Very Low Income, Low Education Level, Unskilled, High Unemployment, Old Housing
46	Very Low Income, Lowest Education Level, Hispanics, Families with Children, Apartment Dwellers, Unskilled Workers, High Unemployment
47	Lowest SESI, Urban Blacks, Very Low Income, Low Education Level, Unskilled Workers, Very High Unemployment, Female Householders with Children, Old Housing

Note: SESI, socioeconomic status index.

Source: Courtesy of Donnelley Marketing Information Services, Stamford, CT.

---

and share similar lifestyles. CACI has developed 13 groups that are categorized into 44 distinct, homogenous market segments based on the characteristics of each area. An Area Profile Report regarding the current situation for a particular geographical area and an Area Forecast Report regarding a five-year forecast of change in the ACORN groups are shown in Table 8-5 and Table 8-6, respectively.

These demographic vendors and their products have widespread use in business, industry and some government agencies. Although hospitals, clinics, HMOs, physicians, and other health lifestyle agencies (e.g., aerobics centers and executive fitness clubs) use demographic and psychographic clustering to enhance their market position, community and public health agencies have not done so. The reasons may include cost, failure to understand the relationship of the data to their health programs, and lack of personnel who are trained in the analysis of such data. In addition, not all administrators see the importance of targeting the appropriate groups for the agency's health programs, as savings are not translated into profit. Any savings that result from efficiency should be translated into resources to permit a wider distribution of the program components, however.

Table 8-5 ACORN Area Profile Report

ACORN Type	ACORN Description	Households			
		1989	Area %	Base %	Area Index
A 1	Old Money	266	0.4	0.5	80
A 2	Conspicuous Consumers	5150	7.1	1.0	710
A 3	Cosmopolitan Wealth	7723	10.6	2.4	441
B 4	Upper Middle Income Families	394	0.5	2.7	19
B 5	Empty Nesters	17165	23.7	2.5	48
B 6	Baby Boomers with Families	0	0.0	3.6	0
B 7	Middle Americans in New Homes	274	0.4	5.3	7
B 8	Skilled Craft & Office Workers	1446	2.0	4.5	44
C 9	Condominium Dwellers	1845	2.5	2.0	125
C10	Fast Track Young Adults	16908	23.3	6.0	388
C11	College Undergraduates	0	0.0	0.3	0
C12	Older Students & Professionals	733	1.0	1.8	56
D13	Urbanites in High Rises	3348	4.6	1.2	383
D14	Big City Working Class	11447	15.8	1.7	929
E15	Mainstream Hispanic Americans	2136	2.9	2.3	126
E16	Large Hispanic Families	0	0.0	1.5	0
E17	Working Class Single Adults	0	0.0	1.5	0
E18	Families in Pre-War Rentals	0	0.0	1.1	0
E19	Third World Melting Pot	0	0.0	1.0	0
F20	Mainstream Family Homeowners	141	0.2	3.1	6
F21	Trend Conscious Families	0	0.0	1.9	0
F22	Low Income Families	0	0.0	0.9	0
G23	Settled Families	0	0.0	3.4	0
G24	Start-Up Families	0	0.0	5.0	0
H25	Family Sports & Leisure Lovers	0	0.0	2.1	0
H26	Secure Factory & Farm Workers	0	0.0	2.0	0
H27	Family Centered Blue Collar	0	0.0	3.1	0
H28	Minimum Wage White Families	0	0.0	4.0	0
I29	Golden Years Retirees	0	0.0	2.5	0
I30	Adults in Pre-War Housing	3324	4.6	5.2	89
I31	Small Town Families	0	0.0	6.2	0
I32	Nostalgic Retirees & Adults	0	0.0	1.0	0
I33	Home Oriented Senior Citizens	0	0.0	2.0	0
I34	Old Families in Pre-War Homes	0	0.0	4.5	0
J35	Resort Vacationers & Locals	0	0.0	0.8	0
J36	Mobile Home Dwellers	0	0.0	1.3	0
K37	Farm Families	0	0.0	0.6	0
K38	Young, Active Country Families	0	0.0	0.3	0
L39	Low Income Retirees & Youth	0	0.0	3.1	0
L40	Rural Displaced Workers	0	0.0	0.1	0
L41	Factory Worker Families	0	0.0	2.7	0
L42	Poor Young Families	0	0.0	0.4	0
M43	Military Base Families	252	0.3	0.5	67
M44	Institutions: Residents & Staff	0	0.0	0.1	0

Base Definition:US   72522

Source: Courtesy of CACI, Inc., Fairfax, VA.

Table 8-6 ACORN Area Forecast Report

ACORN Type	ACORN Description	Households				Annual Growth 89–94
		1989	%	1994	%	
A 1	Old Money	266	0.4	264	0.4	−0.2
A 2	Conspicuous Consumers	5150	7.1	5227	7.0	0.3
A 3	Cosmopolitan Wealth	7723	10.6	7998	10.7	0.7
B 4	Upper Middle Income Families	394	0.5	436	0.6	2.0
B 5	Empty Nesters	17165	23.7	17446	23.2	0.3
B 6	Baby Boomers with Families	0	0.0	0	0.0	0.0
B 7	Middle Americans in New Homes	274	0.4	281	0.4	0.5
B 8	Skilled Craft and Office Workers	1446	2.0	1438	1.9	−0.1
C 9	Condominium Dwellers	1845	2.5	1869	2.5	0.3
C10	Fast Track Young Adults	16908	23.3	17662	23.5	0.9
C11	College Undergraduates	0	0.0	0	0.0	0.0
C12	Older Students and Professionals	733	1.0	750	1.0	0.5
D13	Urbanites in High Rises	3348	4.6	3620	4.8	1.6
D14	Big City Working Class	11447	15.8	12093	16.1	1.1
E15	Mainstream Hispanic Americans	2136	2.9	2125	2.8	−0.1
E16	Large Hispanic Families	0	0.0	0	0.0	0.0
E17	Working Class Single Adults	0	0.0	0	0.0	0.0
E18	Families in Pre-War Rentals	0	0.0	0	0.0	0.0
E19	Third World Melting Pot	0	0.0	0	0.0	0.0
F20	Mainstream Family Homeowners	141	0.2	144	0.2	0.4
F21	Trend Conscious Families	0	0.0	0	0.0	0.0
F22	Low Income Families	0	0.0	0	0.0	0.0
G23	Settled Families	0	0.0	0	0.0	0.0
G24	Start-Up Families	0	0.0	0	0.0	0.0
H25	Family Sports and Leisure Lovers	0	0.0	0	0.0	0.0
H26	Secure Factory and Farm Workers	0	0.0	0	0.0	0.0
H27	Family Centered Blue Collar	0	0.0	0	0.0	0.0
H28	Minimum Wage White Families	0	0.0	0	0.0	0.0
I29	Golden Years Retirees	0	0.0	0	0.0	0.0
I30	Adults in Pre-War Housing	3324	4.6	3437	4.6	0.7
I31	Small Town Families	0	0.0	0	0.0	0.0
I32	Nostalgic Retirees and Adults	0	0.0	0	0.0	0.0
I33	Home Oriented Senior Citizens	0	0.0	0	0.0	0.0
I34	Old Families in Pre-War Homes	0	0.0	0	0.0	0.0
J35	Resort Vacationers and Locals	0	0.0	0	0.0	0.0
J36	Mobile Home Dwellers	0	0.0	0	0.0	0.0
K37	Farm Families	0	0.0	0	0.0	0.0
K38	Young, Active Country Families	0	0.0	0	0.0	0.0
L39	Low Income Retirees and Youth	0	0.0	0	0.0	0.0
L40	Rural Displaced Workers	0	0.0	0	0.0	0.0
L41	Factory Worker Families	0	0.0	0	0.0	0.0
L42	Poor Young Families	0	0.0	0	0.0	0.0
M43	Military Base Families	252	0.3	270	0.4	1.4
M44	Institutions: Residents and Staff	0	0.0	0	0.0	0.0

Total   72522

Source: Courtesy of CACI, Inc., Fairfax, VA.

276

Rapid social change has unraveled markets, and old labels are no longer useful; the context in which things are perceived is becoming more and more of a cultural phenomenon. High-technology and service positions have eroded the differences between white and blue collar; those with a double income and no kids (DINKS) and divorces (both increased) have blurred the difference between the upper and lower classes. Thus, consumers are more difficult to reach. Because of these trends, health agencies must engage in more rigorous marketing approaches by identifying target groups and promoting health programs to these groups.

The cluster analysis that identifies similar or homogenous demographic and psychographic groups can be applied to disease risks and community needs to arrive at a community diagnosis. Correlating infant mortality rates to the demographic/psychographic cluster groups, for example, may elicit one or several clusters in which infant mortality rates are persistently high. The identification of specific lifestyle clusters associated with high infant mortality rates could result in marketing strategies designed for the location and lifestyle of the clusters. Furthermore, forecasting these high-risk infant mortality cluster groups five years in advance would allow health agencies to market infant mortality reduction programs in areas where the potential for success is the greatest. The use of this type of information is unlimited.

As good as their information appears, these demographic vendors have their critics. Certainly, no method is perfect. Merrick and Tordella stated that,"while it is simple to find fault because of the ecological fallacy and the relative crudeness of these systems, they are powerful." [54] The fact remains that most of the demographic vendors' segmentation was done without regard for health, but was developed for general lifestyles.

Several authors have attempted demographic/psychographic segmentation of the health care market. [55-57] Each of the proposals has been developed specifically for the health care market. In addition, Donnelley Marketing Information Services has created a health care package, called Diagnostics, that consists of six comprehensive reports (Fig. 8-5). By combining these reports, a health agency director or manager can target health markets, scan for similar cluster groups, report on trends, predict the morbidity of a geographical area (presently, mostly mortality data is used), determine accessibility of physicians, and use hospital facility data to aid in determining the availability of services and realizing the potential for regionalization. The success of community/public health programs may well be measured by their ability to integrate this information into their overall strategic planning process.

Social Marketing: Ideas and Behaviors

Introduced in 1971,[58] social marketing is defined as "the design, implementation, and control of programs seeking to increase the acceptability of a social

DONNELLEY'S HEALTH CARE PACKAGE INCLUDES:

Trend Report

Key demographic statistics for population, household, age, race, sex, and income. The trend report shows the characteristics of consumers in your market for yesterday (1970, 1980), today (1988), and tomorrow (1993). This demographic data is the most accurate available in the industry today, because it comes from Donnelley's continuously updated database of 79 million unduplicated households (90% of the entire USA).

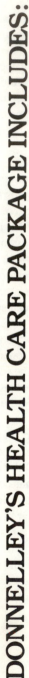

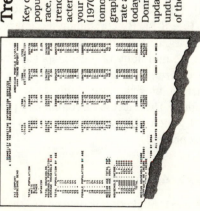

Age/Sex/Race Report

Demographics designed specifically for the health care industry, this report describes population by age, race and sex. The unique aspect of this report is its description of age categories in range from 0 to 85+, in 5-year increments. Since this information is for 1980, 1988, and 1993, you can rapidly assess the dynamics of individual age groups, and clearly understand what is happening to the population in your market.

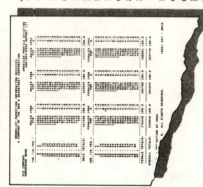

Figure 8-5 Diagnostics Program of Donnelley Marketing Information Services. *Source:* Courtesy of Donnelley Marketing Information Services, Stamford, CT.

Patient Predictive Forecasts

Developed by combining incidence rates for each diagnosis related group (DRG) from Systemetrics/McGraw-Hill and Donnelley current year age estimates, this report provides powerful insight into the demand for specific health care products and services. Choose either a total MDC Report, or one of 23 MDC Reports that include all pertaining DRGs.

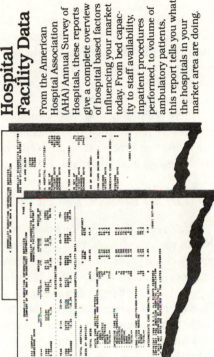

Hospital Facility Data

From the American Hospital Association (AHA) Annual Survey of Hospitals, these reports give a complete overview of hospital based factors influencing your market today. From bed capacity to staff availability, inpatient procedures performed, to volume of ambulatory patients, this report tells you what the hospitals in your market area are doing.

ClusterPlus℠ Area Composition Report

Understand the demographics of any market using the most sought after tool for market segmentation: ClusterPlus. This report classifies the population into 47 lifestyle categories. Clusters are groups of people with similar purchasing and behavior patterns. The ClusterPlus report enhances your understanding of a market's psychographic and socio-economic behavior.

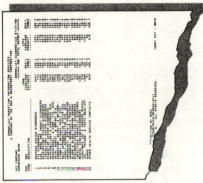

Physician Summary Report

Developed from a national physicians' direct response database, the BMI, Inc., Medec file, this report describes the distribution of physicians in your market, by specialty. Not only will you know the number of physicians by each specialty category, but how that number compares to the country as a whole.

Figure 8-5 continued

idea or cause in a target group(s)."[59] While business marketing aims at satisfying the needs and wants of target markets, social marketing seeks to change their attitudes or behavior. Although the marketing of intangible ideas, including preventive health behavior, is more complex and arduous than marketing a tangible product or service, it is possible and feasible—but only if the marketing process is followed in its entirety.

There seem to be four major reasons that past efforts at social marketing have apparently failed. First, attitudes and behavior are difficult to change. Second, the marketing process is misunderstood. Third, the promotion or communication strategies are misunderstood. Fourth, measures of performance are inadequate.

Attitudes and Behavior: Difficult To Change

Health educators have long been struggling to find effective ways of advancing health messages. Even the experts are not yet sure about how behaviors are set and how they can be influenced, however. It is known that certain types of changes are easier to effect than others. Marketers usually distinguish among four types of social changes in increasing difficulty: (1) cognitive change, (2) action change, (3) behavioral change, and (4) value change.[60]

Cognitive changes, that is, changes in knowledge, are easier to market because they do not require the alteration of any deep-rooted attitudes or behavior. Unfortunately, there appears to be little connection between cognitive change and behavioral change. Although some health educators still hold onto it,[61,62] their traditional model of linear change from knowledge to attitude to practice (KAP) has been proved inadequate and too simplistic many times.[63] Thus, even if they are relatively easy to bring about, cognitive changes may be of little value when the ultimate aim is an attitudinal or behavioral change.

Action changes are considered more difficult to achieve because the target market must understand the reason and then take an action, always at a certain cost of time, effort, or energy. Campaigns for action changes are generally attempts to induce a maximum number of people to take a specific action during a given period. In terms of disease prevention and health promotion, action changes usually involve secondary prevention, such as screening programs and early diagnosis of problems, and can be divided conceptually according to the amount of activity required on the part of the consumer.[64] Some action changes require a one-time act, as in mass immunization campaigns and many screening programs. Others call for repeated, but noncontinuous, acts; annual physical checkups or Papanicolaou smears require the periodic repetition of an action.

Behavioral changes involve repeated and continuous acts. Smoking cessation and improved nutritional habits require repeated and continuous behavioral commitment, for example. Behavioral changes are called for most often in efforts at primary prevention (action designed to prevent the occurrence of disease or injury), although tertiary prevention (rehabilitation and prevention of sequelae, for example, after a heart attack) also require behavioral changes. Not all behavioral changes require the same consumer involvement. A distinction can be made between high-involvement behavioral changes, such as regular exercise and good nutritional habits, in which consumers usually perceive a direct personal benefit (e.g., "feeling better") and low-involvement activities, such as reduced driving speed, in which consumers may perceive more benefits to society than to themselves.[65]

Value changes are alterations in deeply rooted beliefs about some object or situation. Efforts to change people's ideas about abortion, about the "appropriate" number of children, about civil rights, or about race relations are examples of value marketing. These changes are the most difficult to market, and chances of success may be slim.

Health managers may (and perhaps should) be more concerned with action and behavioral changes. The various types of action and behavioral changes require different marketing strategies. In some cases, demand for the product or service offered may be negative.[66] In other words, consumers may be avoiding the required change (service). This is often the case with immunizations, dental services, and treatments for sexually transmitted disease. In such situations, sources of resistance must be identified and eliminated or circumvented.

In other cases, demand may be null, with consumers indifferent to the change (service). This may be the case for road safety or periodic health examinations, for example. In such situations, marketers must increase the public's perception of the benefits associated with the change.

In still other cases, the change involves a reduction in the consumption of a product or service for which demand is positive, such as cigarette smoking or the use of alcohol. Such situations call for a countermarketing strategy because they require not only the abandonment of or reduced adherence to an existing behavior, but also the subsequent adoption of a new behavior. This is a crucial point that is often forgotten in behavior modification programs. Emphasizing the subsequent adoption of a new behavior may facilitate the countermarketing of a harmful behavior, especially in the field of primary prevention where it may be necessary to approximate cause-and-effect relationships through risk (or statistical) relationships (see Chapter 1) because it is impossible to demonstrate them. As Marshall wrote in 1980 concerning smoking cessation programs,

> Essentially, prevention asks the individual smoker to bet that he will develop lung cancer and advises him to avoid this eventuality by giving up cigarettes. In fact, on the individual level, smoking does not guarantee the eventual occurrence of this disease, and abstinence from smoking does not assure its prevention. The ratio of reward to effort is great, and after years or decades the reward is an abstraction involving

a statistical payoff—something bad that might have happened but did not. The modification of life style that is the outcome of successful health education is a "blood, sweat, and tears" approach to prevention. It is not a magic bullet; it is hard work, involving the alteration of old habits and the sustenance of new ones over much of a lifetime.[67]

More emphasis on the benefits of the sustenance of the new behavior, such as increased cardiopulmonary fitness, undoubtedly would increase the effectiveness of the countermarketing.

Marketing: A Misunderstood Process

The lack of success of earlier social marketing programs may be due in part to an incomprehension and misunderstanding of the marketing process itself.[68] Many so-called social marketing (and health education) campaigns have consisted of attempts to sell a predesigned program (i.e., a product orientation). Analyses of the environment and the consumer have been inadequate or nonexistent. Furthermore, many of these programs have merely been advertising campaigns that gave no consideration to the other elements of the marketing mix.

A strategy based on every dimension of the marketing mix is particularly important in health education aimed at behavioral changes. Behaviors are so complex and deeply rooted, and result from the interaction of so many variables, that a narrow approach to change is doomed to failure. Health education literature has emphasized that behavior change requires a comprehensive approach.[69-72] Among other things, this means that a complete marketing process, including a comprehensive marketing mix strategy, is needed.

Preventive health interventions can be broadened to include not only those in which consumers must be active, but also those in which consumers can remain passive.[73-75] Such passive interventions may be of a legal, technological, or economic nature. For example, fluoridation of water and regulation of environmental, chemical, and physical hazards are preventive health measures that do not generally require active consumer involvement. Marketing incorporates these passive approaches through consideration of the marketing mix. Effective preventive health interventions consider service characteristics (product), location of service delivery (place), price, and promotion.

Promotion: Also Misunderstood

The promotion component of the marketing mix is a specialized and complex domain. There are, however, certain basic principles. First, promotion (or communication) is not only advertising, and mass media are not the only promotion channels that marketers consider. As Quelch wrote,

Marketers generally agree that although mass media approaches are appropriate for developing consumer awareness in the short term, face-to-face programs such as workplace encounters are more effective (though not always cost effective) in changing behavior in the long term. In designing any communication policy, the marketer commonly considers the effects that may be achievable through the use of a mix of approaches, capitalizing on the strengths of each.[76]

Second, a promotion strategy should result directly from the previous steps of the marketing process (i.e., from analyses of the environments, the competition, the resources, and the markets). It should always be targeted to specific market segments.

Third, there are three basic conditions necessary for the effectiveness of social communication campaigns.[77]

1. *monopolization of the media*. No counterpropaganda should be present. This obviously is not the case in most social marketing campaigns, a fact that can explain in part their limited effectiveness.
2. *canalization*. There should be an existing attitudinal base for the feelings (ideas) that the social marketer is trying to communicate. When this is the case, it is much easier to promote an idea; all that is required is the canalization (channeling) of these preexisting attitudes in a specific direction.
3. *supplementation*. Mass media campaigns should be followed (supplemented) with other programs, such as face-to-face contacts.

Thus, there should be a comprehensive step-down communication process in which the message is passed on and discussed in more familiar terms and surroundings.

Performance Measurement Inadequacies

It is difficult to measure the effectiveness of social marketing campaigns, because the results are essentially intangible and the relevant time frame is wide and long. In addition, social marketers, particularly health educators, may have unrealistic expectations. In business marketing, companies are usually delighted when a sales increase of 1 percent to 2 percent can be attributed to a marketing campaign.[78] For example, a 1 percent gain is worth millions in sales, even for the less popular brands of cigarettes. On the other hand, many health education campaigns have been judged ineffective and disappointing even if 25 percent (and up to 50 percent) of the target markets have modified a behavior.

For example, when antismoking commercials on television were shown to have reduced smoking in 34 percent of college students and to have led to complete cessation of smoking in 21 percent, at least temporarily, the results were considered disappointing.[79] Similarly, the fact that 25 percent of the public had received the entire series of four polio shots and 60 percent had received at least one after a government publicity campaign was considered disappointing.[80]

Since antismoking campaigns started in Canada in the early 1970s, the proportion of regular smokers decreased from 42.8 percent to 34.2 percent (in 1979), while the percentage of nonsmokers increased from 50.2 percent to 60.1 percent.[81] Furthermore, brands low in nicotine and tar attracted a large proportion of smokers between 1977 and 1979. These modifications of the smoking behavior of Canadians occurred even though cigarette companies continued to spend millions of dollars a year on advertising while the government spent only a fraction of that amount on antismoking promotion.

In the United States, it was estimated that, as of 1975, the cumulative effect of persistent antismoking publicity supported by (a few) other public policies had reduced per capita consumption of cigarettes by 20 percent to 30 percent. This was a conservative measure, as it ignored the potential health impact that could result from a shift to cigarettes low in tar and nicotine.[82] It can be said that "the myth of overwhelming advertiser success has exerted a negative effect on health education (and other social marketing efforts) by encouraging the belief that anything short of a success rate approaching 100 percent is unsatisfactory."[83]

CONCLUSION

Marketing principles and techniques can and should be used to promote health in conjunction with other education methods. The effectiveness of such health marketing depends not only on a thorough understanding of the process, however, but also on the understanding that health (and health-related behaviors) are determined by a wide range of interrelated factors. This moves marketing from its singular focus on changing individual behaviors to the broader context of a healthy public policy that focuses on individual and community concerns.

Marketing concepts for community/public health groups are in their infancy. The challenge of the 1990s and the 2000s will be to expedite the use of these approaches so as to benefit from dwindling resources and respond to the needs of all citizens in a just and equitable manner. Marketing community health can offer solutions to these problems.

NOTES

1. Robin E. MacStravic, *Marketing Health Care* (Gaithersburg, Md.: Aspen Publishers, Inc., 1977), 7.

2. J.G. Keith, "Marketing Health Care: What the Recent Literature Is Telling Us," *Hospital and Health Services Administration* Special 2 (1981): 66–94.

3. MacStravic, *Marketing Health Care*, 16.

4. Peter F. Drucker, *Management: Tasks, Responsibilities, Practices* (New York: Harper & Row, 1973), 64–65.

5. Philip Kotler, *Marketing for Nonprofit Organizations,* 2nd ed. (Englewood Cliffs, N.J.: Prentice-Hall, Inc., 1982), 7.

6. Ibid., 47.

7. H. Mintzberg, "Organizational Power and Goals: A Skeletal Theory," in *Strategic Management: A New View of Business Policy and Planning,* ed. D.E. Schendel and C.W. Hofer (New York: Little, Brown & Co., 1979), 64–80.

8. MacStravic, *Marketing Health Care.*

9. Kotler, *Marketing for Nonprofit Organizations,* 56.

10. MacStravic, *Marketing Health Care,* 20.

11. Kotler, *Marketing for Nonprofit Organizations,* 108.

12. Philip Kotler, *Marketing Management* (Englewood Cliffs, N.J.: Prentice-Hall, Inc., 1980), ch. 3.

13. Ibid.

14. Ibid.

15. D. Finlay, "Geographic Targeting," *American Demographics* 2 (October 1980): 39–41.

16. A.S. Boote, "Mind over Matter," *American Demographics* 2 (April 1980): 26–29.

17. E.J. Forrest et al., "Psychographic Flesh, Demographic Bones," *American Demographics* 3 (September 1981): 25–27.

18. H. Assael, "Segmenting Markets by Groups Purchasing Behavior: An Application of the Aid Technique," *Journal of Marketing Research* 7 (May 1970): 153–158.

19. M.F. Riche, "Psychographics for the 1990's," *American Demographics* 11, no. 7 (July 1989): 25–31, 53–54.

20. J.W. Alley, G.E.A. Dever, and T. Wade, "Social Transformation Model: Human Development and Disease Patterns," SRI International. Datalog File No. 87-1153, 1987. Menlo Park, CA.

21. Arnold Mitchell, *The Nine American Lifestyles* (New York: Warner Books, 1984), 41–43.

22. Ibid., 4.

23. Ibid., 279–280.

24. Ibid., 278–280.

25. Ibid., 63.

26. Ibid.

27. Ibid., 8–9.

28. Ibid., 279–281.

29. P. Francese and B. Edmondson, *Health Care Consumers. Handbook of Trends, Techniques and Information Sources for Healthcare Executives.* (Ithaca, N.Y.: American Demographics Institute, 1986), 68.

30. Mitchell, *The Nine American Lifestyles,* 9–10.

31. Ibid., 279–281.

32. Francese and Edmondson, *Health Care Consumers,* 3–11.

33. Mitchell, *The Nine American Lifestyles,* 11–13.

34. Ibid., 279–280.

35. Ibid., 13–14.

36. Francese and Edmondson, *Health Care Consumers,* 26–48.

37. Mitchell, *The Nine American Lifestyles,* 63.

38. Ibid., 16.

39. Ibid., 279–281.

40. Ibid.

41. Francese and Edmondson, *Health Care Consumers,* 26–48.

42. Mitchell, *The Nine American Lifestyles,* 18–20.

43. Ibid., 279–281.

44. Francese and Edmondson, *Health Care Consumers,* 26–48.

45. Mitchell, *The Nine American Lifestyles,* 20–22.

46. Ibid., 23–25.

47. Ibid., 22.

48. M.F. Riche, "Psychographics for the 1990's," 26.

49. Mitchell, *The Nine American Lifestyles,* 227.

50. Ibid., 218–220.

51. Ibid., 213–215.

52. Ibid., 230.

53. Ibid.

54. T.W. Merrick and S.J. Tordella, "Demographics: People and Markets," *Population Bulletin* 43, no. 1 (February 1988): 30.

55. K.W. Endreson, J.C. Wintz, "Healthstyles: A New Psychographic Segmentation System for Health Care Marketers," *Journal of Medical Practice Management* 3, no. 4 (Spring 1988): 273–277.

56. A.G. Woodside et al., "Preference Segmentation of Health Care Services: The Old Fashioned, Value Conscious, Affluents, and Professional Want-it-Alls," *Journal of Health Care Marketing* 8, no. 2 (June 1988): 14–24.

57. K. Dychtwald and M. Zitler, "Developing a Strategic Marketing Plan for Hospitals," *Health Care Financial Management* 42, no. 9 (September 1988): 44–46.

58. Philip Kotler and G. Zaltman, "Social Marketing: An Approach to Planned Social Change," *Journal of Marketing* 35 (July 1971): 3–12.

59. Kotler, *Marketing for Nonprofit Organizations,* 90.

60. Ibid., 501–510.

61. M. O'Neill, "*Vers une problematique de l'education sanitaire au Quebec*" (Master's thesis, Laval University, Quebec, 1976), 289.

62. "La modification des comportements relies a la sante," *Union Medicale du Canada* 109 (1980): 733–742, 921–928.

63. S. Simonds, "Emerging Challenges in Health Education," *International Journal of Health Education* 19, no. 4, special supplement (1976): 1–18.

64. J.A. Quelch, "Marketing Principles and the Future of Preventive Health Care," *Milbank Memorial Fund Quarterly/Health and Society* 58, no. 2 (Spring 1980): 317.

65. M.L. Rothschild, "Marketing Communications in Nonbusiness Situations; Or, Why It's So Hard to Sell Brotherhood Like Soap," *Journal of Marketing* 43, no. 2 (1979): 11–20.

66. D.A. Lussier, "La sante publique: Est-ce possible d'en faire un marketing," *Les Cahiers de Sante Communautaire,* Association pour la Sante Publique du Quebec, June 1979, 317.

67. C.C. Marshall, "Prevention and Health Education," in *Maxcy-Rosenau Public Health and Preventive Medicine* 11th ed., edited by J.M. Last (New York: Appleton-Century-Crofts, Inc., 1980), 1122.

68. Quelch, "Marketing Principles," 325–331.

69. Amitai Etzioni, "Human Beings Are Not Very Easy To Change After All," *Saturday Review,* 3 June, 1972, 45–47.

70. O'Neill, "Vers une problematique."

71. E.R. Brown and G.E. Margo, "Health Education: Can the Reformers Be Reformed?" *International Journal of Health Services* 8, no. 1 (1978): 3–26.

72. N.D. Richards, "Methods and Effectiveness of Health Education," *Social Science and Medicine* 9 (1975): 141–156.

73. Quelch, "Marketing Principles," 316.

74. J.E. Fielding, "Successes of Prevention," *Milbank Memorial Fund Quarterly/Health and Society* 56 (Summer 1978): 274–302.

75. M. Venkatesan, "Consumer Behavior and Nutrition: Preventive Health Perspectives," in *Advances in Consumer Research,* vol. 5, ed. H.K. Hunt (1978), 518–520.

76. Quelch, "Marketing Principles," 327–328.

77. Paul F. Lazarsfeld and R.K. Morar, "Mass Communication, Popular Taste, and Organized Social Action," in *Mass Communications,* ed. Willard Schramm (Urbana, Ill.: University of Illinois Press, 1949), 459–480.

78. Marshall, "Prevention and Health Education," 1122.

79. M. O'Keefe, "The Antismoking Commercials: A Study of Television's Impact on Behavior," *Public Opinion Quarterly* 35 (Summer 1971): 242–248.

80. R. Bauer, "The Obstinate Audience," *American Psychologist* 19 (March 1964): 319–328.

81. K.E. Warner, "The Effects of the Antismoking Campaign on Cigarette Consumption," *American Journal of Public Health* 67 (July 1977): 645–650.

82. Ibid.

83. Marshall, "Prevention and Health Education," 1123.

Chapter 9

Ethics and Social Justice in Community Health Analysis

The 1990s dawn with some very troubling trends. Basically, these trends reflect a widening gap or increased segregation of many national program and policy efforts. Health care costs are increasing at alarming rates, access to health care is decreasing, the numbers of uninsured and underinsured in the population are increasing, the gap between socioeconomic status and illness has not narrowed, the number of persons living in poverty has not decreased, the educational system is failing, the welfare system is poorly managed and unresponsive to the needs of the population, U.S. national health status compares unfavorably with that of other developed nations, environmental dislocations and disasters are increasingly commonplace, and finally, there is a trend toward hypersegregation of the under class. These trends require a response. Because these issues are bounded by ethical dimensions, dilemmas, and questions, the need for social justice planning and analysis is clear.

Over the next 20 years, there will be a window of opportunity in the United States to change and overcome these inadequacies. The window has been there for the past 20 years, but reaction has been slow. It is essential not to miss this opportunity because of incapability of change and adaption, however, as the postindustrial future called the service and information transfer society is rapidly approaching. It will bring profound changes that must not be ignored. Rather, these changes must be faced, explored, accepted, understood, applied, and resolved.[1]

APPLICATION OF ETHICAL THEORY TO COMMUNITY HEALTH AGENCIES[2]

Most public health agencies have encountered a growing number of questions and conflicts with ethical implications: Should limited resources be allocated for tertiary care or primary prevention? Should agencies be actively attempting to change lifestyles that are considered to be harmful? What are the rights and responsibilities of the client? To address these and other questions, a framework has been developed specifically for solving problems, setting priorities, and developing a healthy public policy that takes into account an ethical perspective. This ethical perspective may be considered from the viewpoints of both the individual (clinical medicine) and the community (community medicine/health). In response to the increasing concern with ethical issues in public health care, an educational model that applies ethical theory to public health practice is proposed (Fig. 9-1).

The ultimate purpose of a health agency is to improve health status. To accomplish this, strategic goals and the parameters to accomplish them must be identified. A goal such as "raising a healthier generation" requires concentrating on improving the health and well-being of infants, children, and adolescents. A goal

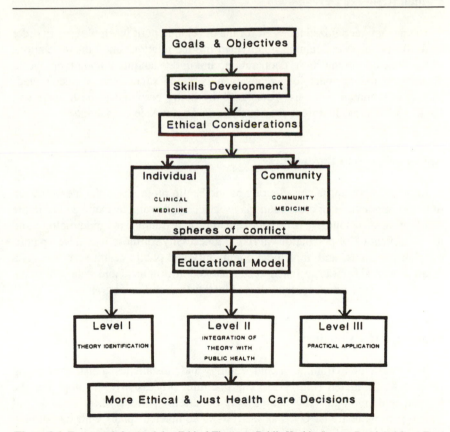

Figure 9-1 Framework for Applying Ethical Theory to Public Health. *Source:* Reprinted from *Family and Community Health,* Vol. 10, No. 1, p. 16, Aspen Publishers, Inc., © 1987.

such as "economic self-sufficiency" requires assisting the disadvantaged to overcome the barriers leading to economic dependency, and a goal of "independence for older citizens" requires allowing the elderly an opportunity for enhanced freedom and health.

To achieve such strategic goals, the Georgia public health agency established five major program elements that have made an impact on the outcome of public health programs: (1) human resource development, (2) epidemiologic and biostatistics approaches to problem identification, (3) planning and evaluation, (4) community resource development, and (5) development in the 1990s—primary prevention. The relationship of these strategic goals to objectives and health status is diagramed in Figure 9-2.

Human Resource Development

The agency recognized the need for the development of its employees in order to fulfill its purpose. Training is provided in race relations and human relations to facilitate communication, cooperation, and understanding among employees. Training in management for agency managers and supervisors is encouraged. Moreover, "human relations specialists" are being prepared to be trainers and facilitators in areas that were previously served by outside consultants.[3]

Epidemiology and Biostatistics

Another important factor affecting public health programs is the identification of target populations in order to market services and promote social equity in the distribution of resources. It became apparent that training in epidemiology and the identification of populations at risk is a necessity for those who develop policy, plan programs, and implement community and public health services. As a result, a workshop was designed to educate and inform local and state staff in the essentials of descriptive epidemiology, biostatistics, and demography.[4]

Planning and Evaluation

As a follow-up to training in epidemiology and biostatistics, a district planning process was initiated (Fig. 9-3). The planning process involves applying the learned epidemiologic skills in analyzing the disease patterns of the areas served by the various districts. Once an analysis is completed, plans with measurable objectives are developed. This planning model is used for the management of local and statewide programs. Evaluation is a major component of the process.[5]

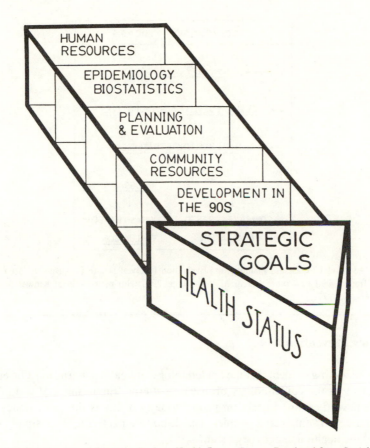

Figure 9-2 Relationship of Strategic Goals to Health Status. *Source:* Reprinted from *Social Indicators Research,* Vol. 19, p. 288, with permission of Kluwer Academic Publishers, © 1987.

Community Resource Development

The agency should work with local communities to identify local needs, get support for services that are provided locally, and develop a plan that includes the delivery of services in an integrated manner, based on identified needs. Thus, working with community groups to promote cooperative activities is essential. In addition, efforts should be made to improve outreach activities; peer counseling for teenagers to address the teen pregnancy problem is an example of a community working toward building capacity and strength. It is believed that more attentiveness to patient needs and to the communities in which they live will result in more efficient and beneficial services.[6]

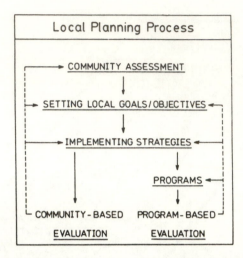

Figure 9-3 Model for Health Planning and Evaluation in Local Health Departments. *Source:* Reprinted from *Social Indicators Research,* Vol. 19, p. 293, with permission of Kluwer Academic Publishers, © 1977.

Primary Prevention

It is becoming evident that the epidemiology of health patterns must be emphasized, as was the epidemiology of disease patterns. Environmental and lifestyle factors have the most impact on people today.[7] If this is the case, policy must concentrate on "enhancing peoples' health-building activities, not simply on repairing the health damage they incur."[8]

The present approach to medical care, concentrating on secondary prevention (immunization) that alters the host and tertiary prevention (treatment), is a misfit for the current disease pattern and the diseases that will predominate over the next two decades. Primary prevention (health promotion and education) is the appropriate response to the current and future disease patterns.[9]

ETHICAL CONSIDERATIONS

In addition to the major elements that have been discussed, a community/public health agency must deal with issues and conflicts that transcend the traditional model of medical care, such as the new economic reality, diminished resources, the limits of medical technology related to life and death,[10] and the lack of a clear definition of the rights and responsibilities of individuals and institutions. As Manga pointed out,

Advances in medical technology, together with economic scarcity, also raise thorny questions of distributive justice. Morally, the choice becomes truly awesome when a decision is fundamentally about whose life is to be saved when the number of patients with fatal or end-stage disease are, as is frequently the case, greater than the available life-saving technology or resources. In the Sixties, this dilemma was illustrated by the allocation of kidney dialysis. Organ transplantation and intensive care units are more recent examples, and the artificial heart looms on the horizon. The sheer magnitude and scope of biomedical research and experimentation is such that we can surely expect further new and expensive treatments that will be available only to a fraction of those in need. The problem of who should benefit will have to be faced squarely and will be a popular concern to the lay public as well as ethicists, physicians, hospital administrators, and government officials. Indeed, new medical technology usually highlights the ever-present dilemma: how should society allocate limited health care resources, knowing that no matter what is finally decided, many needs, both ordinary and desperate, will not be met.[11]

In this context, an agency must examine ethical considerations with respect both to the individual and to the community.

Individual ethical considerations include autonomy, individual responsibility for health, and rights of individuals to health care. Community ethical considerations, including allocation of resources and administration of health care, must be considered in terms of justice and fairness, but applying ethical theory to community and public health programs is not a simple procedure. As Beauchamp, an ethicist from Georgetown University stated, "ethical theory can provide general principles which can then lead to more specific guidelines, such as the principle of respect for autonomy."[12] He cautioned, however, that ethical theory "gives arguments not answers."[13] Finally, he likened moral reasoning to legal reasoning and said that arguments can be made well or poorly and that counterarguments can always be made and are in fact expected.[14]

Individual Considerations

Individual autonomy, the capacity of self-governance or of "being one's own person, without constraints either by another's action or by psychological or physical limitations,"[15] is an important aspect of human resource development plans. Training involves improving the management skills of public health agency staff and emphasizing the development of interpersonal skills. As a result, individual employees increase their ability to make appropriate decisions and to function effectively with others. The recognition of autonomy is also reflected in the emphasis on primary prevention. The basis for primary prevention is behavioral change that can improve health status; the assumption is that individuals are capable of determining their behavior.

The diseases of the next decade will reflect social problems as outlined in the service and information transfer society model. Chronic and/or social disease cannot be controlled by health care providers alone. Individuals must take responsibility for their own health if disease patterns are to be affected. This behavioral change will depend on effective primary prevention. Therefore, health education and health promotion must be marketed in a manner that motivates individuals to take more responsibility for their health.

The language of individual rights is framed in two categories. The first category, negative rights, encompasses the rights of freedom to pursue a course of action without interference. The second category, positive rights, covers the rights to obtain goods or services. Efforts to identify populations at risk and to increase their access to care directly support positive rights to health care. Epidemiological and biostatistics training and the application of these techniques in the planning and evaluation of programs make it possible for individuals to exercise these rights.

Community Considerations

Distributive justice requires the allocation of the benefits and burdens of society according to some fair criterion. Following are some possible formulations of a fair criterion of distributive justice areas:[16]

- to each person an equal share
- to each person according to individual need
- to each person according to individual effort
- to each person according to societal contribution
- to each person according to individual merit

Questions related to distributive justice in the allocation of resources surface when attempts are made to identify the populations' needs (using an epidemiological approach) and determine the best response to such needs.

The inherent danger for community/public health agencies in subscribing exclusively to formulations of distributive justice is the inevitable confrontation with a moral dilemma: having to assign a value and worth to individual persons who may not be considered in the allocation process or who are not members of the group intended to receive the allocated resources. Distributive justice, therefore, must be considered with other ethical principles, such as nonmaleficence (to do no harm) or beneficence (to promote good), as a form of internal critique of policy. Such a mechanism of ethical critique allows for the examination of the fairness of the proposed policy.

In accounting for both the perspective of the individual (clinical medicine) and the community (community medicine/health), three spheres of conflict become evident: (1) health care staff and professional conflicts, (2) conflicts in state and local health policy decision making, and (3) wide-sweeping social policy conflicts. To deal with these conflicts, an educational model has been developed and applied.

IMPLEMENTATION OF ETHICAL THEORY IN PUBLIC HEALTH PRACTICE[17]

An interface exists between ethical theory and health care. Over the years, however, this relationship has assumed different manifestations, ranging from the formation of precise conduct codes for health care professionals to the establishment of review boards that examine specific morally questionable procedures. However, for a community/public health agency, the purpose is to use ethical theory as a form of vision for the development of health care policy for the 1990s and beyond.

Such a vision has the potential to illuminate what the present health care practices are and what they ought to be in light of the ethical considerations already mentioned. As May has written, the use of "ethical theory may not always eliminate moral quandaries, but it opens up a wider horizon in which they may be seen for what they are and thus become other than they are."[18] There are no easy solutions for moral dilemmas. Public health does not seek to provide easy solutions, but to offer a view and an understanding of the ethical implications of public health care practices operating in a modern complex society.

The utilization of ethical theory in public health requires examination at three levels of participation: identification, internalization, and practical application.

Identification of Ethical Principles (Level I)

Since the degree of knowledge and experience with classical ethical theory varies among those persons trained in the health care professions, a basic introduction of the major ethical principles and theories must be provided through group instruction and discussion. The objective of Level I is the creation of a common ethical understanding for the participants, a common underlying structure from which they can view and explore the ethical dimensions of health care.

To achieve this objective, emphasis is placed first on the identification of the major ethical principles associated with health care and second on an understanding of the way in which these principles are assembled into a coherent general ethical theory.

Before the identification process can commence, however, general questions regarding the nature of morality, the different approaches to the study of ethics, definitions of value, fundamental rules of logic, and ways of resolving moral conflicts must be addressed. With this foundation established, the major ethical principles of autonomy, nonmaleficence, beneficence, and justice can be discussed.

These principles can be illustrated in the multiple issues surrounding an infant mortality problem. Autonomy, or self-governance, is addressed when ensuring that a pregnant woman is provided with prenatal care that emphasizes primary prevention. Health education and promotion make it possible for the pregnant woman to control most of the factors that affect the health status of herself and her infant. Approaches that rely on secondary or tertiary prevention place this responsibility in the hands of others, the health care professionals.

The principle of nonmaleficence may be applied by the director of a neonatal intensive care unit who must decide whether to accept or reject an infant that weighs less than 500 grams. Statistically, the infant is unlikely to survive, but the director's decision not to accept it may harm the infant or the infant's family. On the other hand, using scarce resources to care for an infant that is unlikely to survive may harm other infants with a better chance because these resources are denied to them.

The principle of beneficence may be applied when caring for a newborn. Promoting good is ensuring that the infant gets appropriate care that addresses any lifestyle, environmental, biologic, or access-to-care problems.

Justice, or the principle of fairness, is reflected in issues concerning the allocation of funds. Decisions must be made regarding a fair distribution of funds; for example, is placing more emphasis on primary prevention activities, such as prenatal care, more just than emphasizing curative activities, such as neonatal intensive care?

In addition to these principles, the concepts of rights, equality, and respect for persons are examined. Once an understanding of these elements is established, the focus of Level I turns to the historic development of teleologic (consequential) and deontologic (nonconsequential) ethical theories. A teleologic approach to infant mortality is to implement policies that reduce the rate in the most efficient manner possible. A deontologic approach, however, stresses that a policy ought to be carried out because it is the "right" approach, regardless of the outcome or costs.

The identification process also includes an examination of the special philosophical problem areas of absolutism, relativism, and differing theories of knowledge. This level of the educational process concludes with a case study that applies ethical theory in developing a health care policy decision regarding the treatment of a low birth weight infant.

Internalization of Principles (Level II)

Whereas the objective of the first level is the creation of a common ethical understanding through the identification of ethical principles and theories, the second level seeks to expand on those elements of ethical reasoning and their implications for health care. The emphasis of Level II is dialogic and is concerned with creating an in-depth ethical awareness that recognizes the subtleties of complex moral dilemmas. Level I afforded the participants the opportunity of identifying ethical elements; Level II opens the possibility of internalizing these elements. Such a goal is more complicated and difficult, but only when the participants take these elements and concretely apply them to their own experience as health care professionals can the elements assume real meanings and practical uses.

At Level II, topics that have definite moral and practical implications and concerns for health care professionals are examined. Such topics include the nature of individual responsibility for health care, individual rights to health care, and the moral role and responsibility of public health officials. The social and economic content of public health and the idea that public health is an instrument of social justice are also examined.

The issue of infant mortality highlights several of these topics, including the moral role of public health officials and public health as an instrument of social justice. For example, in Georgia, one-half of all infants that die are black and are primarily from low-income families, whereas black births comprise only about one-third of the total births.[19] Questions concerning the role of Georgia's health agency and a just distribution of resources naturally arise from these data.

Through dialogue about these topics, participants are able to build on the foundation established in Level I and integrate those elements of ethical reasoning with the practical problem areas of public health practice. In short, the participants are encouraged to lift up the ethical concerns and consider their implications.

Practical Ethical Applications (Level III)

The final level of the educational model is entirely practical in its scope and emphasis. Level III consists of an intensive review of present agency policies, services, and procedures. From this review, the participants are able to examine the justification for these components and determine their ethical implications within three possible spheres of conflict. As noted earlier, such conflict areas include those between health care staff and agency division leadership, between state level health care objectives and local health policy decisions, and between wider objectives and other social policy initiatives (healthy public policy).

New initiatives taken by Georgia related to infant mortality include a statewide effort to lower the infant mortality rate to 9 per 1,000 live births by 1990. Strategies included not only making the public and health care providers aware of the extent of the problem and groups at risk, but also establishing local district task forces made up of community representatives. This reflects the perspective that the infant mortality problem cannot be successfully addressed by health care professionals alone. The persons affected and the general community share responsibility as well. Therefore, the objective of Level III was to enable the participants to view the present state of public health care from a coherent and consistent ethical foundation.

Crises and Quandaries

Today, health problems, such as infant mortality, are recognized to have multiple causes with multiple effects that encompass biological, environmental, lifestyle, and health care delivery system issues. A possible effect of applying ethical theory to the public health practices intended to deal with this multiplicity of causes and effects is the creation of a health care system that emphasizes the ethical considerations and moves public health away from being merely a technical activity to serving as an instrument of social justice.[20] Considerable difficulty arises in applying ethical theory and social justice principles to the major issues, however, because many of these issues are beyond public health policy alternatives. Thus, the crises and quandaries related to the problems of the poor, illiterate, and unemployed still exist and reflect major societal burdens where gaps exist between the haves and the have nots.

Inability To Close the Gaps: The Burdens

Clearly, the burden of unnecessary illness is encountered in the poor, illiterate, and unemployed population. Each of these components evokes ethical dilemmas and reflects the social inequalities and inequities in our national systems and structure. For example, the United States is known for the best health care system in the world, but the health status of its population does not share the same distinction. Certainly, part of this problem is that there are approximately 37 million U.S. citizens who have no health insurance; additionally, skyrocketing health care expenditures limit access. Coupled with poverty, poor education, unemploy-

ment, substandard housing, poor nutrition, and risk-promoting lifestyle and behavior, the result is social inequalities and inequities.

U.S. Health Care System

Social justice and the health care system are linked. The World Health Organization, as part of its goal of "health for all by the year 2000," provided a vision
based on social equity and noted the urgent need to reduce the gross inequality in
the health status of the people in the world.[21] Sidel posed the problem in this
manner:

> Every two seconds a child dies of preventable illness, preventable by
> safe water supplies, basic immunization, and basic adequate food sup-
> ply. . . . Also, every two seconds, a child is permanently disabled,
> physically or mentally, by a preventable illness—I would like to add
> malnutrition—and is forced to live the remainder of his life with that
> disability. . . . In other words, every second a child is preventably
> killed or maimed. . . . In that same second, the world spends $25,000
> on arms, that is to say $2 billion a day—$800 billion a year. . . . There
> is one soldier for every 43 persons in the world, but only one physician
> for 1,030 inhabitants.
>
> I ask myself whether the Ministries of Health have participated ac-
> tively in the discussion on policies for economic adjustment and on
> sectorial objectives aimed at reducing the negative impact of recession.
> Have they gathered the necessary information showing the effect of the
> crisis—the increase in morbidity and mortality in mothers and chil-
> dren, in malnutrition and low birth weight, among other indicators,
> and the more frequent causes for which there is long-standing and
> proven technology which is very low in cost and has long-term effects
> and is applicable in primary health care? On the basis of the informa-
> tion, have they pointed out the effect of purely economic measures that
> tend to increase income while at the same time reducing the social ex-
> penditure?
>
> In sum, we feel that economic constraints interfere more with human
> development than with the growth of the economy and that shortage of
> resources is relative, given that in most of the countries in the world
> they are *badly allocated and poorly administered*.[22]

In the United States, the health care system has been faced with a multiplicity
of similar problems. National health care expenditures are increasing at alarming
rates (Fig. 9-4). Currently (1990), they are 12 percent of our gross national product (GNP), but they are expected to reach 15 percent by the year 2000. Table 9-1

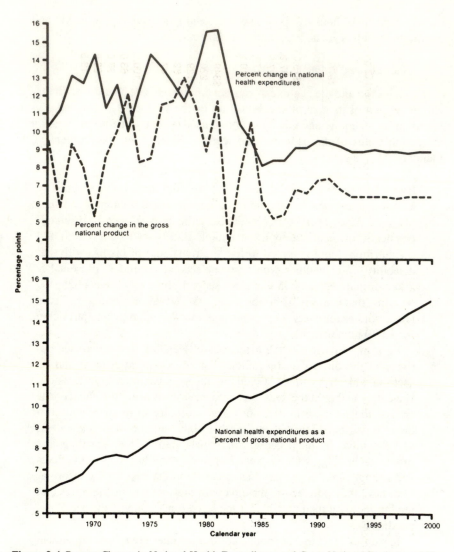

Figure 9-4 Percent Change in National Health Expenditures and Gross National Product, and National Health Expenditures as a Percent of Gross National Product: Calendar Years 1966–1986 and Projections 1987–2000. *Source:* Reprinted from *Health Care Financing Review,* Vol. 8, No. 4, p. 2, HCFA, 1987.

Table 9-1 National Health Expenditures Aggregate and Per Capita Amounts, Percent Distribution, and Average Annual Percent Change, by Source of Funds: Selected Calendar Years 1965–2000

Item	2000	1995	1990	1987	1986	1985	1984	1980	1970	1965
Amount in billions										
National health expenditures	$1,529.3	$999.1	$647.3	$496.6	$458.2	$422.6	$391.1	$248.1	$75.0	$41.9
Private	879.4	575.5	378.2	294.8	268.5	246.6	231.3	142.9	47.2	30.9
Public	649.9	423.5	269.0	201.7	189.7	176.0	159.7	105.2	27.8	11.0
Federal	498.6	317.7	195.5	142.7	134.7	124.5	111.6	71.0	17.7	5.5
State and local	151.3	105.8	73.6	59.0	55.0	51.5	48.1	34.2	10.1	5.5
Per capita amount										
National health expenditures	$5,551	$3,739	$2,511	$1,973	$1,837	$1,710	$1,597	$1,054	$349	$205
Private	3,192	2,154	1,467	1,172	1,076	998	945	607	220	152
Public	2,359	1,585	1,044	802	760	712	652	447	129	54
Federal	1,810	1,189	758	567	540	504	456	302	82	27
State and local	549	396	285	235	221	208	196	145	47	27
Percent distribution										
National health expenditures	100.0	100.0	100.0	100.0	100.0	100.0	100.0	100.0	100.0	100.0
Private	57.5	57.6	58.4	59.4	58.6	58.4	59.2	57.6	63.0	73.8
Public	42.5	42.4	41.6	40.6	41.4	41.6	40.8	42.4	37.0	26.2
Federal	32.6	31.8	30.2	28.7	29.4	29.5	28.5	28.6	23.6	13.2
State and local	9.9	10.6	11.4	11.9	12.0	12.2	12.3	13.8	13.5	13.0

continues

Table 9-1 continued

Item	2000	1995	1990	1987	1986	1985	1984	1980	1970	1965
Average annual percent change from previous year shown										
U.S. population	0.6	0.7	0.8	0.9	0.9	0.9	1.0	0.9	1.0	—
Gross national product	6.4	6.6	6.9	5.3	5.2	6.2	8.3	10.4	7.6	—
National health expenditures	8.9	9.1	9.2	8.4	8.4	8.1	12.0	12.7	12.3	—
Private	8.8	8.8	8.7	9.8	8.9	6.6	12.8	11.7	8.8	—
Public	8.9	9.5	10.1	6.3	7.8	10.2	11.0	14.2	20.4	—
Federal	9.4	10.2	11.1	6.0	8.2	11.5	12.0	14.9	26.1	—
State and local	7.4	7.5	7.6	7.2	6.8	7.1	8.9	13.0	13.1	—
Number in millions										
U.S. population*	275.5	267.2	257.8	251.6	249.5	247.2	244.9	235.3	214.9	204.1
Amount in billions										
Gross national product	$10,164	$7,467	$5,414	$4,433	$4,206	$3,998	$3,765	$2,732	$1,015	$705
Percent of gross national product										
National health expenditures	15.0	13.4	12.0	11.2	10.9	10.6	10.4	9.1	7.4	5.9

*July 1 social security area population estimates.
Note: Figures for 1986 are preliminary and those for 1987–2000 are projected.

Source: Reprinted from *Health Care Financing Review*, Vol. 8, No. 4., p. 24, HCFA, U.S. DHHS, 1987.

illustrates our national health care expenditures by per capita, percent distribution, average annual percent change, and by source of funds for 1965 to 2000. The trends are shocking. We are expected as a nation to spend $1.5 trillion on health care and $5,551 per capita by the year 2000.

Several factors affect these changes in personal health care expenditures: medical care price inflation in excess of the general rate of inflation, economywide price inflation, and population growth, for example (Fig. 9-5). Changes in consumption per capita, intensity as a result of rising incomes, and aging of the population may play a role. Changes in the structure of the delivery system may also affect health care expenditures. For example, the number of regionally consolidated systems that are supposedly addressing issues of indigent care and rural health care is increasing. Hospitals are evolving to emphasize outpatient and diagnostic care, as well as inpatient treatment.[23] Malpractice insurance, reimbursement mechanisms, informed consumers, competitive market places, and the possibility of more government regulations are influencing physician patterns.[24] As important as these trends are to the changes in national health care expenditure, the most significant is demographic change.

EFFECTS OF DEMOGRAPHIC CHANGE

The effects of recent demographic changes—the baby boom, the baby bust, the baby boomlet, and dysfunctional relationships—have only modestly influenced the patterns and expenditures of the health care industry. The greatest impacts will occur in the next century, when the baby boomers reach the age of 65 and over. Before this occurs, however, there will be a temporary reduction in numbers of people aged 65 and over as the smaller Depression cohort of the 1930s reaches age 65. Recognizing and analyzing all these trends has led to the call for a national health care system.

The Health Care Financing Administration has estimated the impact of the aging of the 77 million plus baby boom cohort on the U.S. health care system. Table 9-2 indicates the changes in expenditure patterns to the year 2026, based on the age and sex structure of the population in the selected calendar year; Table 9-3 provides a more specific pattern of expenditures, based on age groups, by category hospital and physician. Clearly, a shift in percent distribution of costs will take place as the population ages.

Although the demographic shift will get the most attention into the next century, there are other significant trends. The most important other issues are intensity of care (i.e., real goods and services provided per inpatient day), 5.7 percent of the GNP; hospital price inflation-1.1 percent of GNP (over and above general price inflation) and, of course, the population .6 percent of GNP. Demographi-

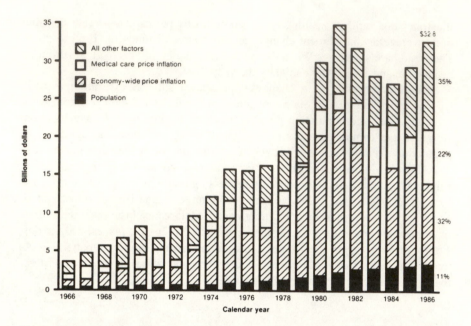

Figure 9-5 Factors Affecting Change in Personal Health Care Expenditures of Billions of Dollars: Calendar Years 1966–1986. *Source:* Reprinted from *Health Care Financing Review,* Vol. 8, No. 4, p. 11, HFCA, 1987. Data from the Division of National Cost Estimates.

Table 9-2 Hypothetical 1986 Expenditures under the Age and Sex Structure of Selected Calendar Years

Type of Expenditure	Calendar Year from Which Age and Sex Structure Is Drawn				
	1946	1966	1986	2006	2026
Total personal	Amount in billions				
health	$356.7	$365.6	$404.0	$449.8	$508.2
Hospital	157.3	161.6	179.6	200.0	230.9
Physician	88.9	87.3	92.0	95.6	105.6
Nursing Home	20.9	26.8	38.1	52.4	64.8
All Other	89.6	89.9	94.3	100.8	106.9

Notes: Figures in this table combine the age and sex composition of selected calendar year populations with 1986 prices and patterns of health care use. Calendar year 1986 spending figures are shown to establish a reference point.

Source: Reprinted from *Health Care Financing Review,* Vol. 8, No. 4, p. 15, HCFA, U.S. DHHS, 1987.

Table 9-3 Hypothetical Distribution of Total Spending among Three Age Groups under the Age and Sex Structure of Selected Calendar Years

Type of Expenditure and Age	Calendar Year			
	1978	2000	2020	2040
Median age of population	29	36	39	41
	Percent distribution			
Hospital				
Total	100	100	100	100
Under 19 years	9	7	6	5
19–64 years	63	61	56	45
65 years and over	28	32	38	50
Physician				
Total	100	100	100	100
Under 19 years	15	12	10	10
19–64 years	60	62	59	54
65 years and over	25	26	31	36

Source: Reprinted from *Health Care Financing Review,* Vol. 8, No. 4, p. 16, HCFA, U.S. DHHS, 1987.

cally, the elderly will demand significant attention; financially, goods and services provided per inpatient day will receive a great deal of the attention.

The other side of the coin in the health care arena is the quality of the health care benefits. As stated earlier, the U.S. health care system is perceived as the best in the world, yet the U.S. health status compares rather unfavorably to that of other nations. Although the United States continues to rank high economically, it ranks 22nd in infant mortality, and life expectancies in the United States are rated 10th and 20th best for females and males, respectively (Table 9-4). Obviously, economics is not the sole solution to improving health status. An interesting comparison of health resources and health status concerning a select number of developed nations is presented in Table 9-5.

A recent study showed that the GNP, as a measure of a country's total wealth, is not necessarily associated with health status.[25] Health status is associated more with the distribution of resources and benefits within a country. In most countries of the world, including the United States, it is not a case of a shortage of resources, but of poor allocations and usually unjust distributions. Furthermore, the administration of programs is often poor because of a service system orientation that builds dependencies and inadequacies rather than a community orientation that builds strength and capacity. Although the study was limited to Latin America, Belmar found a strong correlation between the level of democracy and

Table 9-4 Ranking of Select Variables for Resources and Health Status, United States Compared to the World*

Resources		Health Status	
Variable	U.S. Ranking	Variable	U.S. Ranking
Economic capability assessment	1	Motor vehicle accident death rate	7
Energy production	1	Female life expectancy	10
Energy consumption	9	Heart disease death rate	11
Currency per capita	10	Suicides	12
GNP per capita	14	Cancer death rate	13
		Male life expectancy	20
		Infant mortality rate	22

*All ranks are arranged from high to low. Therefore, number one represents the highest value. However, for health status rankings, high rankings represent poor health status. For example, U.S. has the seventh highest rate for motor vehicle accidents in the world. For life expectancy values, a high ranking is good; the higher the rank the longer life expectancy.

Source: Sciegaj, M.S., Dever, G.E.A., Wade, T.E., Alley, J.W. Public Health as Social Conscience, Paper presented at APHA, Chicago, IL, Oct. 24, 1989; Kurion, G.T., The New Bank of World Rankings. Facts on File, New York, N.Y., p. 487, 1984.

Table 9-5 Comparing Health Care Worldwide

	Health Spending (percent of GNP) 1986	Infant Mortality (per 1,000) 1986	Life Expectancy (in years) 1986	Physicians (per 1,000) 1981–83	Lawyers (per 1,000) 1986
United States	11.1	10	75.3	2.2	2.8
Canada	8.5	8	77.1	1.9	1.9
France	8.5	8	75.7	2.2	0.3
W. Germany	8.1	9	75.8	2.4	0.8
Japan	6.7	6	77.8	1.4	0.1
U. Kingdom	6.2	9	75.1	1.3	1.1

Source: Reprinted from *Health Week News and Solutions for Health Care Management,* Vol. 3, No. 21, p. 33, with permission of Health Investors, Ltd., © 1989..

---

health (see Chapter 6). He stated, "If this [the correlation between level of democracy and health] is found to be generally true, it will have profound implications for health policy and planning experts who now tend to focus on technical medical care and public health measures more than on societal context"[26] [healthy public policy].

Given these facts, it is unlikely that a national health program to provide universal health care for all will have any major impact on health status. Even some

Canadian officials are warning that the provision of coverage alone will not guarantee good health.[27] In fact, two decades after Canada instituted universal coverage, Canada's poor have a life expectancy as much as seven years less than that of their fellow Canadians.[28] This notion of national health care needs more thought. In the meantime, other inequalities and inequities that plague our social systems should receive attention.

Socioeconomic Differentials

Because disease patterns reflect major differences in socioeconomic status, it is critical to assess socioeconomic differentials. The health problems that occur more frequently at lower socioeconomic levels range from some of the most common, such as heart disease, diabetes, and lung cancer, to some of the very uncommon, such as neural tube defects and sinonasal cancer (Exhibit 9-1).

A report prepared by the American Cancer Society on cancer in the economically disadvantaged underscored the fact that major differences in cancer are not due to race, but to poverty and socioeconomic differences.[29] Therefore, the target for correction of these disease variations is not race, but poverty. In fact, Freeman noted that the "significance of race in respect to cancer is generally limited to race as a surrogate for a specific culture and life style."[30] Also, Kaplan noted that

> because socioeconomic position and race are related, racial differences
> in risk factors or medical care are often proposed as explanations for

---

Exhibit 9-1 Health Problems That Are More Frequent at Lower Socioeconomic Levels in the United States

● Total mortality	● Sinonasal cancer
● Heart disease	● Infant and child mortality
● Arthritis	● Neural tube defects
● Diabetes	● Tuberculosis
● Hypertension	● Unintentional injury
● Angina	● Low birth weight
● Epilepsy	● Decreased survival from cancer
● Rheumatic fever	● Decreased survival from heart attack
● Respiratory infections	● Restricted activity and bed days
● Anemia	● Days in short-term hospitals
● Lung cancer	● Number of hospital discharges
● Esophageal cancer	

Source: Reprinted from *Closing the Gap: The Burden of Unnecessary Illness* by R.W. Amler and B.H. Dull (Eds.), p. 126, with permission of Oxford University Press, © 1987.

Table 9-6 Percent Distribution of Uninsured Persons under Age 65 by Selected Population
Characteristics, United States, 1987

Population Characteristic	Population under Age 65 (in thousands)	Percent Uninsured	Percent Distribution of Uninsured
Total*	209,981	17.4	100.0
Age in years			
Less than 6	21,631	16.7	9.9
6 to 18	45,475	16.9	21.1
19 to 24	22,675	30.2	18.8
25 to 54	98,155	15.7	42.2
55 to 64	22,046	13.4	8.1
Sex			
Male	103,607	18.4	52.1
Female	106,374	16.4	47.9
Marital status			
Married	89,502	12.8	31.4
Single/never married	39,336	26.1	28.1
Widowed	3,972	21.2	2.3
Divorced	13,170	23.1	8.3
Separated	3,710	27.2	2.8
Ethnic/racial background			
White	158,656	14.2	61.6
Black	26,028	23.8	17.0
Hispanic	17,888	32.9	16.1
Veteran status			
Yes	25,147	15.1	10.4
No	117,094	18.1	58.2
Place of residence			
20 largest metro areas	60,165	16.9	27.8
Other metro areas	99,874	16.5	45.1
Other	49,942	19.8	27.1
U.S. Census region			
Northeast	43,637	12.8	15.3
Midwest	52,461	12.6	18.1
South	71,163	21.3	41.4
West	42,720	21.5	25.2

*Includes persons in other ethnic/racial groups not shown and persons of unknown ethnic/racial
background, marital status, or veteran status, as well as persons under age 17 for marital status and
under age 19 for veteran status.

Source: Reprinted from *National Medical Expenditure Survey—Household Survey, round 1.* A profile of Uninsured Americans, p. 9, U.S. DHHS, 1989.

gradients of disease associated with socioeconomic position. However,
socioeconomic gradients are found within racial and ethnic groups and
in some cases, socioeconomic position may actually account for what
appears to be racial differences in health.[31]

Thirty-nine million people in the United States are below the poverty level. Of these, 23 million are white, 9.6 million are black, and 6.4 million belong to groups other than blacks and whites.[32] The South has the highest level of poverty in the United States. Of particular importance is the fact that two-thirds of the poor are white and one-third are black, but this one-third is concentrated within only 12 percent of the black population.[33] In addition to the 39 million poor, there are 37 million who have no insurance. The lack of insurance affects access and relates to poverty levels. A profile of the uninsured in the United States for 1987 is depicted in Table 9-6. Thus, a high-risk profile by percent distribution is age 19–24, male, single or separated, black and hispanic, outside a metropolitan statistical area, and located in the south and west. Figure 9-6 shows the ten best and the ten worst states in health rankings based on six factors: life span, disease, lifestyle, access to care, lost school, and lost work time.[34]

Poverty is greater in rural than in urban areas. Both rural and urban poverty have increased during the 1979 to 1986 time period, however (Fig. 9-7). The

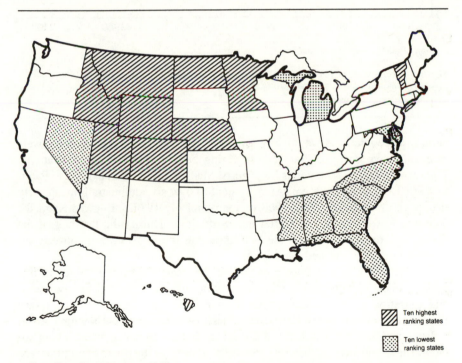

Ten highest
ranking states

Ten lowest
ranking states

Note: Data for 1984 not available.

Figure 9-6 Ten Highest and Ten Lowest Ranking States: Overall Population Health, 1989. *Source:* Reprinted from *The NWNL State Health Rankings: Results, Methodology, and Discussion,* p.18–19, with permission of Northwestern National Life Insurance Company, © 1989.

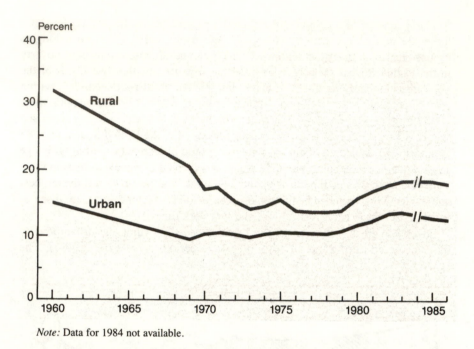

Note: Data for 1984 not available.

Figure 9-7 Percentage of Population in Poverty by Urban/Rural Residence: 1959 to 1986. *Source:* Reprinted from *Population Trends and Public Policy*, No. 15, p. 7, with permission of Population Reference Bureau, © 1988.

number of people living at poverty levels and the number of people on the welfare rolls have changed dramatically during past presidential administrations. Figure 9-8 illustrates the trends for poverty, Medicaid, food stamps, Aid to Families with Dependent Children (AFDC), and SSI over six administrations. Poverty decreased dramatically from 1960 to approximately 1978 during the Kennedy, Johnson, Nixon, Ford, and Carter administrations. During the last half of the Carter administration and all the Reagan administration, however, poverty increased until it approached 1960 levels.

Despite recent gains major gaps remain between blacks and whites in five areas: economic status, residential segregation, health, child and family issues, and education (Table 9-7). The significant gaps in the burdens of unnecessary illness, poverty, education deficiencies, lack of insurance, and unemployment reflect inequities, inequalities, and disparities that are embarrassments to our society. These injustices as they relate to the poor through the prism of culture were best described by Freeman (Fig. 9-9).[35] He stated that "race . . . is a significant proxy for culture, tradition, belief system, and lifestyle. Accordingly, race (culture) becomes a prism through which the effects of poverty are reflected."[36] Fi-

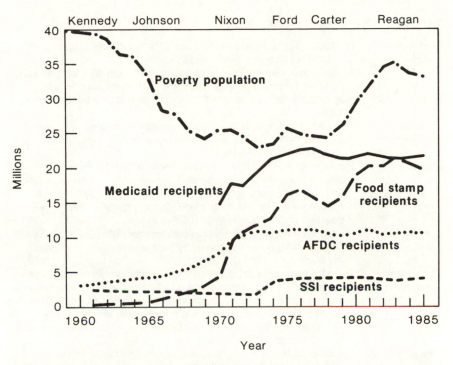

Figure 9-8 Recipients of Major Welfare Programs and the Poverty Population over Six Presidential Administrations, 1960–1985. *Source:* Reprinted from *Population Trends and Public Policy,* No. 13, p. 5, with permission of Population Reference Bureau, © 1987.

nally, the improvement of these inequities or disparities due to poverty requires a sensitivity to cultural issues that the poor endure.

1. Poor people endure greater pain and suffering.
2. Poor people and their families must make extraordinary personal sacrifices to obtain and pay for care.
3. Poor people have substantial obstacles in obtaining and using health insurance and often do not seek care if they cannot pay for it.
4. Current cancer education programs (most health education programs) are culturally insensitive and irrelevant to most poor people.
5. Fatalism about *disease* is prevalent among the poor and prevents them from seeking care.[37]

Thus, a first step to further understanding these problems is to identify and measure the inequities and inequalities that exist for population groups and geographical areas.

Table 9-7 Black-White Gap Persisting Despite Gains

Economic status:	Blacks' per capita income in 1984 was 57% that of whites, up from 39% in 1939 but no higher than it was in 1971.
	Poverty rates, after declining substantially from 93 to 30% for blacks and 65 to 9% for whites between 1939 and 1974, have stopped falling since then—indeed rising to 31% for blacks and 11% for whites by 1986.
Residential segregation:	Black-white segregation in many metropolitan areas is almost as high today as in the 1960s—significantly higher, in fact, than that for hispanics and Asian-Americans.
Health:	Blacks remain behind whites on most health indicators. For example, the black-white gap in life expectancy, although cut in half between 1950 and 1985, has narrowed slowly since 1960—especially among men. At 65.3 years, black men's average life expectancy in 1985 is lower than that of white men in 1950 (66.5 years).
	Access to health care presents another problem, with 22% of blacks and 14% of whites under 65 covered by neither private health insurance nor Medicaid in 1982.
Child & family issues:	Since the postwar baby boom, fertility rates for black and white women have fallen toward replacement level. (Black women's total fertility rate in 1984 was 2.1 children, compared to 1.7 for white women.)
	Black and white children, however, are living under different family structures, with 80% of white children but only 40% of black children under 18 living with both parents.
Education:	In spite of "substantial progress," opportunities for blacks and whites remain unequal. For example, the education level for blacks born in the late 1950s/early 1960s approximates that of whites of those cohorts (medians of 12.6 and 12.9 years, respectively), but the high school dropout rate for blacks, at about 20%, is almost double that of whites.
	Blacks are less than half as likely as whites to enter college within a year after graduation from high school.

Source: Reprinted from *Population Today,* Vol. 17, No. 10, p. 4, with permission of Population Reference Bureau, © 1989.

Measuring Inequality and Social Justice

Issues of inequality and social justice are particularly important to health agencies that are involved in the distribution of resources. Furthermore, health planners, researchers, and policy analysts need measurements to ensure fair and just allocations of available resources. Therefore, they must be familiar with the basic methodological tools that are available to evaluate the existing distribution of resources and to propose a fair and just distribution of future resources.

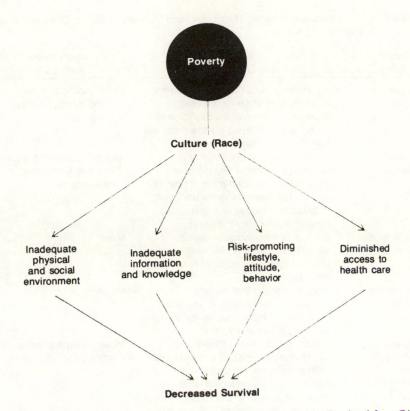

Figure 9-9 Interrelationship between Race, Poverty, and Cancer. *Source:* Reprinted from *CA—A Cancer Journal for Clinicians,* Vol. 39, No. 5, p. 285, with permission of American Cancer Society, Inc., © 1989.

Indexes of Inequality

Many types of indexes have been proposed to measure inequality or social justice. Coulter has divided the inequality indexes into five categories:[38]

1. deviations model
2. combinatorics model
3. entropy model
4. social welfare model
5. inequality, segregation, and interaction model (intergroup indexes)

The logic on which each model is based and its appropriate standard are identified in Table 9-8. Although each of these indexes may be applied to the health

Table 9-8 Types of Inequality Indexes, Their Logic, and Standards Used for Comparison as Delineated by Coulter

Type of Index	Logic	Comparative Standards
Deviations model	Assumes the distributional characteristics of any numerical series are best described in terms of the deviation of each value from some standard derived from the series itself.	Mean, mode, all other components, adjacent component
Combinatorics model	Is concerned with the probability of selecting a subset of two identical (or different) objects from a set of objects as a way of determining the uniformity or diversity of the set with respect to some characteristic of interest.	All pairs, cumulative ogive, temporally adjacent components
Entropy model	Is the sum of the information values of all the individual alternatives, each weighed by its own probability of occurrence.	Mean
Social welfare model	Is a social ordering that permits comparison of alternatives and ranks each one as better than, worse than, or equally good as every other.	Mean
Inequality, segregation, and interaction model	Are based on deviations model and combinatorics model. These intergroup indexes measure inequality in the distribution of (a) members of two social groups, and (b) geographical areas or ordinal classes of some quantity such as income, education, or occupation.	Mean, intergroup pairs, all pairs, cumulative pairs

Source: Adapted from *Measuring Inequality: A Methodological Handbook* by P.B. Coulter, pp. 11, 35, 63, 101, 115, 135, Westview Press, © 1989.

---

field, the most useful of the five are the deviations model; the social welfare model; and the inequality, segregation, and interaction model.

The identification of residential segregation and the components of segregation has far-reaching implications for equitable resource decision making and is very much a significant ingredient in a healthy public policy. Massey and Denton suggested that a high level of segregation is problematic because it may isolate a minority group from amenities, opportunities, and resources that affect social and economic well-being; the result is a low level of health status, poverty, unemployment, and illiteracy.[39] In short, the group may be deprived of mainstream opportunities.

Massey and Denton used five indexes to evaluate the segregation of blacks and hispanics in the United States.[40] These five indexes reflected five distinct dimensions of spatial variation: evenness, exposure, clustering, centralization, and concentration. These dimensions, as well as the definitions, indexes, and interpretation of the indexes used to evaluate residential segregation, are presented in Table 9-9. The analysis undertaken by Massey and Denton is crucial to the improvement of health in the United States, but their analysis and methods may be developed further and/or be applied to health and disease-based variables. For example, it may be possible to determine whether disease patterns, poverty variations, employment differences, illiteracy deviations, and environmental dislocations are hypersegregated. With documentation of these variations, plans and policies can be proposed to provide for a more equitable distribution of resources.

Indexes of Inequity

The group of indexes that identify the distributive characteristics of goods and services in relation to some other distributional standard are called inequity indexes. The philosophical basis of these indexes is that the benefits and burdens of society should be allocated according to some fair criterion, such as equality, need, market forces, demand, or individual merit. Coulter noted that an alternative definition of an equity standard is a minimum level of decency below which a component should not be allowed to fall. He stated that, "according to the above definition, inequity is the extent to which the shares of a given distribution fall below the minimum decency level."[41]

Although indexes of inequality are useful in the health field, indexes of inequity are particularly relevant to health policy and healthy public policy (Table 9-10). The inequity indexes are more complicated than the indexes of equality and segregation, because the inequity indexes involve the comparison of two independent distributions. The differences between the two types of indexes are extremely important to health planners, researchers, and policy analysts, who must be exact in their use of these indexes as they prepare to allocate increasingly limited resources in a fair and just manner.

Coulter identified three indexes of inequity (Table 9-11).[42] Coulter's index of inequity operationalizes the concept of distributing resources to individuals, groups, or geographical areas according to merit in terms of a selected equity standard. Nagel's index of equity distributes resources (societal or governmental benefits or costs) to individuals, groups, or geographical areas according to a minimum decency level of benefits and costs in response to their needs and resources.[43] Finally, like Coulter's index, Nagel's index of proportionality is based on the concept of distributing resources according to some proportional equality or equity (a selected standard), but, because the ratio of the equation is subtracted

Table 9-9 Measures of Residential Segregation: Dimensions, Definitions, Indexes, and Interpretation

Dimension	Definition	Index	Interpretation
Evenness	Degree to which the percentage of minority members within residential areas equals the citywide minority percentage	Dissimilarity Index: $$D = \sum_{i=1}^{n} \frac{t_i|p_i - P|}{2TP(1 - P)}$$	As areas depart from the ideal of evenness, segregation increases.
Exposure	Degree of potential contact between minority and majority members	Isolation Index: $$_xP^*_x = \sum_{i=1}^{n} \left[\frac{x_i}{X}\right]\left[\frac{x_i}{t_i}\right]$$	The extent to which groups are exposed to one another by virtue of sharing neighborhoods in common can be determined.
Clustering	Extent to which minority areas adjoin one another in space	Spatial Proximity Index: $$SP = \frac{XP_{xx} + YP_{yy}}{TP_{tt}}$$	It is maximized when minority neighborhoods form one large, contiguous ghetto and minimized when they are scattered widely in space.
Centralization	Degree to which a group is settled in and around the center of an index area (central business district)	Centralization Index: $$CE = \left(\sum_{i=1}^{n} X_{i-1}A_i\right) - \left(\sum_{i=1}^{n} X_iA_{i-1}\right)$$	The extent to which a group is spatially distributed close to or far from the CBD is reflected.
Concentration	Relative amount of physical space occupied by a minority group	Relative Concentration Index: $$CO = \frac{\left[\sum_{i=1}^{n} \frac{x_ia_i}{X} \middle/ \sum_{i=1}^{n} \frac{y_ia_i}{Y}\right] - 1}{\left[\sum_{i=1}^{n_1} \frac{t_ia_i}{T_1} \middle/ \sum_{i=n_2}^{n} \frac{t_ia_i}{T_2}\right] - 1}$$	As segregation rises, minority members are increasingly concentrated within a small, geographically compact area.

Source: Reprinted from *Demography,* Vol. 26, No. 3, pp. 373–376, with permission of Population Association of America, © 1989.

Table 9-10 Inequality and Inequity Indexes

Inequality Indexes

Definition:	Every component should receive identical shares; the degree to which each component does not receive identical shares is a measure of the inequality of that component.
Standard used for comparison:	In measuring inequality, each share of the actual distribution is compared to the mean, mode, intergroup pairs, adjacent pairs, etc., of the actual distribution. Thus, the standard comes from the existing distribution, which is being analyzed (i.e., it uses some quantitative property of the original distribution itself).
Example:	Components are distributed on the basis of population, which is not evenly or equally distributed (e.g., distributing police protection based on population or distributing fire protection based on home. The basic flaw with this approach is that, as population increases, so do the distributive services. In health, social and environmental situations, this may not be the most advantageous method for distribution.

Inequity Indexes

Definition:	Every component should receive shares based on equality, need, market forces, demand, or social status. Additionally, every component may be set at a minimum level of decency below which a component should not fall. The degree to which shares are not distributed in this manner is a measure of the inequality of that component.
Standard used for comparison:	In measuring inequity, the comparative standard used is an entirely different distribution. It is basically what the researcher wants, expects, or prefers the original distribution to look like. It does not represent some property of the distribution of interest (i.e., it uses some quantitative property of an entirely different distribution).
Example:	Components are distributed on the bases of various factors that are valued more than the simple impact of population distribution. Examples include distribution *according to needs* (in an infant mortality reduction program more assistance is given to higher risk areas, antipoverty programs provide more assistance to poorer persons/areas); *according to ability to pay* (neighborhood property values provide the basis for distributing police protection); *according to demand* (who asks shall receive); *according to social status* (high social status should receive more and better of what is being distributed and those of lower social status should receive less and worse). This inevitably leads to the development of the *"underclass."*

Source: Adapted from *Measuring Inequality: A Methodological Handbook* by P.B. Coulter, pp. 11–34, 161–177, with permission of Westview Press, © 1989.

from 1, it produces an equity index versus Coulter's inequity index.[44] Coulter's index has been used extensively by political scientists (e.g., to distribute public services among subareas) and researchers (e.g., to analyze the distribution of physicians by type among subareas of a state).[45] On the other hand, Nagel's index of equity and Nagel's index of proportionality have not yet been applied to actual distributions.[46]

Table 9-11 Inequity Indexes: Equations and Definition of Terms

Equations	Definition of Terms
1. Coulter's Generalized Index of Inequity $$I_\alpha = \frac{[\Sigma|P_i - Q_i|^\alpha]^{1/\alpha}}{[(1 - minQ)^\alpha - (minQ)^\alpha + \Sigma Q_{i}]^{1/\alpha}}$$ If α is reduced to unity the serialized index becomes: $$I_1 = \frac{\Sigma|P_i - Q_i|}{2(1 - minQ)}$$	where P_i = Proportional share of the component Q_i = Proportional share that should be received by the component; the equity standard distribution $minQ$ = Smallest Q value where P_i = Proportional share of the component Q_i = Proportional share that should be received by the component; the equity standard distribution $minQ$ = Smallest Q value
2. Nagel's Equity $$EQ = 1 - \frac{\Sigma(A_i - M_i)^2}{\Sigma(Z - M_i)^2}$$	where A_i = Actual frequency distribution to the component M_i = Minimum decency level frequency for the component Z = Zero allocation (most inequitable), and when $A_i > M_i$, $A_i - M_i = 0$
3. Nagel's Proportionality $$PR = 1 - \frac{\Sigma(A_i - P_i)^2}{\Sigma(Z - P_i)^2}$$	where A_i = Actual frequency distribution to the component P_i = Distribution of A to each i in proportion to its merit, and Z = Zero allocation (most inequitable)

Source: Adapted from *Measuring Inequality: A Methodological Handbook* by P.B. Coulter, pp. 164–175, with permission of Westview Press, © 1989.

One of the most pressing issues in most health agencies today is the high rate of infant mortality. The health status of the nation, state, or county is often evaluated on the basis of its infant mortality rate. Nagel's index of inequity makes it possible to determine if the number of infant deaths observed in a five-county area is consistent with the expected minimum number as expressed by the goals for the nation in the year 2000. Computing the index from the hypothetical values for an infant mortality program in a five-county area (Table 9-12),

$$EQ = 1 - \frac{\Sigma(A_i - M_i)^2}{\Sigma(Z - M_i)^2}$$

$$= 1 - \frac{69}{1593}$$

$$= 1 - .0433$$

$$= .9567$$

The value .9567, rounded to .96, indicates that the actual distribution of infant deaths is 96 percent of perfect equity, based on the minimum number of infant deaths (minimum decency concept) as proposed by the year 2000 objectives. In this model, 0 represents total inequity and 1 represents total equity. Therefore, the value 96 approaches almost complete equity. Of course, if the minimum decency were considered to be no infant deaths, a 0 value would reflect total inequity. Furthermore, if prenatal care visits were the distribution used to compare to the infant mortality distribution, the answer would surely be different.

Social Vulnerability Index[47]

The social transformation disease model has been developed as a way of responding to problems of inequality and inequity, and as a way of predicting future health care needs. The model provides the framework and the background

---

Table 9-12 Hypothetical Data for an Infant Mortality Program

County	A_i	M_i	$A_i - M_i$	$(A_i - M_i)^2$	$(Z - M_i)^2$
A	12	10	0	0	100
B	23	24	1	1	576
C	4	6	2	4	36
D	30	25	0	0	625
E	8	16	8	64	256
Total	77	81	11	69	1593

where A_i = Number of observed infant deaths
M_i = Minimum number of infant deaths expected
based on the year 2000 objectives
Z = Zero allocation

for a forward-thinking, comprehensive view of societal problems. The next important steps are to identify these problems and to determine what geographical areas and what population groups are most socially vulnerable, as variations in social conditions are important parts of the health planning of the future. Thus, analysis of a state's health patterns, using an index of social vulnerability, may shed light on the injustices in the system and show where resources should be allocated.[48-50]

Based on the previous discussion of the index of inequity, the social vulnerability index becomes the equity standard distribution and the distribution of service delivery resources becomes the actual distribution upon which shares were distributed. In this example, it was based on population (an equality index) or a form of an inequity index only because population is not evenly distributed.

Thirteen variables grouped under five factors were used to produce a social vulnerability index for the total population (Table 9-13). The 13 variables selected were drawn from related studies and detailed papers produced by the Carter Center.[51] The variables were transformed into Z-scores, which were added using the standard score additive model (see Chapter 7). The Z-score is a linear transformation of the original data that does not change the shape of the distribution of the data. When a set of variables is transformed in this way, two parameters of their distributions are equalized (i.e., the mean equals 0 and the standard deviation equals 1), and the units of measurement are eliminated. This allows the

Table 9-13 Factors and Variables Used in the Social Vulnerability Index

Factor	Variable
Social pathology	Percentage of households receiving Aid for Families with Dependent Children (AFDC)
	Female head of household with children under 18 as a percentage of total families
Economic well-being	Percentage of persons below poverty level
	Median family income
Education	Median school years completed by persons more than 25 years of age
	Median cost of education per pupil
	Percentage of free lunches
Health access	Hospital beds per 1,000 population
	Number of total physicians per 10,000 population
	Number of primary care physicians per 10,000 population
Health status	Infant mortality per 1,000 live births
	Percentage of low-birthweight infants (<2500g)
	Teen pregnancy (ages 10–19) per 1,000 female population

Source: Reprinted from *Family and Community Health*, Vol. 10, No. 4, p. 28, Aspen Publishers, Inc., © 1988.

scores on different variables to be combined by simple addition when the signs of those with negative connotation (i.e., high incidence or value is "bad") are reversed. There are several methods of combining and standardizing variables, but the Z-score additive model was used for several reasons.

- practicality
- simplicity
- comprehensiveness
- ease of demonstration
- widespread use
- interpretation of results
- graphic display of information

The standard scores of the 13 variables were combined to produce five factor indexes, each shown in Figure 9-10 as applied to the state of Georgia: (1) index of social pathology, (2) index of economic well-being, (3) index of education, (4) index of health access, and (5) index of health status. The geographical pattern shown is typical for all five maps. Notably, the counties rated "poor" are generally in the south central and southwest sections of the state. The counties rated "excellent" are mainly in the north, with some in the southeast section of the state.

The five factors were combined to produce an index of social vulnerability (the equity standard distribution). The two areas in Georgia that are most socially vulnerable are the southwest and east central sections of the state (Fig. 9-11). Because the north appears to have more counties where the risk level is excellent, the total population is less vulnerable. Each county's ratio of risk (social vulnerability index, an equity standard distribution) to service delivery (the actual distribution) was determined. The scores were compared, with the result being a ratio map that shows where risk equals service, where risk is less than service, and where risk is greater than service (equity index; Fig. 9-12).

To provide a more equitable distribution of resources according to the principle that the most vulnerable should receive the most benefit, it is clear that, where risk is greater than service, some changes must be made. Specifically, the south central and east central sections of Georgia experience the most severe deficiencies. Thus, policies and health plans must be developed to ensure greater consistency and fairness in resource distribution.

The social vulnerability index provides a data base and a mechanism for determining if a standard of justice is being met. While this formulation may be developed further, it can give guidance now for equitable health care planning and resource allocation.

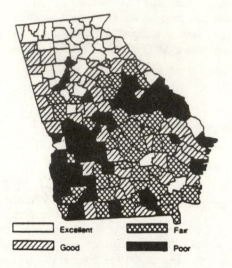

Map of the state of Georgia, showing counties graded excellent, good, fair, or poor as to the level of social pathology.

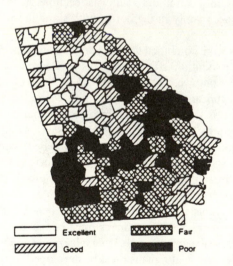

Map of the state of Georgia, showing counties graded excellent, good, fair, or poor as to the level of economic well-being.

Figure 9-10 Factor Index Maps. *Source:* Reprinted from Family and Community Health, Vol. 10, No. 4, pp. 29–31, Aspen Publishers Inc., © 1988.

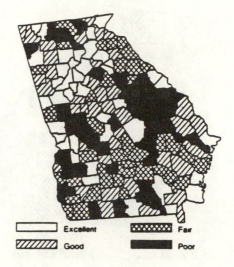

Map of the state of Georgia, showing counties graded excellent, good, fair, or poor as to the level of education.

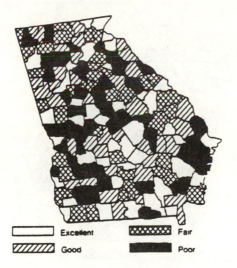

Map of the state of Georgia, showing counties graded excellent, good, fair, or poor as to the level of health care access.

Figure 9-10 continued

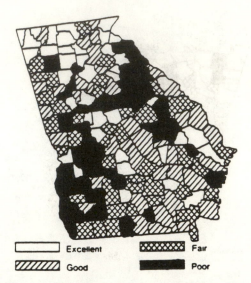

Map of the state of Georgia, showing counties graded excellent, good, fair, or poor as to health status.

Figure 9-10 continued

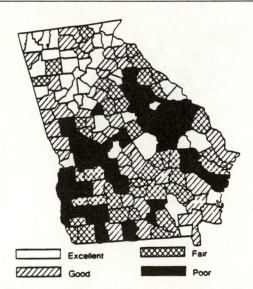

Map of the state of Georgia, showing counties graded excellent, good, fair, or poor as to the index of social vulnerability.

Figure 9-11 Index of Social Vulnerability. *Source:* Reprinted from *Family and Community Health,* Vol. 10, No. 4, pp. 29–31, Aspen Publishers, Inc., © 1988.

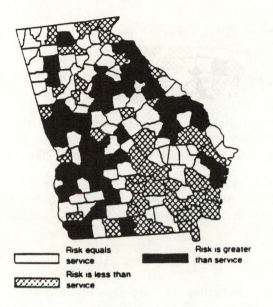

Figure 9-12 Equity Index. *Source:* Reprinted from *Family and Community Health,* Vol. 10, No. 4, pp. 29–31, Aspen Publishers, Inc., © 1988.

NOTES

1. Institute for Health Care Facilities of the Future, "The Post Industrial Future," *Panoramique* 2, no. 4 (Fall 1989): 2.

2. This section of this chapter is abridged from M. Sciegaj, T.W. Wade, G.E.A. Dever, and J.W. Alley, "A Framework for Applying Ethical Theory to Public Health Practice," *Journal of Family and Community Health* 10, no. 1 (1987): 15–23.

3. T.E. Wade, G.E.A. Dever, and T.C. Lofton, "An Epidemiological Model Applied to Planning and Evaluation of Local Health Department Services," *International Journal of Social Indicators Research* 19 (1987): 287–301.

4. Ibid., 289.

5. Ibid., 293.

6. Ibid., 300.

7. G.E.A. Dever, *Community Health Analysis: A Holistic Approach* (Gaithersburg, Md.: Aspen Publishers, Inc., 1980).

8. N. Milio, *Promoting Health through Public Policy* (Philadelphia, F.A. Davis Co., 1987), 4.

9. Wade, Dever, and Lofton, "An Epidemiological Model," 300.

10. P. Manga, "Medical Technology and Ethics," *Panoramique* 2, No. 1 (Winter 1988): 300.

11. Ibid.

12. "Ethics in Epidemiology," *The Epidemiology Monitor* 10, no. 6, special issue (June 1989): 1.

13. Ibid.

14. Ibid.

15. T.L. Beauchamp and J.F. Childress, *Principles of Biomedical Ethics* (New York: Oxford University Press, 1983).

16. Ibid., 187.

17. M. Sciegaj et al., "A Framework for Applying Ethical Theory to Public Health Practice," 20–23. This section is abridged from this article.

18. W. May, *The Physician's Covenant: Images of the Healer in Social Ethics* (Philadelphia, Westminister, 1983).

19. State Data Center, Georgia Division of Public Health, 1986.

20. D. Beauchamp, "Public Health as Social Justice," *Inquiry* 13, no. 3 (1976): 3–14.

21. A.W. Koplin, "A Reminder: Public Health, Social Justice Are Linked," *The Nation's Health* 7 (October/November 1987): 2.

22. Ibid.

23. "Medical Benefits," *The Medical-Economic Digest,* 15 February 1988, 3.

24. Ibid.

25. H.K. Heggenhougen and L. Shone, "Cultural Components of Behavioral Epidemiology: Implication for Primary Health Care," *Social Science and Medicine* 22, no. 11 (1986): 1235–1245.

26. R. Belmar, "Research Statement on Democracy and Other Social Variables as Determinants of Health," *Computer Health System Newsletter* 5 (1989): 1–4.

27. E. Kirshner, "Canadians Say Health System Is No Cure All," *Healthwork News* 3, no. 21 (1989): 11, 31.

28. Ibid., 11.

29. American Cancer Society, *Special Report on Cancer in the Economically Disadvantaged* (New York: ACS, 1986).

30. H.P. Freeman, "Cancer in the Socioeconomically Disadvantaged," *CA. Cancer Journal for Clinicians* 39, no. 5 (1989): 279.

31. G.A. Kaplan et al., "Socioeconomic Status and Health," in *Closing the Gap: The Burden of Unnecessary Illness,* ed. R.W. Amler and B.H. Dull (New York: Oxford University Press, 1982), 125–129.

32. Freeman, "Cancer in the Socioeconomically Disadvantaged," 272.

33. Ibid.

34. Northwestern National Life Insurance Company, *1989 NWNL State Health Rankings* (1989), NWNL, 95.

35. Freeman, "Cancer in the Socioeconomically Disadvantaged," 285.

36. Ibid., 286.

37. American Cancer Society, "A Summary of the American Cancer Society Report to the Nation: Cancer in the Poor," *CA–A Cancer Journal for Clinicians* 39, no. 5 (September/October 1989): 264.

38. P.B. Coulter, *Measuring Inequality: A Methodological Handbook* (Boulder, Colo.: Westview Press, 1989), 1–160.

39. D.S. Massey and N.A. Denton, "Hypersegregation in U.S. Metropolitan Areas: Black and Hispanic Segregation along Five Dimensions," *Demography* 26, no. 3 (August 1989): 373–391.

40. Ibid.

41. Coulter, *Measuring Inequality,* 163.

42. Ibid., 161–177.

43. Ibid., 171.

44. Ibid.

45. Ibid.

46. Ibid., 171–177.

47. This section is adapted from G.E.A. Dever et al., "Creation of a Social Vulnerability Index for Justice in Health Planning, *Journal of Family and Community Health* 10, no. 4 (1988): 23–32.

48. K.C. Land and S. Spilerman, eds., *Social Indicator Models* (New York: Russell Sage Foundation, 1975).

49. J.C. Malney, *Social Vulnerability in Indianapolis* (Indianapolis: Community Service Council of Metropolitan Indianapolis, Inc., 1973).

50. D.M. Smith, "The Geography of Social Well-Being in the United States," in *Territorial Social Indicators* (New York: McGraw-Hill Book Co., 1973).

51. R. W. Amler and H. B. Dull, eds., *Closing the Gap: The Burden of Unnecessary Illness* (New York: Oxford University Press, 1987), 210.

Chapter 10

Computer Graphics in Health Planning

In the 1990s, the focus on the community as the new health care recipient will be crucial to the development of a healthy public policy that includes the precepts of holism and wellness. This new direction may require new approaches to the presentation of community health information. One such approach, computer graphs, is not new per se, but its application to community health has usually been limited. The technological advances since the late 1970s and early 1980s have been remarkable. Even in the later 1980s, however, many public health agencies have not kept stride with this changing technology.

Practical applications of computer graphics have been pioneered predominantly in the aerospace industry.[1] Now, however, some administrative and planning applications of computer graphics have surfaced in the health and health-related literature.[2-7] Researchers, planners, and administrators in the community health field are beginning to use health-oriented, computer-generated graphics for policy planning, evaluation, and decision making. Although few such applications have been documented in the professional literature, they are well represented in a few local and state government publications and in many health agency plans.[8] The latter plans have integrated health planning with health statistics by using computer graphics as a communication format. Thus, they have been able to present basic patterns and trends that aid in evaluation, decision making, and policy formulation. These plans have demonstrated the effectiveness of translating data on health variables into visual information that various levels of management can use to determine future needs.

TRADITIONAL GRAPHICS

The graphic depiction of health data has traditionally taken the forms of tables, hand-drawn charts, graphs, and maps. The laborious accumulation, reduction, and formulation of health data into such finished products frequently consumed many person hours, however. Reproduction of the results was often tailored to meet publication requirements rather than to ensure an adequate graphic presentation of the data. Moreover, the graphics and the accompanying text were often research oriented and, consequently, not immediately applicable to current health program planning or to community health problems.

Graphic displays produced by traditional methods are still useful for some purposes, but they have become essentially obsolete for the communication of data necessary to major planning, policy, and evaluation decisions. For instance, policy decisions in health programming are often based on highly specialized, up-to-date maps of ephemeral subject matter that may be used only a few times. Because of the slow procedures and tremendous costs of producing them traditionally, such maps may not even be available when health decisions are being made. Of course, the availability of 5, 10, or even 15 timely computer maps or graphs does not guarantee improvement over one well-conceived, traditionally produced map or graph. Nevertheless, by automating the graphics process and by improving the material, equipment, and techniques, it has been possible to produce more maps in less time and at a lower cost.

COMPUTER GRAPHICS

The increasing proliferation of health data has made it necessary to present the information, especially the "fragile" information, garnered from such data in a rapid, accurate, and discerning fashion. Administrators in problem-oriented, crisis-producing, health-associated industries, such as health planning, hospitals, health agencies, and community epidemiological programs, must depend upon the absorption and the digestion of precise, opportune information. Computer-generated graphics, presented in quick, accurate, versatile, and interactive formats, is a viable response to this requirement. Before undertaking the expenditure of funds and resources for integrating computer graphics hardware and software into the program mainstream, however, it is important to investigate the advantages and disadvantages of the procedures involved.

Advantages of Computer Graphics

As health problems and the information needed to understand and deal with them multiply in scale, variety, intensity, and complexity, the best possible means are needed to analyze, display, and communicate health information.[9] Computer graphics has distinct advantages because it allows a user to deal with the problems of scale, variety, intensity, and complexity through better visual communication.

- The method is fast, efficient, simple, and economical.
- Computer-generated maps/graphs may provide a clearer view of information than do most tables or charts.
- Data that change with time may be followed with a series of maps.
- Several variables that are spatially identical and contiguous may be analyzed simultaneously.
- It is relatively easy to select and display various sample data sets.
- The scale of the map and the data range levels of the computer graphics may be selected according to the user's need.
- Computer graphics can be interactive; for example, a trial product may be viewed before it is final, thus avoiding costly production errors.
- By mapping, the user is able to visualize large volumes of data rapidly.

These advantages indicate that computer graphics has considerable merit compared to traditional graphics. Of course, the major advantage of computer graphics is its capability for rapid integration of health statistics and health services.

Disadvantages of Computer Graphics

Like most methods or techniques, computer graphics also has disadvantages.

- The majority of time is spent coding the data to be mapped. Furthermore, the "base map" must be digitized. If done by hand, this is time-consuming. Automatic digitizers are available, however, and there are several vendors who sell the digitized geography.
- Considerable initial time may be spent preparing the data to fit available equipment and software programs.
- It is difficult to avoid the pitfall of attempting to map or graph all data.
- Unless a user has a basic knowledge of the techniques of mapmaking and graphic illustration, many problems will arise relative to the scale of the map, choice of symbols, type of map, selection of the legend, and level of measurement (i.e., nominal, ordinal, interval, or ratio).
- The user may not know the usefulness of the output or, for that matter, may not even be aware of the quality of the input.
- It is difficult to select the most appropriate map or graphic for the presentation of data (see Chapter 5).
- Interpretation of data is critical, and caution is warranted at this stage.

- The hardware and software must be tailored to the user's needs, although this problem is diminishing with the advent of several software packages that are multiple-machine compatible.

In light of these disadvantages, it must be stressed that computer-generated maps and graphics are no better than the quality of the data put into them. There will be a major emerging need to recognize the computer professional who produces the graphics as part of an agency's organizational structure for community health in the 1990s. Because the advantages of computer graphics far outweigh the disadvantages, the limitations should not represent insurmountable barriers to implementing computer graphics.

Noise is another aspect of computer graphics that can be considered a disadvantage. Noise may take three forms: statistical, visual, or semantic. Statistical and visual noises are related to the effective presentation of information. For instance, removing various types of statistical noise from the data prior to mapping can often substantially improve the final product. The removal can be done by means of premap operations to reduce or eliminate the excessive statistical presentation that stems from data error. In a strict statistical sense, noise is caused by the use of complex and complicated formulas to convey a point that could, in fact, be conveyed by a simple, uncomplicated procedure.

Visual noise is an excessive accumulation of symbols, patterns, and legends that leads to graphic information overload. In this case, so much information is presented on a map that the result is a poor, cluttered, and unstructured graphic with little communication value. Because the basic reason for using graphics is to present information visually and effectively, the problem of visual noise should be avoided at all costs.

Semantic noise results from verbosity and a language structure that is difficult to comprehend. Computer graphics requires terse and uncomplicated word structures to effect the desired results. The growth of computer graphics may, in fact, be attributed partially to the need to overcome semantic noise. Certainly, one approach toward overcoming this problem is to produce a clear and concise computer graphic.

A GUIDE TO GRAPHIC SELECTION

A public health agency's selection of computer graphic software and hardware depends on the potential use. Riche noted that, "in general, people use computer generated maps because they need to make decisions about many small pieces (areas) of geography."[10] In health planning for facilities, the geography of choice is usually ZIP code, but it could be census tract or county. In community needs assessment, the geographies used reflect a service area or trade area that may encompass several ZIP codes, census tracts, or counties. With such a variety of geographies, demographics, and vendors who sell these products, it is essential to ask pertinent and significant questions to ensure that the needs of the health agency are met. Belcher has suggested at least 15 questions that administrators should ask before they make a decision regarding the purchase of a graphic package and/or system (Exhibit 10-1).[11] Generally, these questions provide guidelines for selecting the appropriate computer graphics package (vendor).

COMMUNITY HEALTH ANALYSIS AND COMPUTER GRAPHICS

There is a clear potential for computer-generated displays in a community/public health agency because it is required to assemble, analyze, communicate, and display data concerning the following:

- the health status, including the determinants of health status, of service area residents
- the status of the health care delivery system and the area residents' use of that system
- the effects of the health care delivery system on the health of area residents
- the number, type, and location of the area's health resources, including services, personnel, and facilities
- the pattern of utilization of the area's health resources
- the factors of environmental and occupational exposure that affect immediate and long-term health conditions

In order to facilitate the manipulation of data in these areas, an agency should exploit its potential for using computer-generated graphics. Not all agencies, of course, will need or want to establish ongoing computer graphics programs. Many resources for completing computer graphics are available through universities and consultants. Indeed, it is frequently advantageous—and advisable—to employ outside resources with experience in the health field.

In some organizations related to community health (e.g., hospitals, health departments, HMOs, insurance companies), computer graphics permits more sophisticated analyses.

- The basic functional aspects of hospital accessibility—time, cost, and distance—can be mapped to show areas of high or low accessibility. This approach is valid for determining patient accessibility of emergency rooms,

Exhibit 10-1 Questions You Should Ask Regarding Selection of a Graphic Package/System

1. **Do you need a mainframe or a microcomputer-based mapping system?**
Large, centralized companies should consider mainframe programs. They store and process large data files, usually offer features supporting more complex problem solving, and can be shared by multiple users. Small organizations will find that microcomputer-based mapping systems offer many of the capabilities of the mainframe packages, but at a much lower cost.

2. **Does the system manage information linked to varied types of geography?**
All mapping programs manage demographic information by census tract and zip code, but the better ones can also manage information such as sales performance by location and traffic counts by street network.

3. **Can you use multiple variables?**
Better systems allow you to use relational ($<$, $=$) and logical (and, or) operators to ask questions using a number of variables. The map shows the geographic areas that satisfy the specified condition. Other programs allow you to identify only one or two variables which are displayed for all areas.

4. **Does the system integrate data from disparate types of geography?**
Programs with this feature allow you to use data referenced by zip code with data referenced by census tract, eliminating the need to geocode to a common geographic type.

5. **Does the system perform density calculations?**
Mapping programs that display only raw counts or percentages can lead to misinterpretation. The best systems perform density calculations that show you, for example, how concentrated an area's population is.

6. **Does it zoom?**
This is important if you're using maps to study sites or street networks that are close to one another. Some zooms only blow up a picture; the better ones will show you greater geographic detail.

7. **How accurate is the system's cartography?**
The most advanced mapping products display longitude and latitude coordinates and a scale that allows you to calculate exact distances between locations.

8. **Can you report information and how flexibly?**
Programs that offer reporting eliminate the need to transfer data to other software packages for calculation. Some programs that offer reporting, however, print out only preselected data in a standardized format.

9. **How good is the quality of details on the finished map?**
Different systems have different types of hatching, cross-hatching, symbols and patterns, texts, and legend boxes. Check them out.

10. **How easy is the system to use?**
A mapping program should include on-line help, fully prompted input screens, and an English-like command language that requires little or no familiarity with programming languages. You should be able to save, recall, and edit your queries and plotting specifications.

11. **How good are the vendor's geographic files?**
Some companies specialize in providing highly detailed map files that include features such as cities, parks, airports, lakes, rivers, bridges, and transportation networks. This eliminates the need to use base maps for further reference.

12. **Can you digitize?**
The mapping products that include digitizing will allow you to add or change map features. This is particularly useful if you're studying markets that are rapidly changing.

Exhibit 10-1 continued

13. **How easy is it to add, delete, and modify data in the system?**
As more information becomes available and other information becomes outdated, it is important that you be able to easily modify your databases.
14. **How supportive is the company?**
The company you buy a complex mapping system from should provide training, installation, testing, tutorials, system documentation, and tollfree telephone assistance. Some companies also offer enhanced versions of software and data through a licensing agreement, helping you stay up to date.
15. **Can you test it?**
Some companies offer potential customers a trial program. Take advantage of these offers to gain hands-on experience with different mapping programs. This will give you confidence that the mapping system you finally choose will be right for you.

Source: Reprinted from *American Demographics,* Vol. 8, No. 6, p. 30, with permission of American Demographics, Inc., © 1986.

---

neighborhood health clinics, county public health departments, patient-physician visits, and nursing homes.

- Medical trade areas or hospital service areas may be delineated through patient origin studies. Such studies may identify patients as points or line flows, indicating volume, or as circles with variable radii or ellipses based on the standard deviation of an areal distribution, indicating area.

- Personnel data may be mapped to illustrate areas of underservice, scarcity, and oversupply. Such a map may be helpful in making decisions about the development and location of satellite clinics and mobile health vans. Moreover, strategies in the recruitment process may be based on locational needs for medical and paramedical personnel.

- Disease patterns may be mapped in relation to facility and personnel distribution. If the health planning organization possesses the appropriate expertise, it may initiate studies to measure and assess the relationship of health status to available resources.

The increasing focus in health planning on population groups in communities rather than on individuals in clinics has facilitated these uses of computer graphics. The shift in disease patterns from infectious to chronic to social diseases has also stimulated more widespread interest in these areas of use.

In the case of morbidity or mortality data, computer graphics has still other functional uses. It can, for example, aid in

- identifying high- or low-risk areas for specified diseases. There is a critical need to reduce random variability in the data in such presentations. This can be accomplished either by prolonging the time period of the study or by aggregating the areal units being investigated.
- rating a community on the health status of its population. This is similar to the identification of high- and low-risk areas, except that periodic community epidemiological studies would be expected.
- setting priorities for the allocation of resources in health programs.
- planning health and social programs.
- making reports or presenting information to state legislators, special governors' councils, boards of health, planning agencies, consumer groups, and news media.
- updating baseline or benchmark health data periodically to indicate changes in evaluation measures from one time frame to another.

In spite of the multiple uses of computer-generated maps and graphics, the technique is by no means the panacea for solving the health problems facing the United States. It is basically merely an efficient and effective way of communicating and displaying pertinent information.

APPLICATION OF COMPUTER GRAPHICS IN COMMUNITY HEALTH

The practical applications of computer graphics in community health can be shown at three scales of analysis: national, state, and city. Appendix 10-A provides a list of vendors, their products (i.e., demography, geography, lifestyle, and health information), and their various computerized mapping and graphing capabilities.

The National Scale

On the national scale, the data are usually aggregated by counties, by state economic areas, or by states to illustrate geographical patterns of health information. The selected administrative units show the relative differences in pattern perception and information content. Computer-generated graphs can further illustrate the data by providing different methods of information display.

Resource Distributions

The maps in Figures 10-1 and 10-2 illustrate resource distribution by state. The two maps illustrate patterns of need for specific types of resources at the national scale. Federal and regional offices may use such spatial portrayals of resource distributions for planning and determining health policy for resource needs.

Mortality Distributions

The Environmental Protection Agency developed an automated cartography system that produces maps of mortality distributions.[12] Such maps appear in the *Atlas of Cancer Mortality for U.S. Counties—1950–1969*,[13] the *Atlas of Cancer Mortality among U.S. Nonwhites*,[14] and the *U.S. Cancer Mortality Rates and Trends—1950–1979*,[15] where they show age-adjusted death rates of various types of cancers for the white and nonwhite population, aggregated by state economic areas and counties, from 1950 to 1979. The maps in these publications are strikingly unique in the method of reproduction and the visual impact. Not only do they demonstrate current descriptive epidemiology, but also they stimulate future analytical investigations. For example, regional and local investigations of patterns of cancer of the lung, mouth, and throat by the Centers for Disease Control

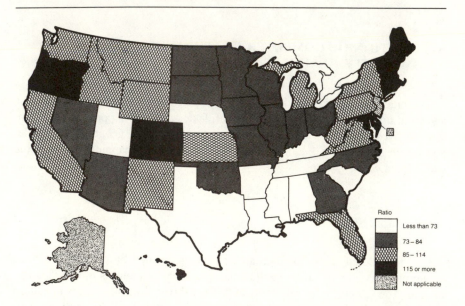

Note: Physicians are active nonfederal doctors of medicine (1980 data) and doctors of osteopathy (1981 data).

Figure 10-1 Patient Care Physicians per 100,000 Resident Population in Nonmetropolitan Areas: 1980 and 1981. *Source:* Reprinted from *Health, United States, 1984,* p. 25, U.S. DHHS, National Center for Health Statistics, 1984.

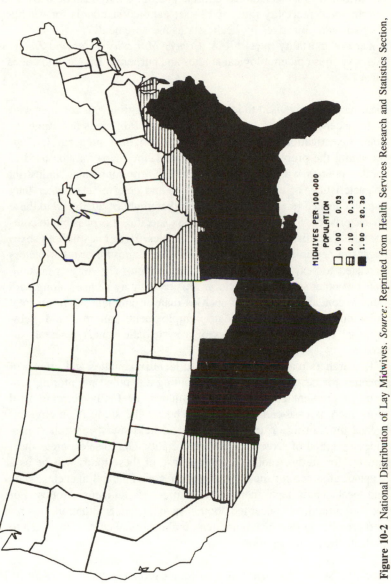

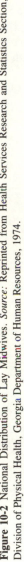

Figure 10-2 National Distribution of Lay Midwives. *Source:* Reprinted from Health Services Research and Statistics Section, Division of Physical Health, Georgia Department of Human Resources, 1974.

may be attributed to these national efforts. The maps may also be used to compare interregional mortality rates and to set national standards for establishing realistic goals and objectives for health status measurement.

The maps of mortality rates in *U.S. Cancer Mortality Rates and Trends* may be used for various epidemiological studies and purposes. Riggan and colleagues stated that

> these maps may be used to identify counties or groups of counties with high cancer mortality rates, large shifts in rank of areas over time, or both. Investigation into possible causes can then proceed. Or, approaching the problem from the other end, the maps may be used to locate counties with unusual demographic, environmental, industrial characteristics, or employment patterns and determine whether they exhibit elevated rates or unusual trends that might be attributed to these characteristics. Since these maps are sex specific, it is possible to compare the mortality among males and females. High rates in both sexes suggest a possible relation to environmental exposure or other factors unrelated to sex, while high rates among men only suggest occupational or other sex-related factors. This report may be used along with other secondary information such as data on ambient environmental pollution levels, emission data, employment patterns, and demographic characteristics as part of a systematic cancer research approach.
>
> Researchers may use this report to identify counties and groups of counties for developing and implementing a detailed monitoring program of ambient environmental pollutants, or for performing field work such as case-control studies. Whether the study is an environmental monitoring or an epidemiological field study, this report provides a method of screening cancer mortality data to select areas most suitable for study. Another important use of these maps will be as a graphic reference for the EPA and other governmental agencies, state and local health departments, universities, and citizens' groups. For local communities concerned about a specific cancer situation, this report provides both a spatial and temporal historical context in which to evaluate the local condition.[16]

Figure 10-3 shows the distribution of lung cancer for white males from 1970 to 1979, and Figure 10-4 shows the relative change in lung cancer for white males between the 1950s and the 1970s. For the rate map in Figure 10-3, the data are divided into five classes based on percentiles and represented by gray tones. A graph of the density distribution, lower left, shows two bars; the lower bar defines the scale by percentiles, and the upper bar gives the actual rates by range

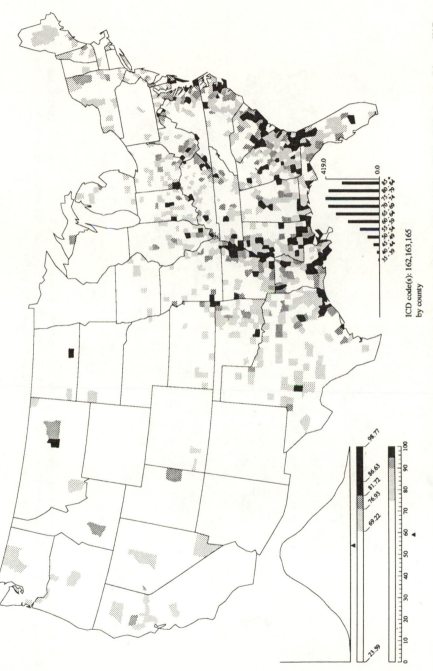

Figure 10-3 Cancer of the Trachea, Bronchus, and Lung, Including Pleura and Other Respiratory Sites, White Males: 1970–1979. *Source:* Riggan, W.B. et al. U.S. Cancer Mortality Rates and Trends, 1950–1979, Vol. IV, MAPS U.S. EPA. Health Effects Research Laboratory. Research Triangle Park, N.C. 27711, Sept. 1987, p. 156. For Sale. Superintendent of Documents. U.S. Gov't. Wash., D.C. 20402.

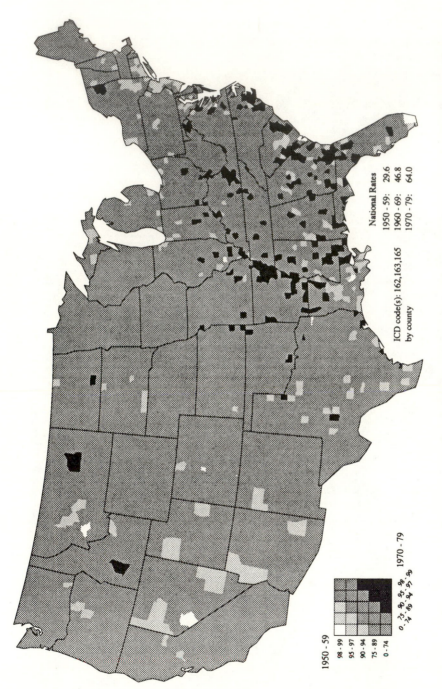

Figure 10-4 Cancer of the Trachea, Bronchus, and Lung, Including Pleura and Other Respiratory Sites, White Males: Relative Change. *Source:* Riggan, W.B. et al. U.S. Cancer Mortality Rates and Trends, 1950–1979, Vol. IV, MAPS U.S. EPA. Health Effects Research Laboratory. Research Triangle Park, N.C. 27711, Sept. 1987, p. 157. For Sale. Superintendent of Documents. U.S. Gov't. Wash., D.C. 20402.

of each class. The black delta-shaped pointers indicate the national rate for the two distributions. In the lower right section of the graph, a bar chart depicts the national age-specific rates.

The trend map (Fig. 10-4) is based on changes in rank of areas between 1950–1959 and 1970–1979. A table in the lower left portion of the map shows the relationship between the two decades in gray tones. White indicates maximum decrease, while black indicates maximum increase between the two periods. Thus, darker colors show relative deterioration over time; lighter colors show relative improvement.

A plotted graph in Figure 10-5 shows age-specific death rates of lung cancer by five-year age groups for white and nonwhite males and females. Figure 10-6 shows age-adjusted death rates for lung cancer for white and nonwhite males and females from 1950 to 1967. These figures illustrate risk factors for lung cancer mortality relative to age, sex, race, geography, and time; they also provide a description of the epidemiology of lung cancer.

Schnell and Monmonier developed an interesting application of computer graphics at the national scale (Fig. 10-7).[17] They demonstrated geographical associations between the birth and death rates; a third category shows the mortality-fertility ratio. The line-plotter maps were produced by SYMVU,[18] a computer program that generates three-dimensional statistical surfaces. Other software packages that produce these three-dimensional graphics, such as SOLO[19] and SYGRAPH,[20] are also available. (Appendix 10-B provides examples of the many and varied types of graphics produced by the SYGRAPH package.)

The maps present four time periods, suggesting change over time and variation in space. These three-dimensional block diagrams (line-plotter maps) show quite vividly the regional pattern of birth and death rates. To allow for comparison among the time periods and between the two rates, the same vertical scale was used for all maps in the first two columns. A constant vertical scale was used for the maps in the third column. The results clearly indicate a decline in the birth rate (as shown by the decrease in height of the graphics), while the death rate remains relatively constant. The ratio between the two increased greatly over the time periods. The application of this kind of three-dimensional map at the national scale can provide the planner with an instant picture of the changing dynamics of demography and its impact on health care.

The State Scale

Data examined on a state scale delineate more precise patterns and relationships. Interpretation at this scale of investigation (i.e., county administrative

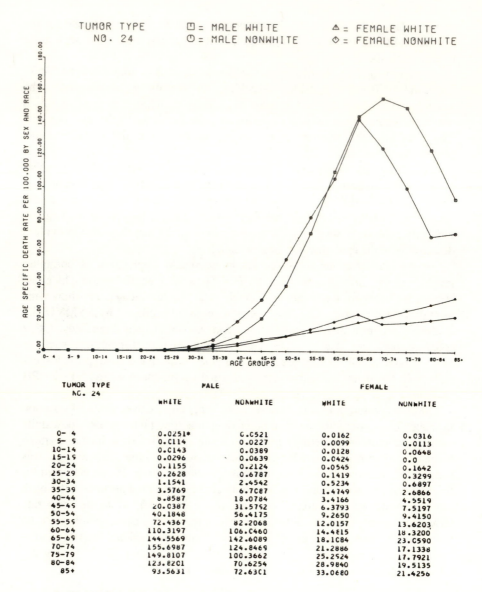

		MALE		FEMALE	
TUMOR TYPE NO. 24		WHITE	NONWHITE	WHITE	NONWHITE
0- 4		0.0251*	0.0521	0.0162	0.0316
5- 9		0.0114	0.0227	0.0099	0.0113
10-14		0.0143	0.0389	0.0128	0.0648
15-19		0.0296	0.0639	0.0424	0.0
20-24		0.1155	0.2124	0.0545	0.1642
25-29		0.2628	0.6787	0.1419	0.3299
30-34		1.1541	2.4542	0.5234	0.6897
35-39		3.5769	6.7087	1.4749	2.6866
40-44		8.8587	18.0784	3.4166	4.5519
45-49		20.0387	31.5752	6.3793	7.5197
50-54		40.1848	56.4175	9.2650	9.4150
55-59		72.4367	82.2068	12.0157	13.6203
60-64		110.3197	106.0460	14.4815	18.3200
65-69		144.5569	142.6089	18.1084	23.0590
70-74		155.6987	124.8469	21.2886	17.1338
75-79		149.8107	100.3662	25.2524	17.7921
80-84		123.8201	70.6254	28.9840	19.5135
85+		93.5631	72.6301	33.0680	21.4256

* AGE SPECIFIC DEATH RATE PER 100,000

Figure 10-5 Death Rates for Lung Cancer, by Age Group, 1950–1967. *Source:* Reprinted from *Patterns in Cancer Mortality in the U.S.: 1950–1967* by F. Burbank, p. 208, U.S. Government Printing Office, 1971.

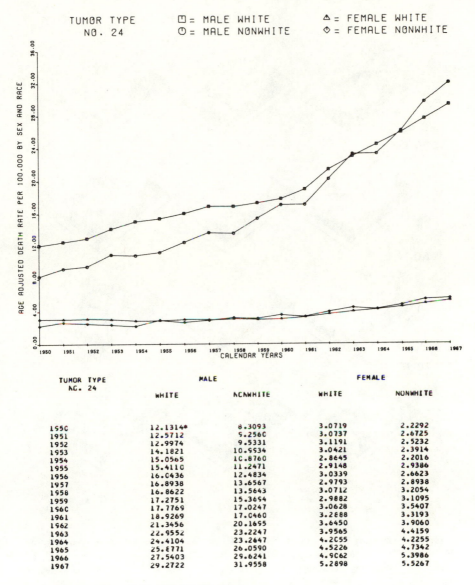

TUMOR TYPE   □ = MALE WHITE   △ = FEMALE WHITE
NO. 24   ○ = MALE NONWHITE   ◇ = FEMALE NONWHITE

TUMOR TYPE NO. 24	MALE		FEMALE	
	WHITE	NONWHITE	WHITE	NONWHITE
1950	12.1314*	8.3093	3.0719	2.2292
1951	12.5712	9.2560	3.0737	2.6725
1952	12.9974	9.5331	3.1191	2.5232
1953	14.1821	10.9934	3.0421	2.3914
1954	15.0565	10.8760	2.8645	2.2016
1955	15.4110	11.2471	2.9148	2.9386
1956	16.0436	12.4834	3.0339	2.6623
1957	16.8938	13.6567	2.9793	2.8938
1958	16.8622	13.5643	3.0712	3.2054
1959	17.2751	15.3694	2.9882	3.1095
1960	17.7769	17.0247	3.0628	3.5407
1961	18.9269	17.0460	3.2888	3.3193
1962	21.3456	20.1695	3.6450	3.9060
1963	22.9552	23.2247	3.9565	4.4159
1964	24.4104	23.2647	4.2055	4.2255
1965	25.8771	26.0590	4.5226	4.7342
1966	27.5403	29.6241	4.9062	5.3986
1967	29.2722	31.9558	5.2898	5.5267

* AGE ADJUSTED DEATH RATE PER 100,000

Figure 10-6 Age-Adjusted Death Rates for Lung Cancer, 1950–1967. *Source:* Reprinted from *Patterns in Cancer Mortality in the U.S.: 1950–1967* by F. Burbank, p. 209, U.S. Government Printing Office, 1971.

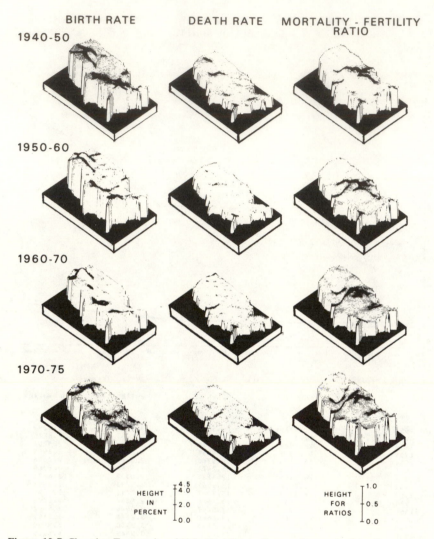

Figure 10-7 Changing Topography of U.S. Vital Rates. *Source:* George A. Schnell and Mark S. Monmonier, *Intercom* 6, No. 8 (Aug. 1978) p. 9; from "The Mortality-Fertility Ratio: A Useful Measure for Describing Demographic Change in the U.S., 1940–1975," *Geographical Survey,* in press.

units) is most beneficial to community epidemiologists, state and local health program managers, community analysts, and health policy formulators.

Resource Analysis

Figures 10-8 and 10-9 show two types of graphics, a three-dimensional map and graduated circles, representing the same set of data. Figure 10-8, a three-dimensional map on primary care physicians in Iowa in 1972, was generated by the mapping program called SYMVU. Three-dimensional maps are useful in showing the relative magnitude of the data. Also, "views" of the data can be "rotated" or "elevated" to produce different perspectives. Because of the complexity of interpretation, however, application of this type of graphic representation to decision making in the health field is quite limited.

Figure 10-9 shows the same data, represented by graduated circles. This map was produced by a mapping program called POWRMAP.[21] Given specified input, the program locates the corresponding place on the map and plots the appropriate size of circle. This graphic is very easily understood by the user and is of considerable use in location/allocation problems involving personnel, facilities, and other health resources.

Mortality Analysis

Figures 10-10 through 10-12 provide the user with a varied information display, demonstrating risk factors for lung cancer mortality by age, sex, race, time, and geographical area. When provided for several disease categories, this information may be used to determine health program policies, fund allocations, and aid in community epidemiological investigations.

Figure 10-10, a plotter map, depicts age-sex adjusted death rates for lung cancer, illustrating the spatial pattern of mortality for 1970 to 1974. The map also shows the rates as above average, average, and below average relative to the state's average. Figure 10-11 is a plotter graph, illustrating male and female crude death rates per 100,000 population for lung cancer for 1950 to 1974. Figure 10-12 is another plotted graphic, a disease pyramid showing lung cancer deaths as percentages by age, race, and sex.

Fiscal Health Analysis

Computer graphics may also be useful in the area of fiscal analysis. Figure 10-13 shows a fiscal analysis of average Medicaid and Medicare payments per vendor in Georgia counties in 1972. The plotted maps show areas of high and low concentrations of average payments to vendors—hospitals, physicians, and nursing homes—in dollar amounts. By showing health-related cash flow in this way, computer graphics can indicate areas in which excessively high payments

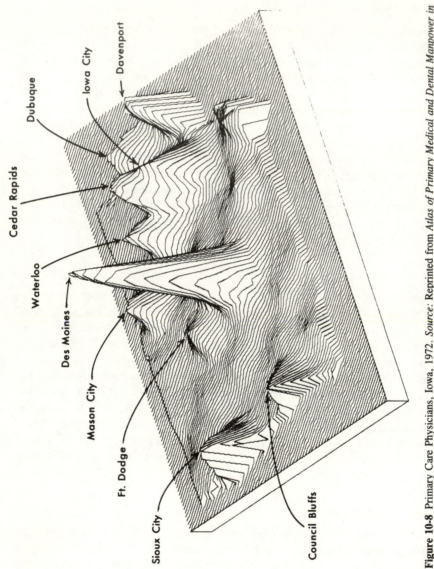

Figure 10-8 Primary Care Physicians, Iowa, 1972. *Source:* Reprinted from *Atlas of Primary Medical and Dental Manpower in Iowa* by P. Frankland, p. 4, Iowa City Center for Locational Analysis, Institute of Urban and Regional Research, University of Iowa, 1976.

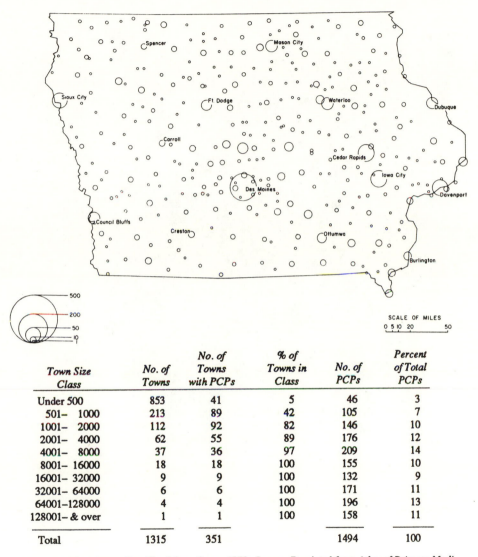

Town Size Class	No. of Towns	No. of Towns with PCPs	% of Towns in Class	No. of PCPs	Percent of Total PCPs
Under 500	853	41	5	46	3
501– 1000	213	89	42	105	7
1001– 2000	112	92	82	146	10
2001– 4000	62	55	89	176	12
4001– 8000	37	36	97	209	14
8001– 16000	18	18	100	155	10
16001– 32000	9	9	100	132	9
32001– 64000	6	6	100	171	11
64001–128000	4	4	100	196	13
128001– & over	1	1	100	158	11
Total	1315	351		1494	100

Figure 10-9 Primary Care Physicians, Iowa, 1972. *Source:* Reprinted from *Atlas of Primary Medical and Dental Manpower in Iowa*, Technical Report No. 50, by P. Frankland, pp. 4–5, Iowa City Center for Locational Analysis, Institute of Urban and Regional Research, University of Iowa, 1976.

to counties or other potential irregularities in reimbursement systems may have occurred. This type of analysis resulted in a strict monitoring of the Medicaid program in Georgia.

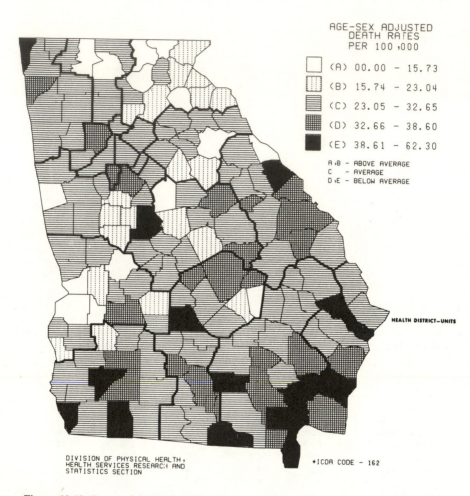

Figure 10-10 Cancer of the Trachea, Bronchus, and Lung, 1970–1974. *Source:* Reprinted from *Disease Patterns of the 70s,* p. 89, Division of Physical Health, Georgia Department of Human Resources, 1976.

The Urban or Metropolitan Scale

Graphic presentations aggregated at the urban, metropolitan, or city scale are useful for intraurban epidemiological investigations to identify city health problems and target areas, to determine appropriate resource placement, and to provide information for program planning. At this scale, it is essential to analyze the data by census tract, ZIP code, block, or even by individual street addresses (i.e., housing units).

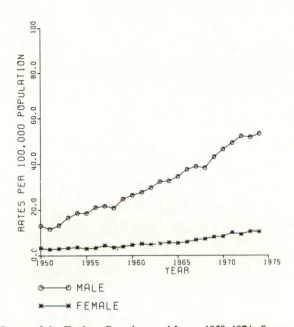

Figure 10-11 Cancer of the Trachea, Bronchus, and Lung, 1950–1974. *Source:* Reprinted from *Disease Patterns of the 70s,* p. 90, Division of Physical Health, Georgia Department of Human Resources, 1976.

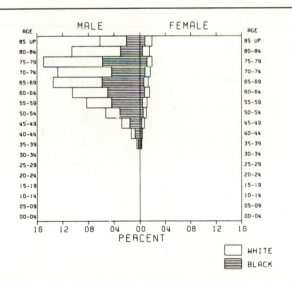

Figure 10-12 Cancer of the Trachea, Bronchus, and Lung, 1970–1974. *Source:* Reprinted from *Disease Patterns of the 70s,* p. 90, Division of Physical Health, Georgia Department of Human Resources, 1976.

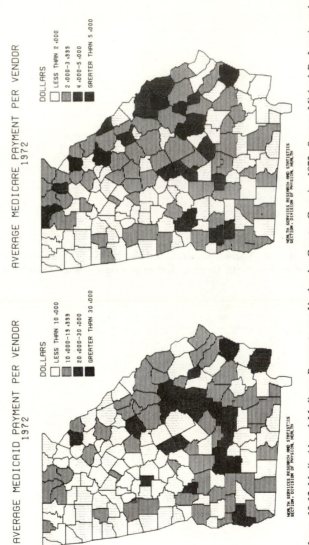
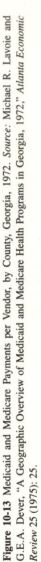

Figure 10-13 Medicaid and Medicare Payments per Vendor, by County, Georgia, 1972. *Source:* Michael R. Lavoie and G.E.A. Dever, "A Geographic Overview of Medicaid and Medicare Health Programs in Georgia, 1972," *Atlanta Economic Review* 25 (1975): 25.

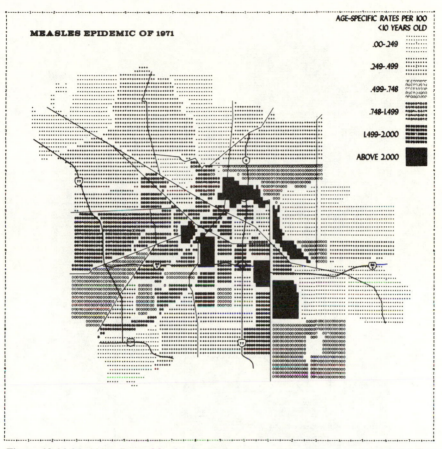

Figure 10-14 Morbidity Rates, Measles Epidemic, Akron, Ohio, 1971. *Source:* Reprinted from *Measles as an Urban Health Problem: The Akron Example* by Gerald F. Pyle, p. 19, paper presented to the 11th Commission in Medical Geography, Guelph, Ontario, Canada, 1972.

Morbidity and Mortality Analysis

Figures 10-14 and 10-15 show data by census tracts. Figure 10-14 depicts age-specific morbidity rates for measles in Akron, Ohio, in 1971; it can define high- and low-risk areas. Figure 10-15 shows the percentage of population five years of age and below in Fresno, California. It may be particularly useful in defining high-risk areas for screening programs for lead poisoning and immunizations, as well as for early and periodic screening, diagnosis, and treatment (EPSDT) programs.

Figure 10-16 is a plotted map of hospital admission data by ZIP code. The map shows the number of admissions by location of the patient's residence in Boston, Massachusetts. The fact that it has only four symbols reduces visual

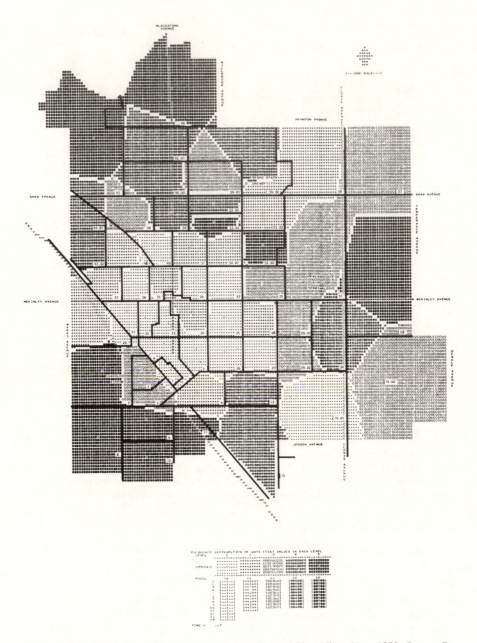

Figure 10-15 Population, 5 Years Old and Below, Fresno Metropolitan Area, 1970. *Source:* Reprinted from *Community Profile, 1973,* p. 9, City of Fresno Administration, Fresno, CA, 1973.

General Hospital Service Area

ZIP Code Boundaries

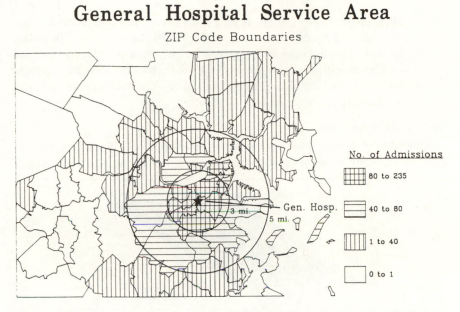

Figure 10-16 Number of Admissions by Patient Residence. *Source:* Reprinted from *Health Progress,* March, 1988, p. 46, with permission of Catholic Health Association of the United States, © 1988. Created with Atlas GIS from Strategic Mapping, Inc.

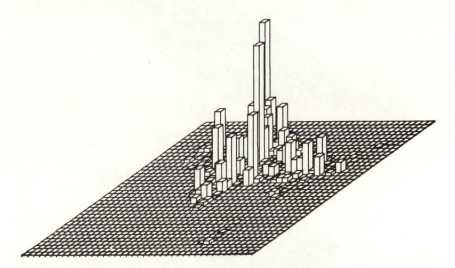

Figure 10-17 Hours Worked by Nurses of a Visiting Nurses Association, New Haven, Connecticut. *Source:* Reprinted from *Census Use Study: Computer Mapping,* Report No. 2, p. 39, U.S. Bureau of the Census, 1969.

noise and facilitates interpretation. A user must always maintain a balance between the number of symbols and the number of units (for example, ZIP codes) to be analyzed. This map can be employed for patient origin studies, hospital catchment area investigations, morbidity analyses, and health policy analyses. The map can also be helpful in determining potential problems connected with hospital availability and accessibility.

Advanced Data Analysis

Although the simple and straightforward presentation of health data should be emphasized, there are more advanced data analysis techniques with which health

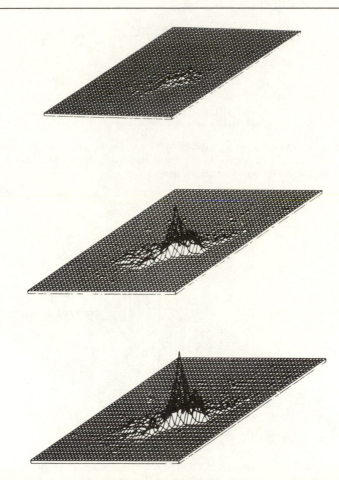

Figure 10-18 Cumulative Spatial Diffusion of a Health Care Plan. *Source:* Reprinted from *Health Care Delivery: Spatial Perspectives* by G.W. Shannon and G.E. Alan Dever, p. 133, with permission of McGraw-Hill Book Company, © 1974.

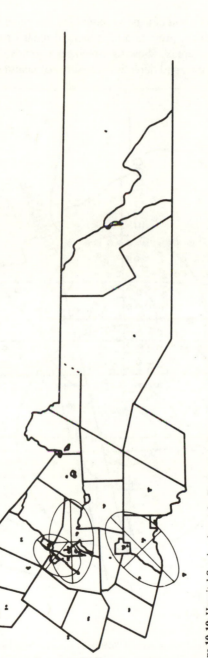

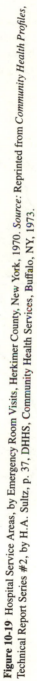

Figure 10-19 Hospital Service Areas, by Emergency Room Visits, Herkimer County, New York, 1970. *Source:* Reprinted from *Community Health Profiles,* Technical Report Series #2, by H.A. Sultz, p. 37, DHHS, Community Health Services, Buffalo, NY, 1973.

planners and analysts should at least become familiar. Such techniques, although more difficult to produce, provide quite practical means for planning facilities, predicting health-poor areas, showing time/space trends, illustrating potential disease distribution areas, and depicting measures of health care effectiveness.

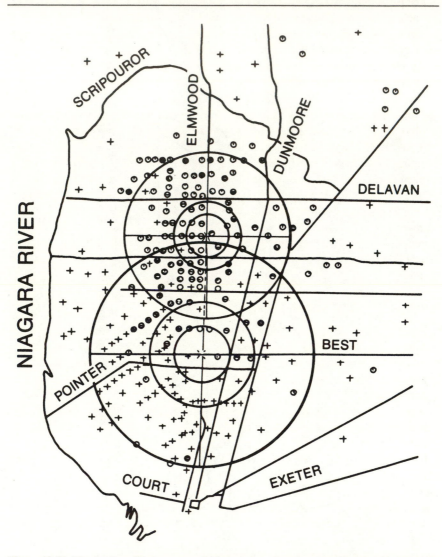

Figure 10-20 Distribution of Patients around Alternate Locations for a Neighborhood Health Center in Buffalo, New York. *Source:* Reprinted from *Community Health Profiles,* Technical Report Series #2, by H.A. Sultz, p. 36, DHHS Community Health Services, Buffalo, NY, 1973.

The map in Figure 10-17, produced by cathode ray tube graphic techniques, shows information through three-dimensional grid cells. It clearly indicates the magnitude of the hours worked by nurses of the Visiting Nurses Association. Because it shows areas of utilization, it may be of value in health program resource planning. It would not be of use in fiscal allocations, however, because of the lack of data that define established administrative units.

Figure 10-18 shows another series of three-dimensional plotted maps. The three graphics show the diffusion of a health care plan, but they could just as easily show the diffusion and magnitude of a disease (e.g., influenza) or predict areas of further diffusion of the selected disease in time and space.

The map in Figure 10-19 employs standard deviational ellipses to define the size and shape of hospital service areas. The ellipses indicate that several hospitals have overlapping or asymmetrical service areas. The ellipsoidal shapes reflect patient preference, facility competition, and barriers to hospital access.

Figure 10-20 shows the distribution of patients around alternate locations of a neighborhood health clinic. Two series of concentric circles have been plotted around alternate locations of the clinics, enclosing the home locations of potential clinic patients at three specified percentage ranges. The map thus shows a considerable difference in the accessibility of the two clinic locations. This graphic can be used in planning the location of facilities, overcoming social or transportation barriers, or assessing clinic accessibility for a specific geographical area.

Patient Origin Data Analysis

Patient origin studies have generally suffered from unimaginative methods to portray the results needed for administrative decision making. Schneider and associates have explored alternatives to origin-destination data in the context of transportation planning.[22] The application of the approach to health planning is remarkably simple. The two graphics in Figure 10-21 were produced primarily by a computer graphic program CENVUE used initially by Tobler.[23] Noguchi and Schneider later developed several innovative approaches to the use of CENVUE.[24]

Figure 10-21 shows two ways to present patient origin data. The upper map illustrates travel by patients to a hospital in Zone 10, using vectors and histograms. In this instance, the height of the histogram shows the volume of the flow. The lower map illustrates the identical data, but the vectors express the volume of the flow. Most individuals seem to find the upper display more clear and comprehensible. The viewpoint from which the graphic is produced is critical to the presentation of these data.

Travel time and accessibility surfaces can be graphically displayed by means of contour maps that show travel times plotted along minimum time paths from a

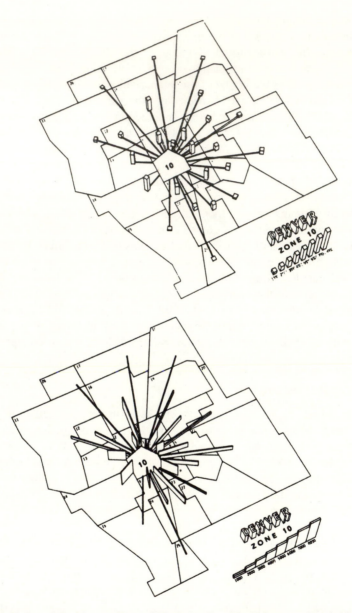

Figure 10-21 Potentially Alternate Ways of Displaying Travel by Patients to a Hospital in Denver. *Source:* Reprinted from *Data Display Techniques for Transportation Planners: Experiments and Applications,* rev. ed., by J.B. Schneider et al., pp. 36–39, University of Washington, Department of Civil Engineering, © 1978.

single origin. Gehner developed a contour line-drawn map by using the minimum path gridding and contouring procedure.[25] This type of graphic can, for example, show accessibility limits of 30 minutes from a primary health care center.

COMPUTER GRAPHICS IN THE FUTURE

The needs of the highly technocratic society of the 1970s and 1980s produced rapid advances in the computer graphics field. Technological advances will continue, as ink jet plotters, line graphics, and equipment with high increment speeds, high resolution, and compactness are being developed and improved. In the 1990s, health managers will utilize computer technology extensively to display health information for community planning, monitoring, and evaluation, and for conducting epidemiological investigations. The judicious and practical application of computer-generated graphics should, thus, ease a health agency's planning and policy problems as the technology enters the mainstream of decision making.

The task of advancing computer graphics in community health does not lie with those who manufacture or develop hardware and software, however, but with those in the health field who must create "peopleware." The contributions that computer graphics can make to community health programs must be determined by health program managers and decision makers. At present, the volume of patient information can be overwhelming and difficult to comprehend. Adequate computer graphics hardware, software, and "peopleware" can help to alleviate this situation. Thus, as the technology of resource persons and computer hardware and software become widespread and more available in the coming years, the practical application of computer graphics will become common practice at all levels of health management.

NOTES

1. R. Eliot Green and R.D. Parslow, *Computer Graphics in Management* (Princeton: Auerbach Publications, 1970), 97, 140.

2. Robert A. Greenes and Victor W. Sidel, "The Use of Computer Mapping in Health Research," *Health Services Research* (1967): 243–258.

3. Robert Lewis and Lawrence Chadzynski, "Evolutionary Changes in the Environment, Population, and Health Affairs in Detroit, 1968–71," *Environmental Changes* 64 (1974): 557–567.

4. Howard Fisher, "The Use of Computer Graphics in Planning" (Paper presented at the National Planning Conference of the American Society of Planning Officials, Harvard University, Cambridge, Mass., April 1970), 7.

5. Dale D. Achabal et al., "Designing and Evaluating a Health Care Delivery System through the Use of Interactive Computer Graphics," *Social Science and Medicine* 12 (1978): 1–6.

6. G.G. Stefansson, "Map Analyses of Psychiatric Services," *Acta Psychiatrica Scandinavica* 70 (1984): 515–522.

7. Niels Keiding, Claus Holst, and Anders Green, "Retrospective Estimation of Diabetic Incidence from Information in a Prevalent Population and Historical Mortality," *American Journal of Epidemiology* 130, no. 3 (1989): 588–600.

8. In an Applied Statistics Training Institute survey of maps on health data, 13 states were found to be using computer graphics (geocoding health data) at the county level or below. See *Applied Statistics Training Institute Series* (St. Louis, Mo.: September 28–29, 1977. A course provided by the National Center for Health Statistics.), 12. Since 1980, simple computer graphics software packages have become available for use in community and public health agencies.

9. R.E. Mytinger and A. White, "Communicating Complexity: A Health Policy Analysis Framework" (Paper presented at the Data Use Conference, Phoenix, Arizona, November 1978), 11.19–11.41.

10. Martha Farnsworth Riche, "Computer Mapping—Takes Center Stage," *American Demographics* 8, no. 6 (June 1986): 26–65.

11. Riche, "Computer Mapping," 30.

12. Wilson B. Riggan et al., *U.S. Cancer Mortality Rates and Trends, 1950–1979*, vol. 4, *MAPS* (Washington, D.C.: U.S. Environmental Protection Agency, 1987), 363.

13. Thomas J. Mason et al., *Atlas of Cancer Mortality for U.S. Counties: 1950–1969*, Department of Health, Education and Welfare Pub. No. (NIH) 75-780 (Washington, D.C.: U.S. Government Printing Office, 1975), 14, 24, 37.

14. Thomas J. Mason et al., *Atlas of Cancer Mortality among U.S. Nonwhites. Counties: 1950–1969*, Department of Health, Education and Welfare Pub. No. 76-1204 (Washington, D.C.: U.S. Government Printing Office, 1976), 142.

15. Riggan, *Cancer Mortality Rates and Trends*, 1987.

16. Ibid., xii.

17. George A. Schnell and Mark S. Monmonier, "The Mortality-Fertility Ratio: A Useful Measure for Describing Demographic Change in the U.S., 1940–1974," *Intercom* 6, no. 8 (1978): 8–10.

18. SYMVU. *Reference Manual for Synographic Computer Mapping* (Cambridge, Mass.: Laboratory for Computer Graphics and Spatial Analysis, Harvard University).

19. SOLO Statistical System, Version 2.0, graphics distributed by BMDP Statistical Software, Inc., Los Angeles, California.

20. SYSTAT and SYGRAPH, Version 1.1, Intelligent Software for Statistics and Graphics, distributed by Systat, Inc. Evanston, Illinois.

21. Phillip Frankland, *Atlas of Primary Medical and Dental Manpower in Iowa*, Technical Report No. 58 (Iowa City; Center for Locational Analysis, Institute of Urban and Regional Research, University of Iowa, April 1976), 103.

22. J.B. Schneider et al., *Data Display Techniques for Transportation Planners: Experiments and Applications*, rev. ed. (Seattle: University of Washington, Department of Civil Engineering, Urban Planning and Architecture, July 1978), 36–39.

23. W. Tobler, "Select Computer Programs" (Department of Geography, University of Michigan, Ann Arbor, 1970, Mimeographed).

24. T. Noguchi and J. Schneider, "Data Display Techniques for Transportation Analysis and Planning: An Investigation of Three Computer Produced Graphics," Research Report 762 Urban Transportation Program, Department of Civil Engineering and Urban Planning, University of Washington, Seattle. (June 1976): 59.

25. C. Gehner, "Utilizing Geographic Benefiles for Transportation Analysis: A Network Benefile System," Research Report 773, Urban Transportation Program, Department of Civil Engineering and Urban Planning, University of Washington, Seattle. (Paper presented at Transportation Research Board, Washington, D.C., 1978), *Transportation Research Record* forthcoming.

Appendix 10-A

Vendors of Computer Graphics

Demographics, psychographics, geographics, lifestyle, buying behavior, media and *direct marketing* will become buzz words in the acquisition, planning, and analysis of data for the development of health care programs in the 1990s. *The Best 100 Sources for Marketing Information—Who's Who from American Demographics* provides the analyst or planner with a compendium of resources of computer data base and graphic information in the United States. A major segment of this document is devoted to the vendors who have produced and supply computer graphics. Table 10-A1 shows the graphic vendor, the products, and a description of the products. In addition to these sources numerous graphic software packages can be purchased separately.

Table 10-A1 Computer Mapping Systems: Vendors and Products

Vendor	Product	Description
Election Data Service, Inc.	Tiger Tamer	Tiger Tamer produces maps and reports to analyze Census Tiger Files for errors and inconsistencies. Tigeredit facilitates the editing of Tiger files. E.D.S., Inc. also provides maps and graphs of demographic and political data.
U.S. Bureau of the Census, Geographic	TIGER Topologically Integrated Geographic Encoding and Referencing system	TIGER is a Census Bureau acronym for the new digital (computer readable) map data base system that automates the mapping and related geographic activities required to support the census and survey programs of the Census Bureau.
		The TIGER File contains digital data for all 1990 census map features (such as roads, railroads, and rivers) and the associated collection geography (such as census tracts and blocks), political areas (such as cities and

continues

361

Table 10-A1 continued

Vendor	Product	Description
		townships), feature names and classification codes, alternate feature names, 1980 and 1990 census geographic area codes, and within metropolitan areas, address ranges and ZIP codes for streets.
		The Census Bureau released a complete set of the precensus version of the TIGER/Line files for the entire United States in July 1989, and the postcensus version of the TIGER/Line files in 1991.
		The TIGER/Line files replace the 1980 GBF/DIME files. The GBF/DIME files covered only the urbanized portions of the SMSAs. The TIGER/Line files cover every county in the U.S. as well as Puerto Rico, the Virgin Islands of the U.S., Guam, American Samoa, the Northern Mariana Islands, and the Pacific territories for which the U.S. Census Bureau assists in the census taking process. However, the address ranges and ZIP codes in the TIGER/Line files will be found only in the areas covered originally by the 1980 GBF/DIME files.
Environmental Systems Research Institute, Inc. (ESRI)	ARC/INFO	The ARC/INFO software is an integrated geographic information system (GIS) and relational data-base management system used to input, manipulate, analyze, and display geographic data through modern computer technology.
Geographic Data Technology, Inc.	GeoSpread-Sheet™	GeoSpread-Sheet™ is a management decision tool consisting of a spreadsheet integrated with a computerized map for site analysis, thematic mapping, and territory planning.
Hawthorne Software Co., Inc.	PINMAP™	PINMAP™ is a computerized version of old-fashioned pin maps which used colored pins to display data on a map. Plots information using colored dots on a map of the U.S. on computer screen or color printer. Shows data values and name of city and ZIP code for any dot on the map. Shows sales territories and market areas using the AREAS function. Plots the whole USA; also has zoom function for a more detailed look. Maps may be customized and saved for a computer "slide show." PINMAP is designed for IBM XT, AT

Table 10-A1 continued

Vendor	Product	Description
		and PS/2 and compatibles running EGA and VGA graphics boards.
Intelligent Charting, Inc.	Intelligent Charting	Intelligent Charting, Inc. produces custom maps to help you develop, implement and manage your marketing and sales programs and conduct site and trade area studies. Their geographic databases are nationwide, right down to the street address level. Available geography includes ZIPs (5-digit, 3-digit, +2, +4), census tracts, counties, carrier routes, MSAs, DMAs, and ADIs. Custom sales, district, franchise and market boundaries can be created. Any data can be displayed, including demographic, business establishment and your own information. All maps are available in full color. Size range of 3 by 3 inches to 3 by 4 feet is available.
National Decision Systems	National Decision Systems	National Decision Systems provides a variety of mapping capabilities. Their customized marketing maps are unique in their ability to display complicated statistical data in an easy-to-understand format. Full color marketing maps make it easy to visualize how various marketing characteristics impact locational analysis and target marketing decisions.
NPA Data Services	NPA Data Services	Periodically publishes atlases and mapbooks of economic and demographic data for U.S. counties and states. Custom maps from own and/or customer data.
Spatial Data Sciences, Inc.		Spatial Data Sciences, Inc., provides software and systems integration for map analysis workstations, and has products and integration experience for all consumer environments.
Spatial Data Sciences, Inc.	Mapstation™	Mapstation™ is a digital map analysis system for such tasks as routing and transportation analysis using network data; terrain and propagation analysis using elevation data; redistricting, demographic and sales territory analysis on thematic displays; and others.
	CustomMaps™	CustomMaps™ is a trip routing system that prints a map atlas with both narrative

continues

Table 10-A1 continued

Vendor	Product	Description
		directions and a highlighted route over a map background.
	MapReader™	MapReader™ is a data conversion system for producing vector data from symbolized linework on a scanned map.
Strategic Mapping, Inc.	ATLAS*GRAPHICS	ATLAS*GRAPHICS creates maps to quickly and clearly analyze and present data by geographic areas such as ZIP code, census tracts or counties. Data can be displayed using hatch patterns, solid colors, or data driven lines, points and symbols. ATLAS*GRAPHICS is easy to learn and use while offering advanced mapping and data handling and graphics capabilities. Boundary files are available for hundreds of geographies. Data can be entered directly or imported from other programs, or purchased from Strategic Mapping, Inc. or other data suppliers. ATLAS*GRAPHICS is menu-driven with on-line help and hands-on tutorial.
	ATLAS*DRAW	ATLAS*DRAW is a program for creating and editing maps, called boundary files, for use with ATLAS*GRAPHICS or a publishing program that uses the HP-GL file format. A map can include geographic areas such as counties, sales territories, and planning districts, as well as roads, rivers, points of interest and other map features. By using a digitized tablet, mouse, light pen, or cursor, new maps can be generated easily and accurately and existing maps can be edited.
	ATLAS*GIS	ATLAS*GIS is a powerful geographical information system with all the features of ATLAS*GRAPHICS and ATLAS*DRAW, plus a number of new capabilities including 256 layers, extensive data management, detailed street mapping, address matching, and import and export of many popular data formats. The program is networkable and allows for easy querying, data aggregation, spatials overlaying, reporting, and annotating. A macro language allows the programming of custom applications.

Table 10-A1 continued

Vendor	Product	Description
TYDAC Technologies	XSPANS	XSPANS is a full functioned, modular geographic information system developed specifically for commercial application such as marketing research, trade area analysis, sales management, target marketing, and site selection. Product features include data modeling, networking, address matching, and overlay analysis as well as interfaces to public and proprietary data sources, statistical software, and database management systems. It has been developed to run on OS/2 under Presentation Manager. XSPANS uses a SQL interface that permits access to single-user DBMSs up to large-scale corporate databases.
Western Economic Research Company, Inc.	WER	WER—the convenience store of the information companies. Their research aids, including five-digit ZIP code maps, ZIP code demographic estimates, ZIP code economic data and specialty maps, are in stock for prompt shipment. ZIP code data may be ordered in small components (even individual ZIP codes).
Claritas	COMPASS	COMPASS is a market analysis and mapping system that can integrate a company's customer database, Claritas databases, and third-party databases. COMPASS users receive comprehensive training and support from Claritas staff and receive pre-built applications custom-tailored for their particular industry or departmental needs. A toll-free number connects users to the Claritas technical support staff who provide unlimited help.
	PRIZM®	PRIZM® is Claritas's demographic segmentation system, which is updated with actual consumer behavior. PRIZM® assignments are available down to the block-group level. The system is backed by ten years' experience with clients nationwide.
	P$YCLE	P$YCLE is a segmentation system developed expressly for use by financial marketers. P$YCLE helps predict use of financial products, especially for high-end investment and banking products.

continues

Table 10-A1 continued

Vendor	Product	Description
	LIFEP$YCLE	LIFEP$YCLE is a similar system for life insurance products.
Donnelley Marketing Information Services	CONQUEST®	CONQUEST® is a personal computer system based on geodemographic marketing information, which provides access to Donnelley Marketing's demographic, economic and geographic databases. CONQUEST can analyze the demographic composition, lifestyle and socio-economic characteristics, business environment and propensity of its residents to purchase specific goods and services for 14 standard areas of geography and geometrically defined market areas including circles, rings, bands, polygons, etc. CONQUEST allows users to include information about their customers, analyze customer characteristics, identify products and services customers are likely to purchase, and determine primary, secondary and tertiary service areas. Other applications include estimating market share, determining market penetration, competitive analysis, and market activity projections based on demographic change. CONQUEST provides access to 1970 and 1980 U.S. Census data, Donnelley's proprietary demographic estimates and projections, Cluster-PLUS lifestyle characteristics and cluster-coded products and services, current year retail expenditure estimates for 21 store types, BusinessLINE business listings and summary data for more than 7 million businesses and shopping center and grocery store information, physician lists and DRG models, auto registration counts and lifestyle profiles, Canadian demographics, and thematic full color mapping boundaries and background reference features.
National Planning Data Corporation	Max Online Demographics	Max Online Demographics, the largest private database of demographic information. Contains: UPDATE—current estimates and five-year projections of demographics; Consumer Clout—purchasing estimates and projections for over 350 consumer categories; YPD—demographics defined by Yellow Pages geographies; DRG Demand—providing health care

Table 10-A1 continued

Vendor	Product	Description
		data on diagnosis categories and medical procedures; and custom reports. Map-Analyst, software for analysis of data and generation of presentation maps. PRIME-LOCATION, featuring demographic data-bases; TIGER street networks and CD-ROM storage combined with satellite images, creating the most advanced desktop analysis system in existence. NPDC also features a wide variety of custom products and mapping.
Urban Decision Systems, Inc.	TELE/SITE	TELE/SITE is a telephone-based order service for obtaining UDS reports, computer-generated maps, and machine-readable databases for customer-defined trade areas—any size or any shape, anywhere in the U.S. Over 100 standard reports on demographics, business, employment, retail potential, lifestyles, shopping centers, and healthcare. Same-day service is available for reports. First orders are prepaid or charged to Visa, MasterCard, or American Express; subsequent orders are billed. Mainframe and PC systems available to generate UDS reports, maps, and databases from an in-house or remote mainframe (ONSITE system) or a PC (Scan/US and ON-SITE/PC systems). Unlimited access licenses available for the entire U.S., any region, state or other geographic subdivision by mutual agreement. ONSITE also available on a pay-as-you-go basis with a single monthly bill from STSC, Inc., incorporating all report and computer resource charges. Manuals and training available. Additional services: consulting, data on diskette, custom reports, maps, databases, and custom site coding and digitizing.

Source: Adapted from *The Best 100 Sources for Marketing Information: Who's Who from American Demographics* by F.J. Charboneau, p. 52, with permission of American Demographics, Inc., © 1989.

Appendix 10-B

Selected Examples of Computer Graphics Generated by SYGRAPH

SYGRAPH is a very useful and probably the most unusual graphics package available. In addition to its stated uses in the technical and business world, it has almost unlimited applications in community health planning. The analysis of demographic, lifestyle, socioeconomic, health, psychographics, marketing, epidemiology, statistical and survey data may be accomplished with ease and a certain degree of creativity. Figures 10-B1 through 10-B3 are examples.

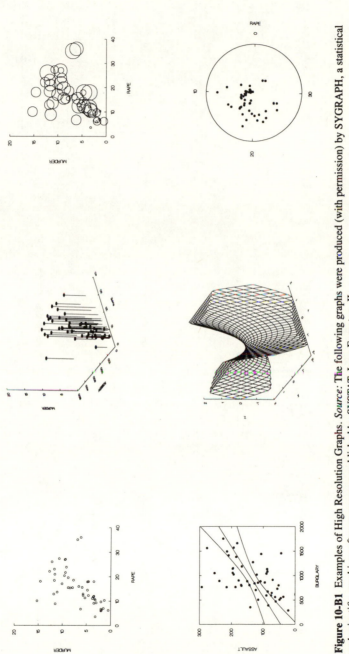

Figure 10-B1 Examples of High Resolution Graphs. *Source:* The following graphs were produced (with permission) by SYGRAPH, a statistical and scientific graphics software program published by SYSTAT, Inc., Evanston, IL.

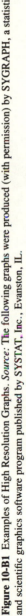

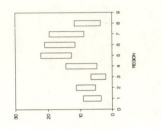

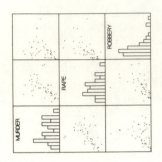

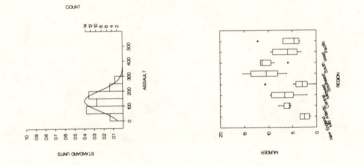

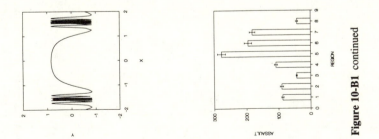

Figure 10-B1 continued

Scatterplot with symbol option.	**Three dimensional scatterplot** with symbol and spike option, to make values more visible.	**Bubble plot** using size and symbol option. The value of the variable can be used to control the size of symbol.
Scatterplot with confidence intervals using smooth option.	**Three dimensional function plot** using hide option. "HIDE" causes portions of the surface face in the background to be hidden behind portions in the foreground.	**Polar data plot** with polar coordinates. The "Y" axis is the distance of a point from the origin of a circle, and the "X" axis is the angle between the horizontal axis and a line from the origin to the point.
Fourier plot, a particularly powerful method for identifying clusters of cases in a multivariate dataset.	**Histogram** plot using smoothing option to show normal density. Thus, a normal curve is superimposed on a histogram.	**Bar chart** with range option. Thus, an interval is plotted using the high and low value.
Bar chart showing standard errors around plotted bars; one may choose standard deviations or standard errors.	**Box plot** shows the range of the data. It is a simple summary of a batch of data.	**Scatter plot matrix.** It is an arrangement of many variables in a row and column order.

* This layout corresponds exactly to the layout of the graphs.

Figure 10-B1 continued

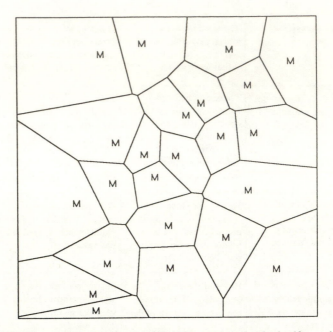

Figure 10-B2 Thiessen Diagram. *Source:* SYGRAPH, a statistical and scientific graphics software program published by SYSTAT, Inc., Evanston, Ill., 1988, p. 584.

The above graph was produced with permission by SYGRAPH, a statistical and scientific graphics software program published by SYSTAT, Inc., Evanston, Ill. "The above figure shows the location of McDonald's restaurants in Memphis, Tennessee. Notice that the smallest polygons are in the center of the map, where population densities are highest. The McDonald's people obviously planned carefully to insure an adequate supply of customers for each restaurant. If you are thinking of opening a chain of stores or restaurants in a uniformly dense area, the Theissen polygons should be relatively compact instead of elongated to provide maximum access to your customers. If you live in Memphis and are looking for the nearest McDonald's from your home (as the crow flies), just find the one inside the polygon containing your house. Every point within a polygon is closer to its corresponding McDonald's than to any other. This is true even when the McDonald's is not at the center of the polygon." This can be an extremely useful technique for location/allocation problems in the delivery of health care services.

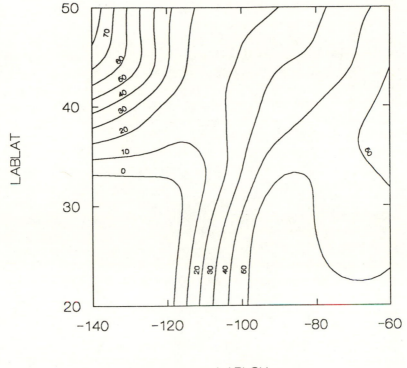

Figure 10-B3 Contour Plot. *Source:* The above graph was produced with permission by SYGRAPH, a statistical and scientific graphics software program published by SYSTAT, Inc., Evanston, Il.

Figure 10-B3 shows a contour plot of rain (average annual rainfall) against latitude and longitude from the U.S. file.

SYGRAPH automatically determines the number of contours to draw so that the surface is delineated and the contour labels are round numbers. This plot is particularly useful for mapping disease patterns in cases where political units inhibit the true pattern. Such contour lines may be labeled isomorts (lines of equal mortality values), isomorbs (lines of equal morbidity values), etc.

Index